Issues in
Health Care Regulation

REGULATION OF AMERICAN
BUSINESS AND INDUSTRY SERIES

Issues in Health Care Regulation

edited by

RICHARD S. GORDON

Director, Regulation as an Instrument of Public Administration,
a program jointly sponsored by
The Kennedy School of Government, Harvard University, and The Health Resources
Administration, U.S. Department of Health, Education, and Welfare

McGRAW-HILL BOOK COMPANY
New York   St. Louis   San Francisco   Auckland   Bogotá
Hamburg   Johannesburg   London   Madrid   Mexico   Montreal   New Delhi
Panama   Paris   São Paulo   Singapore   Sydney   Tokyo   Toronto

Library of Congress Cataloging in Publication Data

Main entry under title:

Health care regulation.

(Regulation of American business and industry series)
"This book synthesizes the major points of discussion and recommendations made at the conference entitled 'Regulation as an instrument of public administration,' held at Harvard University on February 27 and 28, 1978."

1. Medical-care—Law and legislation—United States—Congresses. 2. Administrative procedure—United States—Citizen participation—Congresses. I. Gordon, Richard S. II. Series.

KF3821.A75H37   344'.73'04102636   79-13882
ISBN 0-07-023780-8

1234567890 DODO 89876543210

The editors for this book were Susan L. Schwartz, Robert Rosenbaum, and Susan Thomas; the designer was Elliot Epstein; and the production supervisor was Thomas G. Kowalczyk. It was set in Palatino by The Heffernan Press Inc.

Printed and bound by R. R. Donnelley & Sons Company.

Contents

CHAPTER SIX

Reactions to Breyer's Proposal for Regulatory Reform 275

CHAPTER SEVEN

Issues in Health Care Regulation 331

Richard S. Gordon

Foreword

HEALTH CARE REGULATION AND
THE ROLE OF THE UNIVERSITY

In recent years, we have heard many people deplore the failure of our health care system to control spiraling costs or to provide sufficient access to health services for all areas and economic strata in the United States. Although many of the sharpest critics of health care come from university faculties, universities bear much of the responsibility for these problems. In the last analysis, universities are responsible for the production of knowledge and specialized education, and many of the deficiencies in health care stem either from inadequate numbers of people skilled both in medicine and in administration or from our lack of knowledge about exactly how the health care system works.

The lagging response of the universities has multiple causes. On the one hand, relevant fields such as institutional economics have not enjoyed high academic prestige in recent decades. On the other hand, universities have had a hard time encouraging effective collaboration across disciplinary and faculty lines, and cooperative work of this kind is particularly important in areas such as health policy. Finally, though I regret to say it, universities do not enjoy an exemplary record in anticipating serious social problems. One might suppose that institutions that employ extremely able people and provide them the time and security to study and reflect would be the natural places in which to identify incipient problems and explore them at an early stage. Too often, however, such problems are recognized and dramatized by others in society, and universities begin to develop programs of teaching and research only after the government and foundations have recognized an issue and taken steps to devote resources to it.

Universities have now begun to address the problems of health care with greater vigor. This book, reflecting the work of a two-year program at Harvard, aptly illustrates this trend. Such efforts deserve encouragement. Universities must not fall behind the social issues. Instead, they should lead society in preparing for them. This is our challenge—and the John F. Kennedy School of Government's particular challenge—if we are to render the services of which our institutions of higher learning should ideally be capable.

DEREK BOK
President, Harvard University

Preface

While much public attention is focused on deregulation, it seems unrealistic to expect a reduction in the number of federal health care regulatory programs in the immediate future. Therefore it is assumed that "social" regulation to achieve public purposes in health care will continue but that new approaches are required to improve the quality of that regulation and to foster positive, concordant attitudes in the interaction between regulator, regulatee, and the consuming public.

This volume presents frameworks on which to build improved analyses of any specific regulatory proposal or situation. The goals of this analytical approach are:

1. To suggest alternative means of dealing with a given problem.

2. To predict the consequences of adopting any particular regulatory regime or program.

The general thesis being tested is that experience with economic regulation in nonhealth sectors, as well as a review of some aspects of the implementation of contemporary health care regulation, can provide insights into the problems and pitfalls associated with the burgeoning regulation of the health sector.

This thesis emerged from discussions with senior officials in the Department of Health, Education, and Welfare, who felt that an increasing number of the regulatory proposals being drafted by the Congress as well as by their own subordinates were beginning to move down the same path as those of the Federal Trade Commission, the Federal Communication Commission, and other regulatory agencies. Besides questioning the "fit," or appropriateness, of regulatory regimes from the nonhealth sector to health care, these same officials observed that many such regulatory approaches were under specific attack by a broad range of concerned citizens and even by public officials at all levels of government. New proposals for health care regulation seemed unmindful of the criticisms which analogous regulations in the nonhealth sector were drawing.

A complicating factor in trying to understand the nature of health care regulation is the existence of a welter of overlapping and often contradictory rules under which health care institutions must operate. The ubiquitous nature of health care seems to ensure its oversight by a baffling array of federal, state and local bodies, none of which are able to grapple with the whole system. The picture is further complicated by the continuing polarity between advocates of a "free-market" system and advocates of classic "command and control" centralized regulation, neither of which may speak to the needs of health care over the long term.

A dialogue was started between those interested in analyzing regulatory failure and those interested in improving health care regulation. Over 150 persons with an unusually broad cross-section of interests were involved. The view was developed that health regulatory problems can be categorized and the likelihood of program failure predicted. Moreover, problems, if not outright failure, can be related to the existing regulatory modes the government has at its command to intervene in the health care system. A crucial factor accompanying government involvement is the nature of the bargaining relationship between regulator and regulatee, a matter of relevance to both program design and implementation considerations.

This dialogue, then, led to the preparation of draft papers that were discussed in a number of meetings culminating in a conference convened by the John Fitzgerald Kennedy School of Government, Harvard University, in February 1978. The entire dialogue, paper preparation, meetings, and conference were under the joint sponsorship of the Health Resources Administration and the Alcohol, Drug Abuse, and Mental Health Administration (both of the United States Department of Health, Education, and Welfare) and of the Commonwealth Fund. The papers and the discussion which they generated are the substance around which this book is built.

The specific aim of the chapters that follow is to present some generic guidelines useful in improving the regulation of health care institutions. A particular feature is to suggest approaches to rulemaking which should minimize untoward or unexpected effects. On the other hand, it should be noted at the outset that this book does not consider regulatory problems associated with individual services, such as the patient-doctor relationship, or with such professional questions as licensing and qualifications for practice. Rather, it considers the institutional nature, the quasicorporate arrangements, of most health care providers as the characteristic that seems to invite the translation of regulatory approaches from other sectors.

For example, control of capital expenditures and return on investment is a standard technique employed in the regulation of electric utilities. Control of capital thus becomes an inviting target for the regulation of hospitals, because capital expenditures not only are easy to identify but are already subject to a national Certificate-of-Need review. However, whether or not control of capital spending will prove effective in controlling hospital costs depends on the differences between hospitals and electric utilities: i.e., hospitals have other options for circumventing controls on capital which a utility does not (substituting labor for capital, for one). The untoward consequences of a regulation, then, might be quite different for a hospital and for a utility. Ultimately, the regulator must recognize that hospitals (certainly in the not-for-profit sector) are organized for a different end from maintaining earnings growth or optimizing return on capital.

In order to present such thoughts systematically, the book opens with a review of a few contemporary situations in health care. These situations are related to attempts to control the cost of health care and the writing of meaningful regulations for health maintenance organizations. Chapter Two reviews what is known about how well health care regulations are implemented, relating this to the more generalized sociopolitical process which generated the regulations in the first place. Chapter Three summarizes all the options open to various levels of government in considering how and where to intervene in the planning, organization, delivery, and funding of health care. Chapters Four, Five, and Six are built around attempts to understand some of the generic problems that surround all regulation and to propose some alternatives thereto. Chapter Seven, the final chapter, pulls together the ideas contained in the earlier chapters with the goal of helping the reader develop:

1. A broader perspective concerning the regulatory process.

2. A clearer view of what regulation can "do" to health care.

3. Questions that need to be asked before yet more regulation should be proposed or promulgated.

The development of perspective, view, and questions should result in a better understanding of the nature of regulation itself. The goal of helping one to develop a new approach to rulemaking was deliberately selected by all involved as a more desirable alternative than offering specific solutions to a few current, contemporary health regulatory problems.

Therefore, we will consider what is set forth a success if:

1. This volume guides the reader through the regulatory maze with new insight.

2. This volume helps the reader think through what is required to tie policy objectives to societal outcomes via the regulatory process.

A word of caution Obviously there is no way, no simplistic approach, that guarantees any immediate improvement of the present situation.

RICHARD S. GORDON
Rockport, Massachusetts

Acknowledgments

The editor is grateful to the Health Resources Administration; The Alcohol, Drug Abuse, and Mental Health Administration; and the Commonwealth Fund, all of which gave timely and enthusiastic support to the project from which this book was developed.

Dean Emeritus Donald Price and Dean Graham Allison of the Kennedy School were most supportive of the somewhat unconventional tack that this program took. Doctor Harold Margulies, at the time acting administrator of the Health Resources Administration, provided the philosophical impetus which guided most of our inquiries, while Paul Schwab, the contract officer for the program, was instrumental in shaping its intellectual and logistical organization, as well as the successful execution of what was attempted.

To the contributors to this volume and to the various persons who served as participants and steering committee members, I owe a debt of gratitude matched only by my debt to the graduate students, assistants, and editors who made the entire project possible. In particular, Professors Theodore Marmor and Howard Frazier and Dr. Robert Blendon made many helpful suggestions concerning the shape and content of this book. Professor Linda Cohen of the Kennedy School of Government was instrumental in revising Chapter 2. The constructive editing of Ms. Jane Manilych was an essential ingredient in completing the manuscript. Finally, without the careful and dedicated work, over many long hours, of Ms. Alma Higgins Nahigian, Assistant Editor, this book would not have come into existence.

Issues in
Health Care Regulation

PART ONE

Ferment in the Health Care "Industry"

CHAPTER ONE

Problems in Health Care[1]*

IS GOVERNMENT REGULATION HELPFUL?

Richard S. Gordon, Julianne Howell, and
David Alexander, *Kennedy School of Government*

I. NATIONAL AND LOCAL DEBATES OVER COST CONTROL

MEDIA REFLECTS NATIONAL MOOD OF COST CONTROL IN HEALTH SECTOR

> INITIATIVE TO REGULATE ALL HEALTH CHARGES IS
> NORTH DAKOTA'S HOTTEST ISSUE IN DECADES
> *(The Wall Street Journal[2])*

"It's the biggest turnout we have had in years," chamber of commerce officials remarked as people poured into the high school gymnasium in Hettinger, North Dakota, to attend a debate on a voter initiative that would impose state control on health fees. The editor of *The Adams County Record* explained, "People are just interested in this [measure]. There's just no getting around the fact that something has to be done to slow down spiraling medical costs."

Indeed, as Joann S. Lublin in *The Wall Street Journal* article goes on to report, "The initiative [became] the hottest campaign issue in decades in this sparsely populated, Populist-minded state, even overshadowing a controversial proposal to slash personal income taxes. The health-costs measure won a ballot spot after a group of 19 farmers and other citizens led by maverick state insurance commissioner, Byron Knutson, collected 13,000 signatures in two weeks, a record time."

Of course, "doctors, hospitals and insurance concerns . . . declared war on the initiative with a statewide advertising blitz," the *Journal*

---

* Superior numbers throughout the text refer to notes at the end of the article.

continues, complete with "buttons, brochures, billboards, and bumper stickers." Their theme: The proposal is an antihealth care measure and it "will drive away needed physicians and force some small hospitals to close."

When voters approved the initiative, North Dakota became "the nation's first state to regulate all health charges" (a few states, i.e., Maryland and New York, already control hospital rates). The new law directs the state health officer to "hold public hearings and then set maximum rates for prescription drugs and any service performed by a doctor, dentist, hospital, nursing home, optician, chiropractor, nurse, or physical therapist." The new law also directs "consideration of a [new] state-run health insurance company" (intensifying pressure for national health insurance).

The North Dakota state insurance commissioner estimated that the initiative "might slow the annual growth in the state's estimated $500 million medical bill from 16% to 8%. . . . Then the people of North Dakota will have saved themselves $40 million a year." So, just "as California's Proposition 13 set off taxpayer revolts in other states, passage of the North Dakota measure might spawn similar ballot proposals elsewhere. . . ."

In spite of signs of voter concern over the rising cost of health care, as exemplified by the events in North Dakota, the Carter administration's Hospital Cost Containment bill of 1978 was defeated in the Congress. Why? What was involved in the legislative struggle over this bill?

SCUTTLING OF HOSPITAL-COSTS BILL
(Boston Sunday Globe[3])

The Carter administration's proposed 1978 Hospital Cost Containment bill had won the approval of two House subcommittees, two Senate subcommittees, two Senate committees and the full Senate. But the bill—a proposal to limit increases in hospital costs projected to save the country $60 billion by 1983—did not pass the House as Congress wrapped up for adjournment in October 1978.

Sinclair Ward's article, originally reported in *The Washington Post*, alludes to "those final chaotic hours before Congress adjourned . . . [when] the Carter Administration and an array of powerful private and congressional forces locked into a quiet combat over high stakes." Ward summarizes the health care battleground as follows:

- Americans spend roughly $160 billion a year on health care, about 9 percent of the gross national product. Hospitals take about 40 percent of every dollar.

- At the time Carter came to Washington, medical costs were rising about 15 percent a year, almost twice the overall inflation rate. The cost of hospital services was rising even faster.

- Inflation was adding $1 billion a year to federal, state, and local Medicare and Medicaid expense. It was costing insurance programs and individuals almost that much more every year.

- Most people don't notice that insurance of some form pays the largest share of the nation's hospital bills. Medicare covers the elderly; Medicaid the poor. Third-party carriers insure most of the rest of the public.

- The Carter administration knew all this and recognized there was little public constituency for hospital cost legislation; but it also knew that rising costs threatened Carter's campaign promise to propose national health insurance. Unless cost increases could be curbed, national health insurance had little chance of success.

The administration, through the bill, sought to put a lid of about 9 percent on increases in hospital revenues, place a cap on new capital expenditures for some hospitals, and give incentives to improve the quality of care. The struggle to pass the bill had gone on since its proposal by President Carter in April 1977, and the chance had come to "pass legislation to limit the fast-rising cost of hospital care."[2] Opponents were readying for the House showdown.

Sinclair points to the proposal itself as one reason for House rejection. It posed "a radical solution to a serious problem, a solution that [some felt] threatened the medical industry in America. . . ." On the other hand, the administration said that it had to confront one of the most influential special interest groups nationally—the medical lobby—"which used sophisticated strategy and money to help scuttle cost-containment."

Sinclair reports further that the bill—a "legislative priority" with Carter—was "shepherded by the Health, Education and Welfare [HEW] Secretary, Joseph A. Califano, Jr. . . . Califano wanted the bill passed and he wanted it quickly with as little change as possible. He was in a hurry because the legislation involved billions of dollars—who would spend them, how, when and where?"

The bill was largely drawn up in HEW. Doctors and hospital administrators were not consulted or included in its development. Moreover, Califano "rubbed the medical lobby the wrong way because he [was] outspoken, uncompromising and sometimes abrasive." He stirred up its opposition by accusations of "waste and mismanagement." Even members of key House committees were uncertain about the bill's intentions and the administration's commitment.

The medical lobby, "a formidable influence on Congress" even without provocation, Sinclair concludes, had another important tool at hand—"a custom-built network reaching into every congressional district. . . ." American hospitals are major employers and buyers of services. In most communities they are respected institutions. "[Their] trustees are often the most influential people in town."

Sinclair cites American Hospital Association President J. Alexander McMahon's comments on the bill: "Any time any segment of the economy is threatened with legislation of this kind . . . there is no problem to organize opposition. . . . The bill was so bad, it so misread the problem, that it was relatively easy to attack. And attack we did."

Why was the 1978 Hospital Cost Containment bill seen as "bad" legislation if states such as North Dakota passed even more stringent bills? Was the situation as critical or even as well known as the administration stated? What in the political scheme of things could prevail over continued health care cost escalation? How broad a base could the opposition to the 1978 bill muster?

CAPITAL COST CONTROL THROUGH CERTIFICATE-OF-NEED[4]

In addition to the natural antipathy that those who are still largely unregulated would feel towards imposition of direct intervention by the government (the 1978 bill proposed operating controls through imposition of allowable increases in revenues), perhaps an additional rallying point against the Administration's proposal was that the Administration bill also proposed utilizing existing Certificate-of-Need (CON) machinery to enforce capital spending ceilings. Yet many hospitals were experiencing considerable difficulty operating under existing CON programs. In 1978, these programs were in effect in more than thirty states. Furthermore, the National Health Planning and Resources Development Act of 1974 (Public Law 93-641)[5] requires that all states have CON procedures and programs in place by 1980. Under current CON regulations, hospitals must apply for approval for all capital expenditures that (1) exceed $150,000, (2) increase bed capacity, or (3) substantially change the services of a facility independent of total cost.

If the 1978 Hospital Cost Containment bill had passed Congress, one of the key provisions would have been the imposition of an annual ceiling on the total dollar value of capital expenditures that could be made by the nation's hospitals. A specific total amount would be set nationally, and this would be allocated among the states—at least initially—on the basis of current population. The ceiling would be enforced through existing CON programs. In states lacking a CON program or having one that does not specify a dollar limit on approved projects, it would be administered through review programs established by the Social Security Amendments of 1972 (Public Law 92-603) to control capital expenditures under Medicaid, Medicare, and Maternal and Child Health programs.

In Massachusetts—a state with soaring tax rates, a concentration of excellence in medical teaching/research facilities, and a complex political system—the problems of rising medical costs in general and hospital costs in particular led to passage of the state CON bill in 1972 and a hospital charge control bill in 1976. In many ways Massachusetts has been struggling with the same problems covered by the 1978 Federal Cost Containment bill. Would the experience of Massachusetts' hospital administrators, medical community, regulatory officials, and legislators lead them to support the proposed federal legislation? Let us examine the situation in Massachusetts in somewhat greater detail.

HEALTH CARE REGULATION IN MASSACHUSETTS—
A MEDICALLY SOPHISTICATED STATE

In general, Massachusetts health planning and regulatory structures were established on a more stringent basis than required by the National Health Planning and Resources Development Act of 1974. To date, CON reviews have been conducted on a case-by-case basis, focusing on evaluating the necessity of a specific capital project proposed by an individual institution. In Massachusetts, as in other states, the CON program has not been restrained in the total number or dollar value of projects it can approve. Only in selected instances, such as the review of applications for installations of certain expensive equipment (i.e., computerized axial tomography, the so-called CAT scanners discussed later in this chapter), has the approval of a proposal from one institution required the denial of similar proposals by other institutions. Hence, up to the present, the CON program has served only a limited allocative function.

Nonetheless, CON programs were created to help "rationalize" the health care delivery system by avoiding duplication and assuring that only "necessary" projects are undertaken. This has meant that the state has had to confront such issues as the definition of "necessary" for various categories of health care facilities, equipment, and services as well as to develop criteria for the selection of "qualified" institutions to offer such services.

In terms of the proposed 1978 federal cost containment legislation, has Massachusetts been successful with its cost control efforts? The Massachusetts Office of State Health Planning indicated in 1976 that expenditures for hospital care were continuing to increase by as much as $225 million per year.[6] If a more radical approach is required, where can the state begin?

Before the state legislation was passed, Massachusetts contained 4.9 hospital beds per 1000 of population. That was 10 percent higher than the national average and more than 20 percent higher than the 4.0 beds per 1000 that had recently been proposed as a national goal and deemed "essential" to the containment of hospital cost increases. So the Commonwealth had a problem not simply of controlling further expansion in hospital beds but possibly of reducing capacity as well.[7]

The regulatory machinery which the state has created to deal with capital expansion is headed by the Commissioner of Public Health.[8] The Commissioner chairs the Public Health Council, the nine-member gubernatorially appointed group empowered by statute to make final decisions on all CON applications. William Bicknell, commissioner when the CON legislation was first enacted under Governor Sargent in 1972, saw the CON process as a lever for increasing consumer input into decisions which previously had been the sole province of health care providers. Later, Jonathan Fielding, appointed commissioner by Governor Dukakis, was given a strong mandate by the Governor to control costs and to achieve a more appropriate allocation of health resources in the state. Since that time the CON program has increasingly moved beyond simple evaluation of each application on its own merit to consideration of the regional and statewide implications of a proposed project before making final determinations-of-need.[9]

As will be discussed shortly, this approach necessitated the development of explicit review standards. It has also resulted in a rash of appeals to the Health Facilities Appeals Board[10] (the appellate body created by the Commonwealth's CON statute) challenging the grounds upon which the Public Health Council justified its decision about the use of special exemptive legislation by the state legislature to circumvent CON denials, and, more recently, about endeavors led by the Massachusetts hospitals to get the state legislature to limit the scope and power of the CON programs.

The fact that the CON program has not approved over $20 million in capital projects during the past two years alone[11] probably reinforced opposition to the proposed 1978 federal legislation by the Massachusetts medical and hospital community. At least under present state law there is no dollar ceiling, only a mandate to hold cost increases to some ill-defined minimum. Under both the 1978 and 1979 Hospital Cost Containment proposals, the states would have to hold year-to-year increases in hospital costs to a fixed percentage (about 9 percent in the 1978 bill, somewhat higher in the 1979 bill) or become subject to the provisions of the new law. However, since the imposition of the more restrictive legislation in Massachusetts in 1972, year-to-year increases in costs have been significantly reduced to about 10 percent per year (versus a national average of about 17 percent), so the state is within striking distance of the proposed federal bogie.

Experience with the CON Process in Massachusetts

Since its beginning in 1972, the Massachusetts CON program has approved an average of $96 million in projects annually. Table 1-1 lists projects submitted to the CON program during one six-month period. These projects total close to $90 million, and on the basis of the previous year's experience and the information provided by hospital one-year plans, an equal number of additional applications for CONs could be expected to be filed over the course of the next six-month period. Under the proposed cost containment bill, HEW would have allocated a ceiling of $68 million to Massachusetts, only approximately 70 percent of the annual total previously approved in 1976, the first year that the program under Dr. Fielding had assumed its tough cost-control policy. Such a ceiling would force the Public Health Council to implement fully the regional and statewide resource allocation perspective it had increasingly been assuming.

Yet what about local concerns? The ever-increasing, ongoing need to evaluate, review, and opt for technological improvement in health care delivery and research by the major teaching hospitals is certainly bound to clash with the proposed federal controls as well as the existing state-mandated program. Further, will not rural communities through-

TABLE 1-1 Projects Pending Public Health Council Review by Health Service Area (see Figure 1-1, which outlines Health Service Area Boundaries)

Hospital	Project	Cost
Health Service Area I		
Cooley Dickenson	Replace X-ray; renovate space	$ 484,000
Cooley Dickenson	Expand radiation department, replace cobalt 60 with linear accelerator	818,000
Mercy	Build addition to replace 1927 building; 18 rehabilitation; 25 pediatric eye, ear, nose and throat (EENT); 15 adult EENT; respiratory physical therapy	4,423,000
Providence	Gamma camera and support equipment	155,000
Medical Center of Western Massachusetts	Construct 4-story wing: 117,000 sq. ft. pathology, 24 intensive-care beds, 8 coronary-care unit beds, parking garage, etc.	15,000,000
Health Service Area II		
Henry Heywood	Increase licensed capacity 4 beds: 12-bed psychiatric unit, 6 pediatric, 2 maternity	202,000
Milford-Whittinsville	Replace X-ray equipment; add 5th X-ray room	308,000
Milford-Whittinsville	Convert 14 long-term care to psychiatric, 16 long-term care to acute medical/surgical	160,000
St. Vincent	Lease whole body CAT scanner	471,000
Health Service Area III		
Bon Secours	Air conditioning; replace windows	460,000
Lawrence General	Renovate and expand emergency and X-ray departments and 9-bed intensive-care unit	1,661,000
Bon Secours and Lawrence General	Lease computer to be shared	405,000
Lowell General	Addition: 14-bed intensive-care unit/coronary-care unit, outpatient department, doctor's lounge, modify ambulance entrace	1,425,000
Health Service Area IV		
Boston City	Construct medical office building for labs, X-ray, offices	1,792,000
Boston City	Construct exit stairwells	410,000

TABLE 1-1 Projects Pending Public Health Council Review by Health Service Area (see Figure 1-1, which outlines Health Service Area Boundaries) (*Continued*)

Hospital	Project	Cost	Hospital	Project	Cost
Carney	Build new garage for 375 cars	3,241,000	Marlborough	Effect 19-bed capacity change: 34 medical/surgical to 15 long-term psychiatric	80,000
Charles A. Dana	Expand X-ray department to include angiography, intravenous pylogram, 2 gamma cameras, existing CAT scanner, administration	1,184,000	Waltham	Build 4-level addition: 10-bed intensive-care unit; 6-bed coronary-care unit; 12 progressive care beds, or, recovery room; central supply; outpatient department; 8 medical/surgical beds; 6-level I/II bed; 3-level meal services building	15,747,000
New England Deaconess	Replace and relocate nursing school	4,204,000			
Massachusetts General	Renovate operating room airflow	282,000			
Massachusetts General	Renovate and expand pathology department	955,000	Quincy City	Construct new building, ambulatory care center, garage; renovate existing buildings, increase licensed capacity from 380 to 404 beds	15,659,000
New England Medical Center	Provide emergency electric power per life saving code	250,000			
Mt. Auburn	New radiographic X-ray and chest X-ray to replace 2 radiographic units	362,000	**Health Service Area V**		
Mt. Auburn	Renovate blood bank; expand immunology lab; renovate and expand anesthesia department	571,000	Cape Cod	Construct 1550 sq. ft. and renovate 144 sq. ft. for radiation department	461,000
Watertown Health Center	Establish satellite clinic	17,500	St. Anne's	Demolish 1906 building; build 5-floor, 65,838 sq. ft. tower for 76 medical/surgical beds, emer-	6,750,000

TABLE 1-1 Projects Pending Public Health Council Review by Health Service Area (see Figure 1-1, which outlines Health Service Area Boundaries) (*Continued*)

Hospital	Project	Cost
	gency room, X-ray, physical therapy, EKG, outpatient department, administration, dining room, and kitchen	
Falmouth	Expand laboratory and emergency room; new day surgery; central storage records	1,477,000
Brockton	Construct new emergency facility and new lab; renovate outpatient department, medical records department	6,000,000

Hospital	Project	Cost
Health Service Area VI		
New England Memorial	Replace data processing equipment	700,000
New England Memorial	Replace internal phone system	340,000
Lynn	Lease whole body CAT scanner	496,000
Melrose-Wakefield	Lease minicomputer for bookkeeping	143,000
Salem	Lease and install CAT scanner	497,000

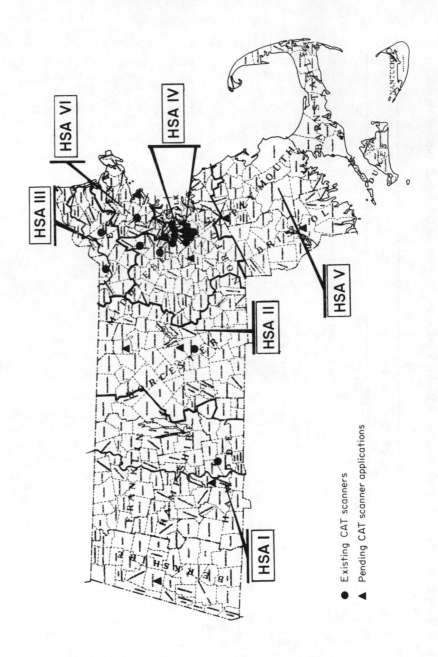

FIGURE 1-1   Health Service Area Boundaries for the Following Health Systems Agencies under Public Law 93-641: (*HSA I*) Western Massachusetts Health Planning Council, Inc., West Springfield; (*HSA II*) Central Massachusetts Health Systems Agency, Inc., Shrewsbury; (*HSA III*) Merrimack Valley Health Planning Council, Inc., Lawrence; (*HSA IV*) Health Planning Council of Greater Boston, Inc., Brighton, and Office of State Health Planning, Boston; (*HSA V*) Southeastern Massachusetts Health Planning and Development, Inc., Middleboro; and (*HSA VI*) North Shore Health Planning Council, Inc., Peabody.

out the state want to take pride in their local hospitals and want them as

complete as possible, facilitating easy access for community residents?
The interests of these hospitals will not always be served by restrictive
cost-control measures. In fact, particularly if such hospitals have
"angels" with money, will they not argue that their patients find it
difficult and costly to go into the "big city" for diagnostic studies? Why
should the state, let alone the federal government, tell them what they
can and cannot do to improve the efficiency and efficacy of diagnosis or
treatment? There really is no clear answer to these questions. Therefore,
it would appear that most state health professionals (except state regulatory officials) seem to have continuing objections not just to further
reduction in capital availability but to the CON process itself.

The CAT Scanner Controversy

To illustrate the nature of the controversies likely to arise under the
proposed federal legislation, let us examine the history of a Massachusetts CON application which involved making a choice between two
major Harvard teaching hospitals.[12]

HOSPITAL A

In 1976 the Public Health Council, acting on the advice of the director of
radiation control, authorized the installation of only one third-
generation total body (CAT) scanner at a research institution, and the
authorization was on condition that carefully developed research protocols be devised to determine the efficacy of total body scanning.

Hospital A had made an initial application for a CAT scanner in 1975
and had been working with planners to establish satisfactory research
protocols. As a result, both the Health Planning Council of Greater
Boston (HSA)[13] and the Department of Public Health of the Commonwealth of Massachusetts CON office endorsed the application.

Hospital A made what the state planners regarded as a strong case for
a CAT scanner. The hospital argued that:

1. There was good reason to believe that full-body scanning would be of
   tremendous medical value.

2. On the basis of previous research experience the hospital was uniquely
   qualified to undertake the project.

3. The hospital had worked with state planners to develop satisfactory
   research protocols and referral arrangements.

4. The financing scheme was both sound and reasonable.

The medical argument was based primarily on diagnostic value
rather than expected improved-patient outcome. This emphasis de-
parted somewhat from the criteria advanced by the director of the Office
of Radiation Control and usually accepted by the Public Health Council.

In his advice to the council, the director had said, "The Council should consider an application for one third-generation body scanner within the State provided that such a machine is located in a research institution and is installed under rigid research protocols to determine the efficiency of the whole body CAT scanner on patient outcome."[14]

Nevertheless, the argument for diagnostic value alone was a strong one.[15] The list of possible medical applications was long and included liver tumors, bile duct obstructions, spleen enlargement, pancreatic tumors, blood clots, and various types of lesions. The expectation was that physicians would be able to plan much more accurately for therapeutic treatment and that they would be able to do so based on improved diagnostic information from tests that were noninvasive, safer, and more efficient.

Hospital *A*'s staff also predicted that the demand for body scanning would be considerable. They argued that judging from the demand for brain scanning, demand for body scanning was assured.

The planners accepted the argument that Hospital *A* was well qualified—if not uniquely qualified—to conduct CAT scanner research. Five years of experience conducting utilization studies of radiological diagnostic procedures for the National Institutes of Health buttressed the hospital's claim.

The planners also accepted the hospital's proposed research protocols and were encouraged by its willingness to accept patients from a number of Boston hospitals and community clinics.

Finally, the planners accepted the hospital's financing for the $570,000 machine (later upgraded in a separate CON approval to $625,000) and the projected total charges of $260 per scan ($200 technical component; $60 professional component).

HOSPITAL B

While Hospital *A*'s CON request was pending before the Public Health Council, Hospital *B* moved to acquire a research CAT scanner of its own. It was able to do so without going through the CON process by entering into an arrangement with the manufacturer, E.M.I. Ltd. of England, whereby E.M.I. would install a CAT scanner at Hospital *B* for demonstration purposes for one year only. Massachusetts law requires a CON only when a facility makes a major capital expenditure. E.M.I. classified the costs associated with the CAT scanner as "inventory costs chargeable against current operations and, therefore, not as capital expenditures."[16] Thus, neither the hospital nor E.M.I. had made a capital expenditure. A CON was not technically required.

The HSA and state planners were confronted with a special issue. Although the E.M.I. loan was for only one year, planners regarded the hospital's CAT scanner as more permanent. They expected the hospital, with a sophisticated research program already well underway, to file for a CON at the end of the one-year period. Indeed, the hospital had successfully worked just this strategy some years earlier when acquiring a brain scanner.

But both state and HSA planners had determined that only a single third-generation CAT scanner could be justified for research purposes in the Boston area. They strongly urged that proliferation of new technology should await further investigation of its merits. The planners had worked closely with Hospital A to develop a research plan. To deny Hospital A's application would, they felt, reward Hospital B for circumventing the CON processes and disregard Hospital A's efforts to work within the planning process. To grant Hospital A a CON on the other hand, would be to allow the installation of one more CAT scanner than they believed could be justified by sound planning. The CON staff phrased the dilemma clearly in its report to the Public Health Council:

> Staff has recommended that only one scanner is necessary to determine the efficacy of the procedure but staff notes that it may not be fair to deny an applicant who has, in good faith, undergone the rigors of the CON process because another institution has been successful in bypassing the very same process without violating the statute. In addition, would a denial encourage other institutions to follow the path of the bypasser? Staff is very concerned that a denial would be a clear incentive to all other institutions to exhaust all possibilities of bypassing the CON process. [17]

Thus, what the planners had initially regarded as a clear and reasonable planning decision, to grant a single CON to Hospital A to evaluate full-body scanning, had become a much more complicated problem. Rational planning principles had to be balanced against concern for the question of equity and for the integrity of the planning process.

In June 1976, the Public Health Council approved the acquisition of a CAT scanner by Hospital A. In January 1977 Hospital B formally requested a CON for the CAT scanner it had been operating on loan from E.M.I.

By August 1977 Hospital B had not acquired a CON for its CAT scanner. When informally advised by the HSA that the CON request would not be approved, Hospital B arranged to table the application. It considered extending the E.M.I. loan while organizing a new CON strategy. In September 1978 it submitted a new application for a CAT scanner to the CON office. Meanwhile a moratorium had been declared on scanner applications pending completion and approval of new guidelines for CAT scanner CONs. The new guidelines were approved by the Council in October 1978 and published for distribution in December 1978. These guidelines are more flexible and liberal and could allow Hospital B to obtain its request; therefore it is possible that the matter will come again to the Public Health Council. Recently, there were seventeen pending CAT scanner CON applications. [18]

Appealing and Circumventing the Massachusetts CON Procedures

One can see that even without new federal legislation there is every reason for a hospital to fight for a long period of time for a CON. The hospital must have the certificate in order to receive approval from the

Department of Public Health to operate any new facility as well as to
receive reimbursement for interest and depreciation.

The Department of Public Health licenses all health care facilities in
the Commonwealth. In conjunction with this responsibility, the Department conducts periodic surveys and inspections of the number of
beds of various types in a facility and of the specific services offered. An
institution denied a CON, therefore, could not proceed with the project
because it would be denied the necessary operating license. Further,
the Rate Setting Commission (RSC), in establishing each institution's
allowable charges, recognizes capital expenditures requiring CON review only if a CON has been obtained. Some institutions may seek to
avoid the CON process entirely by packaging some intended capital
projects in ways that will avoid the $150,000 threshold. A major expan-
sion or renovation, change in service, or acquisition of high technology
equipment cannot be long disguised in this manner.

The extensive auditing of hospital financial records by the RSC as
part of Blue Cross and Medicaid cost analysis also tends to deter such
behavior. Hence, as long as the CON process exists, institutions are
constrained to abide by its decisions.

Institutions whose applications have been denied must, therefore,
obtain a reversal of the final council decision if they are to proceed with
a desired project. Two basic mechanisms have been employed by institutions seeking to override application denials: appeals to the Health
Facilities Appeals Board (HFAB), the legitimate route sanctioned by the
CON process; and exemptive legislation introduced by sympathetic
legislators, the *end-run* to which Massachusetts hospitals and other
health care institutions increasingly resorted during 1976 and 1977.

APPEALS TO THE HEALTH FACILITIES APPEALS BOARD

There were forty-six appeals through December 1977 to the HFAB.
Eighteen of them related to applications from acute-care hospitals.
Seven appeals were filed in 1976, three in 1974, and two in each of the
other years with the exception of the first year of the program (1972).
Three of the appeals were made by ten-taxpayer groups,[19] the rest by
hospitals themselves.[20]

Most of these appeals were remanded to the Department of Public
Health for correction of procedural errors. The rash of appeals in 1976,
however, challenged the grounds upon which the Public Health Council made and justified its decisions.

In 1976, under the leadership of Dr. Fielding, the council began to
apply regional considerations to the evaluation of applications from
individual hospitals, rather than simply considering an application on
its own merit. Hence, for example, in the case of an application from
Children's Hospital to renovate its neonatal intensive care unit (NICU)
and simultaneously to expand the capacity of the unit from twelve to
eighteen bassinets, the council denied that portion of the application
involving expansion, stating:

There is a current maldistribution of NICU bassinets in the Commonwealth
so that any increase of NICU bassinets in the Boston area would further
exacerbate the concentration of NICU bassinets in Boston. As such, the
applicant should not be allowed to expand the proposed NICU from twelve
to eighteen beds.[21]

In denying the New England Medical Center application to rebuild
the Floating Hospital, the Council noted, among other reasons:

Although the applicant made a sizable effort to work with state and regional planning agencies, the Council felt that further expenditure in the
Boston area, without a joint regionalized planning effort, represented a poor
allocation of health care resources.[22]

In denying the Mt. Auburn application for a linear accelerator to be
used in radiation therapy, the Council listed as its first reason for
denial:

There was no demonstration of need for an additional supervoltage unit in
the Greater Boston area.[23]

The responses of the HFAB in these three cases provide important
insights into the board's evaluation of what constitutes the necessary
standards, circumstances, and evidence to support such denials.
Both the Children's Hospital and the New England Medical Center
cases were remanded[24] to the Department of Public Health because of
abuse of administrative discretion on the part of the Public Health Council. Regarding the *Children's Hospital* case, the HFAB stated:

The Department relied upon the fact that proportional to population there
is a relative overabundance of NICU bassinets in the Boston Metropolitan
area. In making that argument we cannot find that the Department ever
determined whether the number in the Boston Metropolitan area is excessive relative to what the Department judges it should be.[25]

In regard to the relevance of a lack of comprehensive planning in
Boston to review the New England Medical Center application, the
HFAB noted:

In light of the applicant's acknowledged willingness to engage in such
planning as required by the Regulations, we agree with the inference
drawn by the applicant that the Department is concerned that needed
regional master planning has not been done. But we also agree that the
burden cannot be placed upon any single applicant to undertake joint
planning for all hospitals in its region. To impose such a requirement on an
applicant which has clearly made a good faith attempt at joint regional
planning, while granting determinations to other institutions in comparable situations, is arbitrary, capricious, and an abuse of discretion.[26]

The HFAB, however, denied the Mt. Auburn appeal, noting that a
Department of Public Health study on the number and utilization of

supervoltage radiation therapy units in the Greater Boston area, considered by the council in reaching its decision, constituted appropriate evidence. Further, the HFAB found that the council's conclusion that the hourly use of the current machines in the Greater Boston area could be increased was "a consideration within its discretion in determining need for another supervoltage unit in the Region."[27]

Progress now being made in the development of criteria and standards for various categories of application may serve to limit the number of appeals for *abuse of discretion* in future years.

"END-RUNS" THROUGH EXEMPTIVE LEGISLATION

Exemptive legislation introduced in 1973 on behalf of the Bessie Burke Memorial Hospital in Lawrence, an industrial town outside of Boston, marked the first of several attempts to supersede Public Health Council determinations by action of the Massachusetts Legislature.

Passed over the Governor's veto, Chapter 923 of the 1973 statutes directed the commissioner of public health to issue a CON to the Burke Hospital. Chapter 923 was challenged by the Department of Public Health before the Massachusetts Supreme Judicial Court as being unconstitutional, but the court upheld the constitutionality of the statute in a ruling in 1975.[28]

During 1974 and 1975 no legislative exemptions were filed. In 1976 bills were introduced in the legislature on behalf of the St. Joseph's Manor Nursing Home, the St. John of God Chronic Disease Hospital, and the New England Baptist Hospital, each of which had been denied CONs for major construction projects. The Legislature passed bills for St. Joseph's and St. John, both of which were vetoed by Governor Dukakis; only the veto for St. Joseph's was subsequently overridden.

During 1977, bills were introduced on behalf of seven institutions denied CONs: New bills for St. John of God and the New England Baptist; a bill for the Amesbury Hospital, denied a CON for expansion of its emergency room; and bills for a chronic disease hospital, two nursing hospitals, and a freestanding kidney dialysis unit. The bills for St. John, Amesbury, one nursing home, and the New England Baptist were passed by the Legislature and vetoed by the Governor; with the exception of the New England Baptist bill, all of these vetoes were overridden. Bills for two other institutions also passed the Legislature but were pocket-vetoed by the Governor.

FIGHTING THE "END-RUNS"

In response to these bills, the Department of Public Health, the Office of State Health Planning, and the Greater Boston HSA undertook aggressive campaigns to inform the Legislature and the public about both the CON program in general and the reasons for each of the specific CON denials. Papers were prepared and presentations made explaining the basic purpose and functioning of the CON program, and an economic

analysis was developed to demonstrate the cost savings that had been
achieved as a result of its presence. Fact sheets were prepared on each of the institutions involved explaining why the proposed projects had been denied and stressing the importance of not circumventing the CON process.

The Boston press provided extensive coverage of the bills and wrote editorials on the necessity of maintaining the integrity of the CON program given the very high cost of health care in Massachusetts.

Blue Cross, the Associated Industries of Massachusetts, the Hospital Insurers Association of America, and segments of organized labor all lobbied hard, first against the passage of the bill for the New England Baptist Hospital and then to assure that the Governor's veto of it was sustained. This bill in particular was singled out because the Baptist project involved a $30 million replacement and expansion of the current facility that would have had a significant cost impact on private insurance. That this veto alone was sustained probably reflects both the success of these extensive lobbying efforts and the fact that the Baptist, unlike other institutions, had traditionally drawn its patients from all around the country and thus lacked the local constituency and support typical of the community-based facilities.

The impact of the successful "end-runs" on the ability of the CON programs to continue and to advance a stringent cost containment policy has yet to be evaluated. As a *Boston Globe* editorial in early January 1978 noted:

> Efforts to control medical costs in Massachusetts were unquestionably hurt during the just-concluded session of the state legislature, and the prognosis for their survival is at best guarded. Only strong support for the cost control program efforts which every sector of the Commonwealth's populace should support, can assure its return to full health.[29]

By continuing to press for full and public participation by all affected institutions, the hope within the Office of State Health Planning is to obviate the end-run or due process challenge to the CON process (see Appendix 1-C *infra*). However, by 1979, the Massachusetts Legislature had again passed a number of bills seeking either to overrule the Public Health Council or to circumvent the CON procedures entirely, and by year end, Governor King had vetoed most of these.[30]

NATIONAL IMPLICATIONS

Accordingly, if state and local consensus concerning definition-of-need is so difficult to achieve, securing similar agreement at a national level would seem to be much more difficult. In particular, the allocation of a scarce resource tends to encourage both overt and covert adversary proceedings.[31] Thus passage of the 1978 Federal Cost Containment bill, with its proposed emphasis on the CON process, would have exacerbated in Massachusetts what already seemed to be a difficult situation.

Similar difficulties could be expected to occur in every state with an established CON program, as the process embraced by the proposed 1978 National Hospital Cost Containment bill would be cumbersome at best. Losers, probably unable to make congressional end-runs as easily as they could in a state legislature, could still appeal adverse decisions through the courts. Therefore, it is possible that such an appellate process would also delay approvals, given the fact that if available monies were spent during the appeal, the question would become moot. Clearly, the whole process could take an unconscionably long time.[32]

In short, without some ready way for all interested parties to negotiate before regulations are written, one would predict difficulty in regulatory implementation. Moreover, remoteness of federal regulation drafting from the give-and-take of the local scene must have fueled the opposition to the 1978 Hospital Cost Containment bill.

II. OBTAINING CLEAR FEDERAL REGULATION: HEALTH MAINTENANCE ORGANIZATION (HMO) IMPLEMENTATION[33]

Clearly it is difficult to translate legislative mandates into a list of rules and regulations which can be applied uniformly across the nation. Furthermore, the continuing failure of HEW agencies to promulgate useful regulations and guidelines expeditiously following congressional action is a constant annoyance to those operating health care institutions. One glaring example, fresh in many minds, is the difficulty HEW experienced writing regulations for the Health Maintenance Organizations (HMOs).[34] This section will examine problems encountered in attempts to draft regulations for the particular section of the original 1973 act as well as the amendments thereto passed in 1976 covering reimbursement for the treatment of chronic alcoholism.

RELEVANT LEGISLATION

It should be noted that three pieces of legislation define the range of federal structural intervention in the health sector: The Professional Standards Review Organization (PSRO) program, the National Health Planning and Resources Development Act of 1974, and the Health Maintenance Organization (HMO) Act of 1973.

The PSRO program is at one end of the range. It was established by the Social Security Amendments of 1972. PSRO programs emphasize self-regulation by hospital physicians and involve a minimum of structural change. They address action within the profession to reduce costs and improve quality.

At the other end of the spectrum is the National Health Planning and Resources Development Act of 1974 (Public Law 93-641)[35] which mandates that each state have a CON program in effect by 1980. This law

provides strong federal direction and support for state and local planning and regulatory activities, to be conducted by a set of newly created
organizations. It replaces a number of outmoded health planning activities embodied in the Hill-Burton Hospital Construction Act, the
Regional Medical program, and an earlier comprehensive health planning law.

Somewhere in the middle is the Health Maintenance Organization
Act of 1973. HMOs, of which the best known is the Kaiser Plan, are
largely organized around prepaid fixed fees covering all essential medical services.[36] The 1973 act was designed to offer a market solution to
the nation's health needs; presumably publication and marketing of a
prepaid plan would stimulate competing groups to try to offer equivalent services for less (evidence that this actually occurs is cited by
Enthoven, Chapter Six *infra*[37]). Consequently, at the core of the act is
the belief that competition among health care delivery organizations
should produce more efficacious structural reform. The result should be
a health financing and delivery system to be preferred over either
"reversion" to self-regulation or increased federal control.

HMOs do not have to be federally certified. However, if they wish to
qualify for certain benefits to remain competitive, they frequently elect
to meet the conditions required and become subject to regulation by the
federal government.

So the puzzle is that if competition is to be fostered by both qualita-
tive and quantitative differences among competing institutions, how
are regulations to be drafted that would foster these differences (i.e.,
promote competition) rather than lock in uniformity and, supposedly,
freeze or fix cost?

Persons struggling to decide whether or not to support the 1978 cost
containment proposals do so against a background of massive federal
involvement in health care, with regulatory responsibility divided
among several agencies. It is reasonably certain that most health care
professionals (within and without the federal government) knew, or
could have guessed, the difficulty HEW staffers were having with
rulemaking for the HMO services mandated by Congress. Health care
professionals had to be concerned with the difficulties and delays that
each new congressional health care legislative act entailed.

THE HMO REGULATORY SETTING

Why Is It So Difficult to Come Up with Guidelines for Reimbursement for Treatment of Chronic Alcoholism?

The HMO program was designed as a conditional grant and loan program. Through the dual-choice mechanism, however, the statute's impact goes beyond the federally qualified HMOs to the rest of the medical
marketplace.

The purely conditional requirements of the HMO Act placed extraordinary burdens on the regulation writers in HEW. The legislation specified a wide range of required practices and services for any HMO that seeks to gain federal certification and eligibility for federal financial assistance. The wide range of required services called for regulation which would affect the stakes and interests of a large number of governmental and nongovernmental parties (e.g., the National Institute for Alcohol Abuse and Addiction (Public Health Service)), many of whom had only nominal previous interaction with the heretofore nonregulated, prepaid health plan industry. While the statute specified controversial conditions such as community rating for federal qualification, the development of regulatory options—or, indeed, even a single regulatory definition—demanded high levels of expertise requiring outside consultants. In addition, other statutory requirements such as family planning were left so vague that there were large numbers of parties whose stakes and interests might be affected by the regulatory language and who could (and did) propose an endless number of regulatory alternatives.

An intent of the statute was that the regulations should induce market demand for federally qualified HMOs. This aim involves both labor and business interests in bargaining for medical benefits.

WRITING THE REGULATIONS FOR THE 1973 ACT

Several months before the HMO Act was finally passed and signed in 1973, HEW began the process of drafting the regulations. George Zenk,[38] in the program division, was given the responsibility to write an implementation plan for the promulgation of regulations. In regulatory parlance, an *implementation plan* is a timetable for writing and publishing regulations. Zenk reported to Paul Chandler, the director of the Bureau of Community Health Services in which the HMO program division then resided.

Chandler organized and headed a policy work group made up of high-level HEW staffers to oversee promulgation of the regulations. This group would review the issue papers that were to be developed by the task groups (the staff within HEW assigned to HMOs is hereinafter referred to as HMO/HEW). The task groups consisted of representatives from HEW and from potentially affected interest groups and private consultants. Based on the recommendations of the task-group reports, the policy work group was charged with writing the final language of the proposed regulations and forwarding them to the Secretary of HEW for approval before publication as proposed rules in the *Federal Register*.

In early November, 1973 Zenk began to organize eight task groups to prepare issue papers for various sections of the anticipated legislation. The task groups were organized to deal with issues as follows:

Task group 1	HMO data and evaluation
Task group 2	HMO loan program
Task group 3	Medical quality

Task group 4   Insurance, rates, and regulatory matters
Task group 5   Services and benefits
Task group 6   Enrollment
Task group 7   HMO administration, management and funding procedures
Task group 8   HEW administrative issues

Zenk issued the implementation plan, the timetable for the eight task forces. According to this *Butterfly Plan* (so-called because of its appearance on paper), the task groups would do preliminary work before the legislation was finally passed and signed, and would begin work on issue papers shortly after the signing of the legislation. The regulations were to be published nine weeks later, after the policy decision group made its final recommendations to the Secretary.

The Alcoholism Regulations: Task Group 5

The first formal meeting of Task Group 5 in November 1973 did not discuss alcoholic services directly, but the members did discuss general strategies for specifying required services. According to an interesting set of minutes from the meeting:

> On the subject of Basic Health Services there seemed to be a consensus that it would be preferable to be general rather than specific in describing the services which an HMO must offer. It's difficult when writing a national program to mandate a minimum set of benefits for the entire nation. If the Government makes HMOs offer a nice package at $75 a month, but lets the HMO competitors offer less than $50 per month, "you're pricing us out of the market."

After this general discussion, an issue paper on a minimum benefits package was assigned to a subgroup. Treatment of the issue of specificity, discussed again by the subgroup, indicated that it was difficult to tailor a plan for a national program that could be applied locally.

An information memorandum was prepared for Task Group 5 by Jack Blackman of the Kaiser Hospital Foundation Health Plan. In essence, the memorandum served as a preliminary issue paper on the minimum benefit package. It stated:

> The benefit package(s) presently offered by the older more mature prepaid group practice plans have evolved in response to the demands of major purchasers and have been tailored to meet their needs and requirements. The primary objective in the development of a minimum benefit package is to devise a benefit structure that provides a reasonably broad spectrum of benefits at a cost that is competitive in the marketplace.[39]

Based on the House bill, Blackman proposed seventeen "permissible limitations and/or exclusions" from the required services package, including "limitations upon and/or treatment for acute and chronic alcoholism and drug addiction."

At this time, neither the House nor Senate HMO bill called for mandatory services for alcoholism as a requirement for HMO qualification.
The House HMO bill and the Senate HMO bill were passed in December 1973. The Senate and House formed a conference committee for
the bills that met late in December.

Senator Hughes (D-Iowa) was able to induce the conference committee to include alcoholic services as a mandatory benefit. Discussions
with a Senate staffer indicate that Hughes's concern was that alcoholism
be defined as a *mainstream* medical problem and be so recognized in the
expenditure of federal dollars; inclusion as a mandatory service would
enhance that objective by providing precedentary value.

What emerged from the conference was a compromise between the
Senate bill's broad range of requirements and high subsidies, and the
House bill's less comprehensive range of services and lower financial
support. The compromise statute was characterized by a broad range of
required services, extraordinary specificity, a low level of funding, and
a designation as a "five-year demonstration project."

The first draft of Task Group 5's issue paper, adopting the point of
view expressed in Jack Blackman's memorandum, recommended that
the primary objective in the development of a minimum-benefit package be to devise a benefit structure that provided a reasonably broad
spectrum of benefits at a cost that was competitive in the marketplace.

Dr. Joseph L. Dorsey, based upon his experience running the Harvard Community Health Plan, responded that it would be a mistake to
require comprehensive services for alcoholism:

> The precise intent of the Senate lawmakers in adding this section to the
> definition of "basic health services" is not self-evident, thus, it appears
> both necessary and appropriate to interpret this section in the context of
> current arrangements for handling patients with the problems described.[40]

Dorsey recommended that the regulation require federally qualified
HMOs to diagnose and treat organic complications which arise from the
abuse of or addiction to alcohol or drugs, such as gastrointestinal
bleeding or skin infections. However, the HMO should be responsible
only for referring patients to traditional medical and psychiatric resources for help in dealing with the underlying abuse or addiction
problems:

> Services for dealing with alcohol abuse and drug addiction require highly
> specialized resources which cannot be developed within most HMOs. In
> this area, it is much more appropriate to develop linkages to existing
> community programs rather than to require their direct provision by the
> HMO.[41]

Up to this point, there was no organized participation by the Alcohol, Drug Abuse, and Mental Health Administration (ADAMHA) in the writing of any of the minimum-benefits package regulations. The National Institute for Alcohol Abuse and Addiction (NIAAA) is the agency within ADAMHA with the responsibility for program planning and research on alcoholism. It is also the strongest organizational advocate for strengthening the alcoholism treatment components of HEW programs.

As Task Group 5 was completing its report, NIAAA finally mobilized itself to make an organized effort to affect the regulation. The NIAAA position was decidedly opposed to the Dorsey position:

> [As] part of the basic benefits package, HMOs should provide "medically supervised withdrawal from prolonged or acute intoxication and other accepted therapies appropriate to the treatment and medical management of alcoholism and drug abuse."

The Task Group 5 Report noted:

> This is an unresolved issue with obvious differences in the point of view. The primary difference of opinion centers around the NIAAA language which would have the HMO responsible for "medically supervised withdrawal from prolonged or acute intoxication . . . ." Consultants of Task Group suggest that the NIAAA approach to this part of the legislation would not be workable "in the real world."

Although the report noted that it was an unresolved issue, the leadership of the task group had already decided to recommend a regulation to the policy work group that would not require long-term alcoholism services. The subtask group on minimum benefits had already decided, before the verbal objections to the Dorsey position, that to require comprehensive alcoholism benefits would place unreasonably heavy economic burdens on federally qualified HMOs.

NIAAA finally assigned a staffer to write a memorandum explaining fully its position in late January 1974. The first sentence in this memorandum capsulizes the NIAAA position on what the regulations should require:

> Medical treatment and referral services for alcohol related problems must be comprehensive. [42]

The NIAAA recommendations were made too late to affect the regulations. The HMO program staffers and outside members of the task group felt that to require comprehensive long-term alcoholism services would wipe out the HMOs. By the time the work policy group had received the NIAAA memorandum it had already decided the language of the HMO regulation that would be published in the "Notice of Proposed Rulemaking" in the *Federal Register:*

Section 1302(E) of HMO Act

Requires federally qualified HMOs to offer as basic health services, "medical treatment and referral services (including referral services to appropriate ancillary services) for the abuse of or addiction to alcohol and drugs.

Proposed Regulations Published in Federal Register, May 8, 1974

110.108 Health benefits plan; basic health services.

(a) Each health maintenance organization shall have the capacity and capability to deliver or arrange for the delivery of the basic health services, as follows . . .

(5) Medical treatment and referral services (including referral services to appropriate ancillary services) for the abuse of or addiction to alcohol and drugs. The diagnosis and medical treatment of alcohol and drug abuse and addiction shall be provided to health maintenance organization members. Screening, referral, and followup of patients with alcohol or drug problems to appropriate ancillary resources also shall be provided.

(b) The following are not required as basic health services:

(6) Treatment for chronic alcoholism and drug addiction, except as required by section 1302(E) (1) of the Act and paragraph (a) (5) of this section.[43]

Drafting Guidelines

By mid-February 1974, the task groups were no longer meeting on any sort of systematic basis; their work was largely done. The next task facing the group, still under the purview of Paul Chandler, was to write and promulgate guidelines. The guidelines for the alcoholism regulations would have to resolve several policy issues that were left quite vague in the regulations. For example, what exactly did Section 1302(E) (1) of the statute require? What were the exact distinctions between the services for which the HMO remained at full financial risk and those for which they could refer patients to other facilities without assuming financial responsibility? What constituted *treatment*?

According to plan, these guidelines would be published concurrently with the publication of final regulations in the *Federal Register* in October 1974, after a public comment period on the proposed regulations presented *supra*. Chandler was pushing hard to keep to this timetable; as the head of the Bureau of Community Health Services, he felt that timely promulgation of regulations and guidelines for the HMO Act would help him in his fight to keep control of the HMO program.

Zenk was faced with the task of formulating a wide-ranging set of other guidelines for this extremely detailed statute. In addition to having a small staff, Zenk had no insurance experts or medical doctors on his staff.

Janet Smith, a HMO/HEW staffer, was given the responsibility for writing the alcoholism guidelines. Since she had no alcoholism experts or medical doctors on her staff, Smith asked NIAAA to write a set of guidelines based on the proposed regulations published in the *Federal Register* (May 8, 1974). According to Zenk's original *Butterfly Plan*, the guidelines were to take from four-to-six weeks for writing and an additional two weeks for review and approval by Chandler. After a higher review process, the final guidelines would be ready for HEW regulation in October, when the final regulations were published.

It soon became clear through an exchange of memoranda that NIAAA was determined to write extremely detailed guidelines based on the somewhat vague regulations. This would force HMOs to adopt a sweeping and comprehensive program of alcoholism services. Not only did NIAAA write proposed guidelines that would require long-term and chronic care, it also specified in great detail what was acceptable medical practice for treatment. The position of the HMO/HEW staffers was that overspecificity in defining the required services for any single item in the required benefits package would introduce rigidity that could not account for differences in geography, socioeconomic characteristics of the population to be served, and the normal variations in medical practices among doctors. In addition, highly detailed guidelines would not account for the differences in available resources in potential federally qualified HMOs. Smith said in a later interview, "We [HMO/HEW] wanted to write guidelines that would allow them [the HMOs] to make scarce resources equitably available for treatment of their enrolled patients."

The NIAAA-proposed guidelines on alcoholism were far different from what the HMO/HEW program staffers wanted. The final regulations were published in October 1974 with the guidelines on the required-benefits package far from ready even for consideration by Chandler. The final regulations on alcoholism published in October of 1974 were slightly changed from the May 8, 1974, version. The final regulations *deleted* the requirement for screening, as it was not required by the statute. The regulations *added* language requiring detoxification services. They also specified that referral services could include referral for medical services, although the HMO would remain financially responsible for paying for medical services on referral. The final regulations kept the language, "Treatment for chronic alcoholism and drug addiction, except as required by section 1302(E) (1) of the Act and paragraph (a)(5) of this section are not required to be provided as basic health services."

An Outside Expert to Resolve Conflict

Faced with steady pressure by Chandler to produce guidelines, Smith decided to hire Dr. Jack Criley—director of a Kaiser Foundation hospital in San Francisco. He had a wealth of experience with a long-operating and heavily subscribed prepaid health plan, and he was a medical doctor. Criley, according to Smith, reflected the Kaiser position on alcoholism, which is generally one of trepidation about providing comprehensive services under their basic contracts.

Criley, after reflecting on a set of guidelines written by ADAMHA— the umbrella organization in which NIAAA resides—stated:

> When I began to read them [ADAMHA guidelines] I realized that they were totally inappropriate. First of all, they were so detailed and rigid that they went well beyond the intent of the statute in telling the federally qualified HMO doctors how to do their jobs. Secondly, in some sections they conflicted with the law. Third, it appeared that ADAMHA really did not understand the HMO concept.
>
> The guidelines were entirely too prescriptive. For example, they not only told a doctor in very specific terms what to look for during a physical examination of an alcoholic; they even specified which tests to order. This is not appropriate for guidelines.
>
> In addition, in other sections the guidelines conflicted with the law. They [ADAMHA] simply did not realize that under the statute a federally qualified HMO was allowed to refer patients out to other treatment facilities. The law only required treatment of medical emergencies, detoxification, and referral for long-term rehabilitation and care. As one example, the proposed guidelines would prohibit an HMO from contracting with another commercial services for detoxification services. They simply did not understand that this was acceptable under the law, as long as the HMO paid for it. In addition, the guidelines prohibited referral for long-term rehabilitation services. This runs counter to the law; in addition, ADAMHA did not seem to understand that most M.D.s, in an HMO or not, would accept the ethical responsibility to make sure a referral agency could be found.
>
> Other sections of the guidelines reflected the fact that they [ADAMHA] did not understand the intent of the law or the concept of the HMO in the medical marketplace. For example, one section of the proposed guidelines mandated that before any HMO patient could be released from the facility after a detoxification, he would have to be interviewed by a social worker retained by the HMO. Can you imagine how that would work in practice? Let's say a mineworker in east Kentucky comes into an HMO late on a Saturday night, drunk as a lark, and the HMO detoxifies him. By 3:00 a.m. Sunday morning he may be ready to go home to his wife and children. Just how is the HMO supposed to find a social worker at 3:00 a.m. on Sunday morning to interview him? Should we simply require that he stay there, rather than go home to his family, until Monday morning?[44]

The Argument Unresolved

Criley decided that he should try to educate NIAAA on the HMO concept and on the need for flexibility in the guidelines in order to preserve economic incentives for prepaid plans to become federally qualified.

NIAAA staffers reportedly knew that they would have a tough fight

on their hands to have their guidelines approved for publication by
Chandler. They considered Criley to be fairly negative about the appropriateness of prepaid health plans providing long-term alcoholism
treatment.

The HMO/HEW, according to a spokesman, was fearful that "if you opened the doors for wide-ranging alcoholic services, 9 million alcoholics would come streaming through their doors and financially devastate the HMOs."

Criley sent memoranda to NIAAA trying to convince it of the need for flexibility on the part of HMOs; NIAAA sent memoranda back to Criley and HMO/HEW restating the need for comprehensive guidelines. Above all, NIAAA tried to convince HMO/HEW that the contractual promise for comprehensive alcoholic services would not financially devastate the HMO.

By this time it was December 1974, nearly one year after the HMO Act was passed and signed, and there were still no published guidelines for Subpart A which included the benefit package. Although guidelines for several other sections were at least in the clearance process by this time, Subpart A guidelines—in many respects the most crucial, since they would specify exactly what a prepaid plan had to provide in return for qualification—had not yet even been sent to Chandler's office.

Pushing the conflict up the Bureaucratic Ladder

Criley, Zenk, and Smith finally went to Chandler and explained their lack of progress in reaching a compromise with NIAAA. Chandler, however, was under strong pressure to produce guidelines for higher-level review in HEW. He asked Zenk, Criley, and Smith to explain the nature of the issues yet to be resolved for Subpart A, not only for alcoholism but also for mental health, family services, child services, and several other categorical types of services. They explained to Chandler that organizational advocates of the categorical services in HEW were putting a great deal of pressure on them for "pages and pages" of guidelines for each required service.

Chandler decided that he would resolve the policy differences by acting as an arbiter. In late December 1974, he set up a meeting concerning alcoholism guidelines with Zenk, Criley, Smith and representatives of NIAAA and ADAMHA. According to Zenk, "Chandler used his muscle as bureau chief to carry the weight of the argument that flexibility was needed for the HMO concept."

As an example of one of Chandler's decisions, the guidelines mandated the HMO to be responsible financially only for the first three detoxifications in any one year for a patient; after that, it was no longer required as a service. This standard was accepted at the suggestion of Criley—it was the standard he employed at Kaiser in San Francisco.

Similar meetings were held by Chandler for most of the individual items in the required benefits package, and under pressure from his superiors, Chandler arbitrated between HMO/HEW and the categorical program units in HEW and decided on a complete set of Subpart A regulations.

The next step in the process for guidelines was to send them to the Office of the General Counsel (OGC) for legal clearance and to clarify redrafting where necessary. The OGC attorneys assigned to review the guidelines read the first 18 pages (out of over 200) and finally gave up in frustration. They returned the guidelines, largely unread, to Chandler saying the HMO/HEW would have to resolve policy issues fully in the formulation phase before OGC could clear the guidelines.

The guidelines have never been published. After the OGC rejection of the guidelines, there was never again a concerted effort to write them.

1976 AMENDMENTS—HMO ALCOHOLISM BENEFITS

In 1976 the Congress considered a series of amendments to the HMO Act of 1973 that would remove some structural constraints and economic disincentives contained in the original act. Many HMO advocates urged that requirements for services for alcoholism be stricken from the statute altogether.

HEW submitted a package of proposed legislative amendments early in 1976. In preparation for the HMO package, HMO/HEW staffers were asked to draft a set of recommendations. When completed, these recommendations suggested that the alcoholism benefits be stricken from the original 1973 statute. HMO/HEW staffers believed that the existing alcoholism benefits were impeding HMO growth. This recommendation was accepted by HEW and forwarded to the Office of Management and Budget (OMB) for clearance. However, under intense pressure from organizational advocates such as NIAAA, the OMB rejected the recommendation to delete alcoholism benefits. At the hearings on the 1976 amendments to the HMO Act, HEW representatives therefore urged in their testimony that the alcoholism benefit *not* be dropped.

Because of differing views on how best to help the HMO program through statutory amendments, the House and Senate reported HMO Act amendment bills with widely varying provisions. The House bill dropped alcohol and addiction services from the required basic health services and added to the optional supplemental health services "referral services and medical treatment for the abuse of or addition to alcohol or drugs." This would completely remove the requirement for any kind of mandatory alcoholism services at a federally qualified HMO. The Senate amendment did not change the alcoholism provisions.

The House-Senate conference committee met in September 1976, and it was widely assumed by the members and staffers that the House position on alcoholism would be accepted. The conference committee had to consider controversial measures on a number of requirements, such as community rating; dual choice (i.e., a requirement that all employees of an organization be offered membership in an HMO as

part of their medical benefits plan, if there were a qualified HMO in **31**
their area); methods of tying Medicare and Medicaid into dual choice; *Is Government*
and open enrollment. A basic issue was how much the conference *Regulation*
Helpful?
part of their medical benefits plan, if there were a qualified HMO in
their area); methods of tying Medicare and Medicaid into dual choice;
and open enrollment. A basic issue was how much the conference
committee would be willing to relax federal requirements in order to
stimulate greater growth in the number of federally qualified HMOs.
Deleting alcoholism requirements might be one way to stimulate
growth.

However, Dr. Daniel Duffy, a Senate staff member who had been a
member of the 1973-to-1974 task group charged with writing recommendations for regulations for HMO services and benefits, fought to
retain the alcoholism requirements in the statute. He was able to form a
coalition, and the conference language, in the final report of the conference committee, "conforms to existing law because of indications that
provision of alcohol and addiction services as part of basic services, is
not an economic burden on the HMO."

After passage of the HMO amendments of 1976, HEW was faced with
the task of writing new regulations. At that time five major areas
needed rewriting in order to conform with the amended statute. Even
those regulations that were not directly affected were being reviewed
for possible rewriting.

Five task forces had been established to accomplish the rewriting.
One of them (headed by Gary Tolbert) was to have reviewed and
rewritten completely the regulations on the required and supplemental
benefits package by August 26, 1977. It missed the completion date, and
HEW authorities reviewing the matter concluded that the group had
been unable to resolve a number of key issues, in particular the issue of
reimbursement for treatment of chronic alcoholism.

Historically, the guideline assignment has been ill-fated. Deadlines
seem to come and go with little success in drafting regulations for
reimbursement for the treatment of chronic alcoholism or for other
controversial matters. The problem regulatory bodies have in converting regulations into workable sets of rules for the implementation of
mandated programs can be virtually insoluble. Table I-2 illustrates this
problem by summarizing the status of rule and guideline publication
for the several sections of the HMO Act.

NATIONAL IMPLICATIONS

The question, then, is how different is the drafting of health care
regulations compared to regulation writing for other sectors of society?
Are rate-setting via the CON process and rulemaking for the HMOs
examples of particularly cumbersome processes created only to resolve
complex health issues? Or, rather, is regulation, which has become
prevalent in other societal sectors, still unfamiliar to most involved in
health care? Consider the following health care examples drawn from all
levels of government. Are they generally parallel or different from
regulatory issues in other sectors of the economy? Assuming the con-

TABLE 1-2 Regulation Timeline and Status for Health Maintenance Organization (HMO) Act of 1973 before the Passage of the 1976 Amendments (information current as of June, 1978)

Major area	Publication of proposed rules	Publication of final rules	Publication of guidelines
Subpart A Requirements for an HMO	May 8, 1974	October 18, 1974	Never published
Subparts B, C, D, E Federal financial assistance; grants for feasibility; grants and loan guarantees for planning, initial development, and loans; and loan guarantees for initial operating costs	May 8, 1974	October 18, 1974	1975
Subpart F Qualification of HMOs	December 9, 1974	August 8, 1975	1975
Subpart G Restrictive state laws and practices	May 8, 1974	October 18, 1974	1975
Subpart H Employees' health benefit plans	February 12, 1975	October 28, 1975	1975
Subpart I Continued regulation of HMOs	September 17, 1976		1975

cerned administrators are acting in good faith, will resolution of these problems lead to reasonable programs?

- An analyst in a state health planning and development agency struggles to develop a scoring system to rank sixty proposed projects, only half of which can be accepted. The task seems overwhelming. No procedure exists for making the necessary trade-offs. How can one compare two ultrasound machines in a local community hospital to a physical therapy room addition in an urban teaching institution? What is in the public interest? What can be defended? What system will stand the test of time?

- A joint meeting of HEW and Federal Trade Commission (FTC) lawyers quickly reaches a deadlock. The FTC lawyers believe that physician licensure is a fertile area for an antitrust investigation. But according to their counterparts from HEW, more doctors appear to push prices up rather than down through competition. How can government address the rising costs of physician services? Where and how should traditional models be amended or new ones developed?

- A PSRO committee attempts to establish guidelines for reviewing patient records, but finds criteria running off into infinite detail as it encounters the uniqueness of nearly every patient treated. Each case reviewed costs twelve dollars. Is there a better way to provide incentives to conserve resources throughout the health care provision system? How can this be done? Is this difficulty insurmountable in health care because of the doctor's need to do all he can for the sick?

- A member of a state RSC ponders the problem of establishing fair rates for reimbursing hospital services. A patient-based system is appealing— this much for inguinal herniography, that much for cholecsytectomy. Yet the large teaching hospital or referral center receives the most diagnostically and therapeutically complex patients and might deserve a premium. But how much should that premium be? Should rates differ from institution to institution? How do we measure cost when even the hospitals do not know the economic cost of treating a disease?

TOO MUCH HEALTH CARE REGULATION?

With all the national focus on deregulation in other societal sectors, why is it that Congress and the Executive Branch consider governmental intervention in health care as the preferred regulatory mode? Is it possible that the conflict inherent in such seemingly contradictory goals as containing health-care cost escalation while increasing access to quality health care does not lend itself to monolithic federal resolution? Toward the end of the current decade (the seventies), is there a growing disenchantment with the nation's ability to convert "simple," general health directives into practicable cost-effective programs?

If the situation in North Dakota represents a first step toward a "Proposition 13" equivalent for health care, then why did the 1978 Cost Containment Bill not pass Congress? It seems much too simple to ascribe the defeat of the legislation to a "small, narrowly based medical lobby." Perhaps the formulation of health care policy and health care regulation in the United States is no longer susceptible to sweeping mandates which are difficult to implement and enforce. Certainly the North Dakota and Massachusetts examples illustrate the pervasiveness of government in the organization and delivery of health care in the United States. The question is has this governmental intervention improved the quality or reduced the cost of health care?

Chapter Two by Professors Feldman and Roberts examines what happens when regulatory proposals and programs confront local, state, and national political realities. One usually assumes that the United States constitutional process encourages actions based on enlightened self-interest rather than quiet acquiescence to some central authority. Unless some sort of bargaining process is set in motion to accompany regulatory design and implementation and to encourage this enlightened self-interest, Feldman and Roberts argue, regulatory attempts will encounter grave difficulties. This seems particularly true for health care.

NOTES

1. This chapter is based on case studies developed by the authors preparatory to the conference organized by the Kennedy School of Government, Harvard University, pursuant to Contract No. HRA 230-77-0037 with the Health Resources Administration of HEW and with additional support from ADAMHA and the Commonwealth Fund.

2. The following text is extracted from J. Lublin, "Initiative to Regulate all Health Charges is North Dakota's Hottest Issue in Decades," *The Wall Street Journal*, Oct. 31, 1978, p. 19.

3. The following text is extracted from W. Sinclair, "Scuttling of Hospital-Costs Bill," *Boston Sunday Globe*, Nov. 19, 1978, p. 70.

4. The material in this section is taken from "Certificate-of-Need in Massachusetts," a case prepared by Julianne R. Howell, with the assistance of Cynthia J. Dahlin under the supervision of Dr. Richard S. Gordon, Kennedy School of Government, Harvard University, pursuant to Contract No. HRA 230-77-0037 (Copyright © 1977, The President and Fellows of Harvard College). The material in this case will be incorporated into Howell's Ph.D. dissertation for the Kennedy School of Government, Harvard University. For reference purposes the case as originally prepared has been deposited in the Kennedy School Library. Ms. Howell is now on the faculty of the Department of Community Medicine, University of California San Diego School of Medicine.

5. See Appendix 1-B *infra* for information concerning the provisions of Public Law 93-641.

6. *White Paper: Health Care Expenditures in Massachusetts*, Health Planning & Policy Comm., Commonwealth of Mass. (Apr. 30, 1976). See also M. L. Ingbar and L. D. Taylor, *Hospital Costs in Massachusetts: An Econometric Study* (Harvard Univ. Press, 1968).

7. *A Policy Statement: Controlling the Supply of Hospital Beds*, Inst. of Medicine, Nat'l Academy of Sciences (Oct. 1976); W. McClure, *Reducing Excess Hospital Capacity*, Contract No. HRA 230-76-0086, Bureau of Health Planning &

Resources Dev., HEW, Excelsior, Minn. (Oct. 15, 1976). Obviously it was

difficult in this broad study to recognize that major teaching centers attract a significant number of patients from outside the state for which provision of beds must be made.

8. See Appendix 1-A *infra* which describes "Key Participants in the Massachusetts Certificate-of-Need (CON) Program" and includes Figure 1-A-1 depicting the CON process in Massachusetts.

9. The Certificate-of-Need (CON) Program is officially called the Determination-of-Need (DON) in Massachusetts. The terms are interchangeable, and for the purposes of this book the acronym for the federal program (CON) is used in all references to the program.

10. The Health Facilities Appeal Board (HFAB), a five-member body, is independent of the Department of Public Health. It is empowered by statute with authority to review questions of procedure. In the course of a CON determination, it does not render judgment concerning the need for particular projects or the appropriateness of Public Health Council decisions. It can rule only on whether the Department of Public Health has adequately adhered to procedures dictated by statute and regulations, and thus has a scope no greater than that normally given the courts. Observers of HFAB action have noted that the merits of a particular case can informally influence the board's ruling. (See Appendix 1-A *infra* for further details.)

11. See Appendix 1-C *infra*, "Update Concerning the Massachusetts Certificate-of-Need Experience," written by Getson, Director, OSHP, DPH, Commonwealth of Mass. (May 1979).

12. Howell, n. 4 *supra* at Appendix B, "C.A.T. Scanner Policy in Boston," taken from the Codman Research Group, Inc., *The Impact of Planning and Regulation on the Pattern of Hospital Utilization in New England* #108–126, Progress Report No. 3, Contract No. HRA 291-76-003 (Apr. 1, 1977). By permission of Codman Research Group, Inc.

13. There are six Health Systems Agencies in Massachusetts, and each is located within one of six Health Systems Areas in the state. See Appendix 1-A, "Key Participants in the Massachusetts Certificate-of-Need Program" and Appendix 1-B, "The Provisions of Public Law 93-641."

14. N. 12 *supra* at 123.

15. Full-body scanning became feasible when technological advances reduced the scanning time from the two-and-a-half minutes necessary for a CAT brain scan to under twenty seconds. As a result, it became possible to obtain a clear image of particular organ tissues. Thus, organs with different attenuation coefficients and different tissue densities are candidates for brain and body scanning.

16. N. 12 *supra* at 125.

17. N. 12 *supra* at 126.

18. The Commonwealth of Mass., DPH, *Determination of Need Guidelines for CT Scanners*, Boston (Oct. 24, 1978).

19. Ten-taxpayer groups are a unique part of the Massachusetts CON process. The group can be an established organization or an *ad hoc* association of any ten people who register with the Department of Public Health to participate in a given determination.

20. In the early years of the program, most appeals dealt with basic procedural issues in the conduct application review by the CON staff and the Public Health Council: Provision of adequate notice and opportunity for comment to the planning agencies and to other concerned parties, observation of the time limits during which project review was to be completed, and provision of adequate opportunity for the applicant to present its case before Public Health Council.

21. Children's Hosp. Medical Center v. The Department of Pub. Health, HFAB *Final Decision* 2 (Dec. 22, 1976).

22. New England Medical Center Hosp. v. The Department of Pub. Health, *HFAB Final Decision* 2 (Aug. 10, 1976).

23. Mount Auburn Hosp. v. The Department of Pub. Health *HFAB Final Decision* 1 (Aug. 10, 1976).

24. The cases were each returned to the Department of Public Health for review and reconsideration based on the HFAB's evaluation.

25. N. 21 *supra* at 2.

26. N. 22 *supra* at 4.

27. N. 23 *supra* at 2.

28. A. E. Reider, J. R. Mason and L. H. Glantz, "Certificate of Need; The Massachusetts:", *American Journal of Law and Medicine I* 32 (1975).

29. "End-Run on Medical Costs," *The Boston Globe*, Jan. 9, 1978, p. 14. Cited with permission of *The Boston Globe*.

30. Editorial, "Health Facilities: Plans or Politics?" *The Boston Globe*, Aug. 10, 1979, p. 12; "Mahoney Urges King to Veto Some Medical Certificate Bills," *The Boston Globe*, August 17, 1979, p. 35; S. Cohen, "King Plans Veto for Most Special Health-Care Bills," *The Boston Globe*, Aug. 18, 1979, p. 13.

31. See S. Breyer, Ch. 5 *infra*.

32. Nevertheless, while the Hospital Cost Containment Act of 1979 as passed eliminated mandatory limits on the annual increases in hospital inpatient revenues, a separate bill containing proposals to limit capital expenditures, as in the 1978 Bill, was still pending when this book went to press.

33. The material in the following section is based on "HMO (Case B), Section III: The Reimbursement of Chronic Alcoholism," a case prepared by David Alexander under the supervision of Dr. Richard Gordon pursuant to Contract No. HRA 230-77-0037 (Copyright © 1977, The President and Fellows of Harvard College). Section III has been deposited in the Kennedy School Library for reference purposes. Some of the memoranda cited in this section are taken from the case. Alexander is now with American Management Systems, Inc., Arlington, Va.

34. The Health Maintenance Organization Act of 1973 provided a mechanism to certify health care delivery organizations. HMOs are prepaid medical care plans in which a fixed fee is paid for medical and hospital treatment. The oldest and best known HMO was founded by Henry J. Kaiser and now operates as the Kaiser-Permanente Foundation in the United States and Hawaii. See also Alain C. Enthoven's discussion of alternative health care financing and delivery systems (prepaid group practice, individual practice association, health maintenance plan, and health care alliance and variable

cost insurance) in "Consumer-Centered vs. Job-Centered Health Insurance," *Harvard Business Review* 143 (Jan.–Feb. 1979). See A. Enthoven, "Consumer-Choice Health Plan—A National-Health-Insurance Proposal Based on Regulated Competition in the Private Sector," 298 *The New England Journal of Medicine* 709–720 (March 30, 1978).

35. See Appendix 1-B *infra*.

36. See Enthoven, "Consumer-Centered vs. Job-Centered Health Insurance," n. 34 *supra* at 144.

37. See generally Enthoven, "Consumer-Centered vs. Job-Centered Health Insurance," n. 34 *supra*.

38. Pseudonyms have been used at the request of several persons interviewed for this case to allow for a more candid exchange of information.

39. N. 33 *supra*.

40. *Ibid.*

41. *Ibid.*

42. *Ibid.*

43. "Notice of Proposed Rulemaking," *Federal Register* (May 8, 1974).

44. N. 33 *supra*.

APPENDIX 1-A: KEY PARTICIPANTS IN THE MASSACHUSETTS CERTIFICATE-OF-NEED PROGRAM

The central actor at the state level in the Certificate-of-Need (CON) program is the Department of Public Health, which by statute has authority to make all final determinations of need. Actual decision-making power resides with the Public Health Council, chaired by the commissioner of public health.

The responsibility for analysis of all applications and for development of recommendations to the Public Health Council has been placed in the CON program within the Office of Health Facilities Development. Other staff offices such as the Division of Radiation Control and the Office of Emergency Medical Services may also be called upon if their expertise is relevant to the assessment of a particular application or to the development of requisite review standards and criteria. Since 1976, the Office of State Health Planning (OSHP), the former Comprehensive Health Planning (CHP) "a" Agency, has also resided within the Department of Public Health, and the Department of Public Health as a whole has been designated the State Health Planning and Development Agency (SHPDA) for Massachusetts under the provisions of Public Law 93-641.

The one other participant in *all* determinations of need is the Health Systems Agency (HSA) responsible for regional planning in the health service area in which the particular applicant is located. Depending upon the application, various ten-taxpayer groups and the state Rate Setting Commission (RSC) may also be involved. If there is disagreement with the final determination, then the Health Facilities Appeals Board (HFAB), the Legislature, the courts, and the Governor may also enter the CON process. Figure 1-A-1 outlines the various steps in the Certificate-of-Need process for the Commonwealth of Massachusetts.

The Public Health Council

The Public Health Council is a nine-member body chaired by the commissioner of public health that was established by statute to exercise the decision-making authority of the Department of Public Health for all determinations of need. All nine members are gubernatorial appointees and with the exception of the chairman or chairwoman serve for six-year terms. By law, three must be pro-

	1. Application	2. Review and recommendation	3. Decision	4. Appeal*
Specified procedure (by statute)	Office of State Health Planning ↑ Hospital	1. CON Program Staff 2. Health Systems Agency 3. Rate Setting Commission	Public Health Council	1. Health Facilities Appeal Board 2. Judiciary
Public action	↓ Newspaper announcement	10-taxpayer group (if organized)	Approval without appeal-project proceeds	Legislature Governor

* By applicant, HSA, or ten-taxpayer group.

viders of health services (two physicians) and five, nonproviders; the ninth member, the commissioner, has traditionally been a physician. In addition to rendering final judgment on all CON applications, the council must approve all regulations issued by the CON program and is the source of appeal for procedural decisions rendered by the director of the CON staff office.

While the council as a whole has played an active and central role in the CON program from its earliest days, it has also been subject to the influence of the commissioner of public health.

Staff Support

The CON program within the Office of Health Facilities Development of the Department of Public Health is responsible for conducting a detailed analysis of each CON application, receiving comment from the relevant HSA and ten-taxpayer groups, and making a recommendation to the Public Health Council. The director and staff of the program include members with backgrounds in health services administration, law, third-party reimbursement, and public administration.

The CON program is a regulatory one that derives its ultimate authority from the law. Therefore substantial legal expertise is required within the department to develop procedures that can eliminate the need for appeals to the greatest extent possible. The legal staff has worked closely with the CON staff in developing regulations and has issued advisory opinions on request of CON applicants and other participants in the CON process. The general counsel of the Department of Public Health serves as the counsel to the Public Health Council.

The development and maintenance of reliable baseline data on the availability and utilization of health care resources within the Commonwealth are essential to the assessment of "need" for proposed projects. These functions are being performed with increasing precision by the Office of Health Statistics within the department.

The Office of State Health Planning (OSHP)

The role of OSHP has gradually evolved into one of coordinating the development of the standards and criteria required to provide an objective and consistent basis for determining need and of serving as a liaison between the regional HSAs and state-level review and planning activities. OSHP rarely exercises the right of comment upon individual applications accorded it by the CON statute. Under the provisions of Public Law 93-641, OSHP is also responsible for developing the State Health Plan, State Medical Facilities Plan, and Annual Implementation Plan, which ultimately should provide an important foundation both for institutional planning and for CON evaluations.

The Health Systems Agency (HSA)

The six HSAs in Massachusetts all derive from regional CHP "b" agencies originally created by Public Law 89-749 in the late 1960s. Hence, the HSAs are well-versed in the "doctrines" of planning and are familiar with the various health care institutions in their geographic areas. Although the original CON legislation gave the regional CHPs only a review and comment role, the regulations effective in November 1976 made consultations with the HSAs mandatory in the development of all capital projects and in the preparation of all CON applications. Hospitals must also seek advice from the relevant HSAs in the preparation of one- and five-year plans mandated by this set of regulations. Copies of all CON applications must be filed with the relevant HSA, and HSA review proceeds simultaneously with the evaluation by the Department of Public Health CON staff. HSAs submit written recommendations to the department on all applications, and while the Department of Public Health is still free to make CON decisions that run counter to the recommendations of the HSA, it must state in writing its reasons for doing so. Under the provisions of Public Law 93-641, HSAs are now engaged in the development of health services plans for their regions. When completed, these plans could potentially play an important role in guiding CON implementation and further strengthen the role of the HSA in the CON process.

Ten-Taxpayer Groups

Unique to Massachusetts' CON process, any ten residents of the Commonwealth are provided the opportunity to participate in the review and evaluation of any CON application. The ten-taxpayer group can be an established organization or an ad hoc association of any ten people who register with the Department of Public Health to participate in a given determination. Such groups may register with the department at any time during the tendency of an application and have the right to comment during the review process, to request a public hearing on an application, to appear before the Public Health Council when it is considering the given application, and to appeal a final determination. Ten-taxpayer groups thus have standing equal to that of the applicant and the HSAs.

The ten-taxpayer mechanism was created to increase the leverage that consumers could bring to bear on the further development of the health care system in the Commonwealth. Ten-taxpayer groups have been active in many of the most controversial applications in recent years; the extent to which ten-taxpayer groups have represented health care consumers versus competing providers and the roles they have played in shaping the ultimate CONs have not as yet been systematically evaluated.

The Massachusetts Rate Setting Commission (RSC)

The RSC was created in 1968 with the merger of previously existing hospital and long-term care rate-setting bureaus. The RSC is now responsible for implement-

ing and administering a comprehensive charge control program for all Massachusetts hospitals. The RSC is also the recipient of one of six Social Security
Administration contracts under Section 222 of Public Law 92-603 to develop a
statewide prospective reimbursement system for hospitals. With three full-time
commissioners and a staff of more than a hundred, the RSC is the primary locus
in Massachusetts state government of expertise in hospital financial analysis.
Since January 1976, the RSC has conducted the requisite financial analysis on all
major applications for CONs submitted by hospitals. The RSC's input has
greatly increased the sophistication of CON financial review and has insured
that issues such as the eligibility of proposed expenditures for reimbursement
under Blue Cross, Medicare, and Medicaid regulations, and the impact of a
proposed project on a hospital's per-diem costs and charges are given the
necessary attention both by the applicant and the Public Health Council in
making its CON determination. The participation of RSC in the CON process
has also improved the linkages between the commission and the Department of
Public Health, and hence between the regulation of capital expenditures and of
hospital reimbursement.

The Health Facilities Appeals Board (HFAB)

As established by statute in Massachusetts General Laws, Chapter 6, Section
166, the HFAB is a five-member body placed within the Executive Office of
Human Services, the executive office under the aegis of which the Department
of Public Health also resides. Of the five members, three must be consumers not
associated with any provider of health care services. One of these consumers
must be a member of the bar of the Commonwealth and serves as chairman or
chairwoman of the group. All members are appointed by the Governor for
three-year terms on a staggered basis and are to be selected from persons
"knowledgeable in matters pertaining to the delivery of health care services."
Despite this presumed knowledge of health care issues, however, Massachusetts General Laws, Chapter 3, Section 25E limits the board's review authority
to questions of procedure in the course of a CON application. The scope of
review over Department of Public Health actions is thus no greater than that
normally given the courts. The HFAB does not render judgment on the need for
a particular project or on the appropriateness of the Public Health Council's
decision, but instead rules only on whether the department has adequately
adhered to the procedures dictated by the CON statute and regulations. Some
observers have noted, however, that an assessment of the merits in a particular
case may well be a factor in determining the board's ruling.

The Massachusetts Legislature

The CON program is a creation of the Legislature through whose efforts the
basic structure and purpose of the program were framed. However, while the
majority of legislators supports the general principles underlying the CON
program, it has found the translation of this policy into denials of specific CON
applications much less palatable. As a result, since the earliest days of the
program, institutions denied CONs have upon occasion sought exemptive
legislation to override the decisions of the Department of Public Health. The use
of this "appeal mechanism" has escalated in the past few years as the Public
Health Council has increased the stringency of its review and hence the rate of
application denials.

APPENDIX 1-B: THE PROVISIONS OF PUBLIC LAW 93-641

Public Law 93-641, the National Health Planning and Resources Development Act of 1974, was signed into law by President Ford on January 5, 1975. The Act established the framework for the creation of a new system of regional and state agencies intended both to rationalize the existing health care delivery system and to guide the development of future services. As stated in Section 1502, the priorities to be emphasized in the development and operation of federal, state, and area health planning and resource development programs are:

1. The provision of primary care services for medically underserved populations

2. The development of multi-institutional systems for coordination or consolidation of institutional health services

3. The development of medical group practices

4. The training and increased utilization of physician assistants

5. The development of multi-institutional arrangements for the sharing of support services necessary to all health service institutions

6. The promotion of activities to achieve needed improvement in the quality of health services

7. The development by health service institutions of the capacity to provide various levels of care . . . on a geographically integrated basis

8. The promotion of activities for the prevention of disease

9. The adoption of uniform cost accounting

10. The development of effective methods of educating the general public concerning proper personal health care

The fundamental geographic unit within which planning and resource development is intended to occur is the "health services area,"

[a] geographic region appropriate for the effective planning and develop-

42

ment of health services, determined on the basis of factors including population and the availability of resources to provide all necessary health
services for residents of the area.[1]

As required by the Act, health service areas must have a population between 500,000 and 3,000,000 (with certain exceptions), include at least one center offering tertiary care services (to the extent feasible); and, again to the extent possible, reflect existing "medical trade areas." With the assistance of the governors of the various states, the Secretary of HEW is required by the law to designate health services areas encompassing the entire United States. By the end of 1975, 202 health service areas had been designated.

The fundamental organizational unit created by Public Law 93-641 is the Health Systems Agency (HSA), the body intended to be responsible for health planning and development within a health service area. As provided by the Act, the Secretary of HEW, after consultation with the governor of the appropriate state, must designate either a private nonprofit corporation or a public entity operating under the aegis of a local governmental unit as the HSA for each health service area. The law requires each HSA to:

- Gather and analyze data regarding the health status of the residents of its health service area and the status and utilization of the health care delivery system in the area.

- Establish health systems plans stating the long-term goals for health service development in the area and Annual Implementation Plans (AIPs) stating the ways to achieve these goals and the priorities among them.

- Provide technical and/or limited financial assistance to organizations seeking to implement these plans.

- Coordinate activities with Professional Standards Review Organizations (PSROs) and other appropriate planning and regulatory agencies.

- Assist states in the review of CON applications for proposed capital expenditures by health care facilities within their health service area.

- Assist states in reviewing the appropriateness of existing institutional health services offered in the area.

- Review and approve or disapprove applications for federal funds sought for health programs within the health service area under various federal Acts.

- Recommend annually to states projects for modernizing, constructing, and converting health facilities in the area.[2]

Each HSA must have a governing board of ten to thirty members, the majority of whom must be consumers and the rest providers within the health service area. The governing body must also include appropriate elected officials and other government representatives. Each HSA is initially given conditional designation for up to two years, followed by permanent designation after the agency has submitted a Health Systems Plan acceptable to the Secretary of HEW. Funding for HSAs is provided by the federal government under a formula that provides up to 50 cents per capita in the health services area to a maximum of $3.75 million, subject to the annual appropriation of funds by Congress.[3]

To provide necessary planning and coordination at the statewide level, Public Law 93-641 established State Health Planning and Development Agencies (SHPDAs). These were intended to be state governmental agencies that would, among other things, (1) integrate the Health Systems Plans of the state's HSAs into a State Health Plan, taking appropriate cognizance of statewide as well as regional considerations and priorities; and (2) develop an annual State Medical Facilities Plan providing an inventory of existing facilities and services and a survey of the need for and proposed distribution of new or modernized facilities and services. This plan is to serve as the basis for distributing federal dollars for modernization, renovation, and development of facilities and services authorized by Title 16 of the Act.[4]

An SHPDA is to be selected by the governor of each state and designated by the Secretary of HEW. Annual grants to cover as much as 75 percent of the operating costs of these agencies are provided under the law. States which fail to participate by 1979 preclude any institution or agency within the state from receiving any form of assistance under the Public Health Service Act.

To provide advice and guidance to the SHPDAs comparable to that given HSAs by their boards, Public Law 93-641 created Statewide Health Coordinating Councils (SHCCs) to be composed of at least sixteen members appointed by the governor. The SHCCs are required annually to review and approve or disapprove the Health Systems Plans, Annual Implementation Plans, and the State Health Plan; to review the budget of each HSA; to review applications for the allotment of funds provided by several federal programs; and to advise the SHPDA on the performance of its functions.[5]

The National Health Planning and Resources Development Act thus created a new organizational framework within which both health planning and facilities regulation are to take place and mandated the development of four new and hopefully complementary plans: Health Systems Plans and Annual Implementation Plans to be generated at the HSA level and State Health Plans and State Medical Facilities Plans to be developed at the state level.

The Act also called for the establishment of national guidelines for health planning to provide the state and regional planning agencies standards to be used in plan development, on which to evaluate need for a wide range of medical services and facilities, and on which to act to control excess capacity in the health care industry. Guidelines for acute care services were first issued for comment on September 23, 1977, and amid a storm of controversy and debate, more than 55,000 comments were sent to the Secretary of HEW. On January 18, 1978, revised guidelines proposing the following national standards were issued:

- A maximum of 4 hospital beds per 1000 people

- An average annual occupancy rate of at least 80 percent for hospitals in a health service area

- At least a 75 percent average occupancy rate and at least 15,000 births annually for hospitals that provide care for complicated obstetrical problems

- No more than 4 neonatal intensive and intermediate care beds per 1000 live births

- A minimum of 20 beds for pediatric units in urban areas

- Average annual occupancy rates ranging from 65 to 75 percent for pediatric units, based on their size

- At least 200 open-heart procedures annually in any institution in which open-heart surgery is performed for adults, and at least 100 heart operations annually in any institution in which pediatric open-heart surgery is performed

- At least 300 cardiac catheterizations annually in any adult cardiac catheterization unit, and at least 150 cardiac catheterizations annually in any pediatric catheterization unit

- A service area with a population of at least 150,000 persons, or treatment of at least 300 cancer cases annually for megavoltage radiation therapy units

- At least 2500 procedures per year for each CAT scanner

- Plans consistent with already established HEW standards and procedures for suppliers of end-state renal disease services[6]

Public comment was once again sought on these standards. Additional guidelines to establish national health planning goals, to provide better access to health care, and to promote preventive services are now in preparation. HSA plans must be "consistent with" these guidelines; however, if a particular standard is felt to be inappropriate, given regional circumstances, an HSA may apply to the SHPDA, SHCC for a special exemption. Under the provisions of Public Law 93-641, the federal government is thus beginning to establish the quantitative standards that many states will require to operate stringent and effective CON programs.

The Implementation of Public Law 93-641 in Massachusetts

Massachusetts is well advanced in the development of both the organizational and the conceptual framework mandated by Public Law 93-641, and in many realms has established a planning and regulatory structure more stringent and sophisticated than that required by the Act. The Commonwealth's six HSAs, its SHPDA (the Department of Public Health), and its SHCC (State Health Coordinating Council) have all been functioning under conditional designation from HEW for several years; acute care standards and criteria more stringent than those proposed by the federal government have been in force since late 1976; and draft Health Systems Plans and Annual Implementation Plans have now been developed by each of the HSAs.

The Commonwealth is taking great pains to develop the coordination and linkages among the various regional and state actors necessary to make health planning and regulation effective forces in shaping the health care system. Among other developments, OSHP has established close linkages with the six HSAs. Monthly meetings are held between the director of OSHP and the six HSA directors as well as among the state and regional directors of planning and implementation. The task forces established for developing standards and criteria include representatives from the HSAs. An HSA/SHPDA Plan Development Coordinating Committee developed statewide guidelines to provide a uniform framework for the development of the Health Systems Plans and the State Health Plan. These guidelines were formally accepted by the six HSA boards of directors, the Health Policy Group, and the SHCC. The final plans ultimately developed will also be brought to each of these groups for ratification. A common basis upon which coordinated planning and regulation can proceed is thus being established.[7]

NOTES

1. The National Health Planning & Resources Dev. Act, P.L. 93-641, U.S.C. § 1511(a) (1) (1974).

2. *Health Planning and Resources Development Act of 1974* 7–8, Contract No. HRA 76-14015, HEW (1976); *ibid.* at § 1513.

3. *Health Planning and Resources Development Act, ibid.* at 8–9.

4. *Ibid.* at 10–13; n. 1 *supra* at § 1523.

5. N. 1 *supra* at § 1524(c).

6. "Statement by Joseph A. Califano, Jr., Secretary of Health, Education, and Welfare," *HEW News*, Jan. 18, 1978, pp. 3–4.

7. Interview with J. Getson, Director, OSHP, Commonwealth of Mass. (Jan. 4, 1978).

APPENDIX 1-C: UPDATE CONCERNING THE MASSACHUSETTS CERTIFICATE-OF-NEED EXPERIENCE

Jacob Getson, *Director, Office of State Health Planning,*
The Commonwealth of Massachusetts, Department of Public Health

I think it is particularly important to note the strong linkages which now exist among the planning and the regulatory agencies, specifically, the Office of State Health Planning (OSHP), the CON program, and the Rate Setting Commission (RSC). These forces have made a significant impact on containing health care costs in Massachusetts.

During the time that the RSC has been in place, the percentage increase in hospital costs has slowed from 14 percent to less than 10 percent. This is well below the present national average of 17 percent. In addition to using their authority to review and approve prospectively all hospital budgets, the RSC limits unnecessary expenditure growth by disallowing charges for any new service that has not been granted a CON by the Department of Public Health or by disallowing any operating charges which exceed the limits originally stipulated in a CON approval.

Complementing the RSC's effort to limit charge increases is the CON program which has had a slight but noticeable impact on limiting bed expansion. From 1973 to 1976, the overall ratio of hospital beds per 1000 population has dropped from 4.6 to 4.5. At the same time, however, the national average has increased from 4.3 to 4.6. In addition, the CON program has disapproved over $20 million in capital projects during the past 2 years alone. The increases in hospital costs that we have experienced are largely due to the increased intensity of ancillary service usage and outpatient department activity.

Underlying all of this regulatory activity is the planning function. Responsible for identifying unmet need and expensive programs, developing least costly alternatives, and promoting their implementation in a rational and orderly manner, the planning function is both a driving and guiding force behind the regulatory structure. Much of this direction and guidance is embodied in the State Health Plan which Massachusetts adopted in March of 1979.

Jointly, the three agencies have worked to improve the planning performance of hospitals through the development of hospital long-range plans and a new CON application form. In the long-range plan, hospitals must list all anticipated CON projects and address how each project relates to national, state, and regional health planning priorities. In the new application kit, hospitals must project the financial impact that a proposed project will have on operating costs. With the aid of changes like the ones I have just mentioned, I think we in Massachusetts have made great strides toward improving provider awareness of the importance to address cooperatively the problems of spiraling health costs.

The Massachusetts Legislature has also become more acutely aware of the impact that growing health care expenditures has on the tax dollar and therefore of the need to control them. Consequently, there have been no hospital CON exemption bills passed in the last two years. These events, I believe, point out the changing sentiment in Massachusetts toward the importance of the regulatory and planning process.

Two papers were developed by our office which might be useful references. One is a "Funds Flow"[1] report of hospital expenditures in Massachusetts. It compares the relative magnitude and trends among categories of health expenditures and provides a profile of the sources and uses of funds for all health care expenditures in the state. The second paper, "Determination of Need Guidelines for CT Scanners,"[2] is an updated version of the earlier position papers used by the department to evaluate CAT scanner CON applications. It is currently being used to assess some seventeen pending applications.

NOTES

1. Available upon request to the Office of State Health Planning, Department of Public Health, Commonwealth of Mass., 600 Washington St., Boston, Mass. 02111.

2. *Determination of Need Guidelines for CT Scanners*, Department of Public Health, Commonwealth of Mass., 600 Washington St., Boston, Mass. 02111 (Oct. 24, 1978).

APPENDIX 1-D: THE PURPOSE OF THE CONTRACT

INTRODUCTION

Upon his return to Harvard from service as Secretary of Labor (March 1975–February 1976), Professor John T. Dunlop was instrumental in developing a university-wide seminar and program devoted to the study and reform of the regulatory process. At about the same time, Professor Stephen Breyer of the Harvard Law School, a key member of the seminar, was commissioned by the American Bar Association to draft a book dealing with the reform of economic regulation. A few months later (in early 1977) senior officials of the Health Resources Administration (USPHS-HEW), learning of this activity, approached Harvard University with the idea of asking a task force—drawn from the seminar—to take a broader look at the regulatory morass in which health care agencies seemed to have become engulfed. The request was made not with the idea of analyzing any particular program or problem, but with the hope of developing an analytical approach or a "roadmap" that would help regulatory officials and interested parties work their way through the myriad pitfalls and quicksands associated with improving the regulation of health care.

THE CONTRACT

The contract[1] between the Health Resources Administration and Harvard University was made with the purpose of developing materials which would advance the following goals:

1. To study the changing character of regulation as it increases in amount and changes in type from distributive to redistributive

2. To improve the understanding of the regulatory process in order to maximize the opportunity for thoughtful approaches to future regulation

3. To reap experience from the more "traditional" regulator agencies which

might be useful in considering future approaches to regulation in health care

4. To stimulate large numbers of people, institutions and agencies to think broadly about regulation

5. To consider ways to maintain a continuing overview of the use of regulation at all levels of government

6. To find a systematic approach to regulation which would predict the likelihood of success, of failure, or of untoward and unforeseen consequences of proposed regulatory approaches

7. To develop a scholarly publication which can stimulate further inquiry and support initiatives to continue what the project began

Accordingly, the contract provided for the preparation of a series of core papers which evolved into:

1. An analysis of the nature of governmental intervention to improve health resource allocation (the Weinstein-Sherman paper).

2. Two "synthesis papers": Breyer's work examining problems generally associated with regulatory strategies in all fields, and the Feldman-Roberts paper establishing an analytical framework for the orderly examination of problems associated with implementation of regulation in health care. The papers were generally to address problems associated with program design and implementation.

3. A number of short papers reacting to the synthesis papers. Alain Enthoven, Theodore Marmor, Lawrence Brown, and Caspar Weinberger address Breyer's work and Roger Noll and Harold Cohen react to the Feldman-Roberts paper.

4. Two case studies ("Certificate-of-Need in Massachusetts" and "The HMO Case: The Reimbursement of Chronic Alcoholism") keyed to the major papers, were used to supply a setting, to validate principles, illustrate conclusions, expand theoretical frameworks, or develop prospective approaches to possible alternative regulatory strategies.

A steering group and a special planning session were used to help develop the thrust of the papers. (Separate summaries and proceedings are available for review.) The contract also provided for a conference if the steering committee and special planning session so recommended. As a result of a positive recommendation, a group of leading public administrators, health professionals, lawyers, sociologists, political scientists, and economists were convened in Cambridge, Massachusetts on February 27–28, 1978.

The purpose of the conference was to examine the current state of health care regulation in light of the experience of regulation in other sectors of the economy. Organized to bring together experts in "traditional" regulation with experts in the field of health policy, the conference sessions were devoted to discussion of the ideas and problems illuminated by the papers and case studies. The papers made no attempt to prescribe what the future course of health policy should be. The conference was viewed as an opportunity for informed persons in the health area to review and improve the material developed in the project.

1. Contract No. HRA 230-72-0037 between The Health Resources Administration, HEW and the John Fitzgerald Kennedy School of Government, Harvard University, with additional support from ADAMHA and The Commonwealth Fund. Paul Schwab, Health Policy Analyst, served as Project Officer for the Health Resources Administration. Dr. Richard S. Gordon was Principal Investigator and Project Director and Graham T. Allison, Dean, Kennedy School of Government, was co-Principal Investigator. Schwab is now Director, Office of Program Coordination, Health Resources Development.

APPENDIX 1-E: REGULATION AS AN INSTRUMENT OF PUBLIC ADMINISTRATION

CONFERENCE[1] AGENDA

Session I

A. Welcome, History of the Project, and Plan for the Conference

  1. Graham Allison, Dean, Kennedy School of Government
  2. Harold Margulies, Deputy Administrator, Health Resources Administration
  3. Richard Gordon, Project Director, Kennedy School of Government

B. Lessons to be Learned from the Regulatory Experience in Non-Health Care Sectors

  Discussion Focus: Does the Breyer paper[2] serve as a useful "roadmap" to guide regulatory experience in health care?

  1. Don Price, Dean Emeritus, Kennedy School of Government, Session Chairman
  2. Howard Berman, Vice President, American Hospital Association
  3. Stephen Breyer, Harvard Law School
  4. Lawrence Brown, Brookings Institution
  5. Alain Enthoven, Stanford University
  6. Theodore Marmor, Yale University (formerly University of Chicago)
  7. Caspar Weinberger, Bechtel Corporation (former Secretary, HEW)

Session II

Certificate-of-Need Case[3] Discussions

A. How Should One Proceed If A Capital Lid is Imposed on Expenditures?

   1. Harvey Fineberg, Harvard School of Public Health, Session Chairman

   2. Jonathan Fielding, Commissioner of Health, Commonwealth of Massachusetts

   3. John Hill, Chairman of the Board, Hospital Corporation of America

B. The Weinstein and Sherman Paper[4]—What Alternatives to the Certificate-of-Need Process Does it Suggest to Accomplish Certificate-of-Need Objectives?

   1. Graham Allison, Kennedy School of Government, Session Chairman

   2. James Kimmey, Director, Midwest Center for Health Planning, Inc.

   3. Roger Noll, Department of Economics, California Institute of Technology

   4. Herbert Sherman, Center for the Analysis of Health Practices, Harvard School of Public Health

   5. Milton Weinstein, Center for the Analysis of Health Practices and the Kennedy School of Government

Session III

A. Health Care Regulation and the Role of the University

   1. Derek Bok, President, Harvard University

B. The Role of Consensus in Regulation Writing

   1. John Dunlop, Lamont University Professor, Harvard University

Session IV

A. The Effect of Program Implementation on Regulatory Outcomes

   Discussion Focus: How does the Feldman and Roberts paper[5] focus in useful ways on the problems of implementing health care regulation?

   1. Robert Blendon, Vice President, Robert Wood Johnson Foundation, Session Chairman

   2. Harold Cohen, Executive Director, Maryland Health Systems Cost Review Commission

   3. Penny Feldman, Harvard School of Public Health

   4. Jacob Getson, Assistant Commissioner of Health, Commonwealth of Massachusetts

   5. Lawrence Huston, Group Division, Aetna Life and Casualty Company

   6. Roger Noll, Department of Economics, California Institute of Technology

7. Mitchell Rabkin, General Director, Beth Israel Hospital

8. Marc Roberts, Harvard School of Public Health

B. Health Maintenance Organization Case Discussion: Would Knowledge of the Feldman and Roberts Bargaining Model Have Speeded The Regulation Writing Process—What Other Approaches Might Have Been Desirable?

1. Marc Roberts, Kennedy School of Government, Session Chairman

2. Scott Fleming, Senior Vice President, Kaiser Foundation Hospital Plans, Inc.

3. Lee Cummings, Legislative Services Unit, the Alcohol, Drug Abuse and Mental Health Administration

Session V

A. Insights, Hunches, and Bets About Regulatory Directions—Reflections on the Sessions

1. Henry Foley, Administrator, Health Resources Administration, Session Chairman

2. Don Price, Kennedy School of Government

3. J. Skelley Wright, United States Court of Appeals

B. Synthesis of Preceding Discussions

1. Howard Hiatt, Dean, Harvard School of Public Health

2. Howard Frazier, Center for the Analysis of Health Practices, Harvard School of Public Health

C. Future Agenda, Discussion and Closing Remarks

1. Harold Margulies, Health Resources Administration, Session Chairman

2. Graham Allison, Kennedy School of Government, Harvard University

CONFERENCE PARTICIPANTS

Henry Aaron
Assistant Secretary for Planning and Evaluation
Department of Health, Education and Welfare
David Alexander
Research Assistant
Kennedy School of Government
Carl Allen
Chief, Policy and Data Analysis Branch
Medical Bureau
Department of Health, Education and Welfare

Graham T. Allison
Dean, Kenndy School of Government
Robert Baitty
Program Analyst
Bureau of Health Planning and Department of Health, Education and Welfare
Katherine Bauer
Harvard Center for Community Health and Medical Care
John F. Bean
Principal Regional Official
Boston, Department of Health, Education and Welfare

Sally Berger
Chairwoman, National Council on Health Planning and Development

Howard Berman
Vice President
American Hospital Association

Robert Blendon
Vice President
Robert Wood Johnson Foundation

Derek Bok
President, Harvard University

Stephen Breyer
Harvard Law School

Lawrence Brown
The Brookings Institution

Philip Caper
Vice Chancellor for Health Affairs
University of Massachusetts Medical Center

Harold Cohen
Executive Director, Health Systems Cost Review Commission
Maryland

Earl Collier
Executive Deputy Director
New York Office of Health Services Management

Cheryl Conner
Kennedy School of Government

Lee Cummings
Legal Assistant
Legislation Services Unit
The Alcohol, Drug Abuse and Mental Health Administration

John T. Dunlop
Lamont University Professor
Harvard University

Christopher Edley
Kennedy School of Government

Paul Ellwood
Interstudy

Alain Enthoven
Graduate School of Business
Stanford University

Penny Feldman
Harvard School of Public Health

Jonathan Fielding
Commissioner of Health
Commonwealth of Massachusetts

Harvey Fineberg
Harvard School of Public Health

Reginald Fitz
Vice President
The Commonwealth Fund

Scott Fleming
Senior Vice President
Kaiser Foundation Hospital Plans, Inc.

Henry A. Foley
Administrator
Health Resources Administration

Howard Frazier
Director
Center for the Analysis of Health Practices

Jacob Getson
Assistant Commissioner of Health
Commonwealth of Massachusetts

Lee Goldman
Chief
Planning, Evaluation and Legislative Branch
Health Resources Administration

Richard S. Gordon
Project Director
Kennedy School of Government

Robert Graham
Deputy Director
Bureau of Health Manpower
Health Resources Administration

David A. Hamburg
President
Institute of Medicine
National Academy of Science

Ron Harm
Assistant to the Regional Administrator
Kaiser-Permanente Medical Center

James Haughton
Executive Director
Cook County Hospital

George Heitler
Senior Vice President for Legal Affairs
Blue Cross Blue Shield

Howard Hiatt
Dean
Harvard School of Public Health

John Hill
Chairman of the Board
Hospital Corporation of America

Julianne Howell
Research Associate
Kennedy School of Government

Laurence B. Huston
Assistant Vice President
Group Division
Aetna Life and Casualty

John Iglehart
Contributing Editor, National Journal

Glenn Kamber
Director
Regulation Management Unit
Department of Health, Education and Welfare

James Kimmey
Director
Midwest Center for Health Planning, Inc.

David Kinzer
President
Massachusetts Hospital Association

Richard Lee
Chief
Shortage Area Designations Section
Bureau of Health Manpower

Harold Margulies
Deputy Administrator
Health Resources Administration

Theodore Marmor
Center for Health Administration Studies
The University of Chicago

Libby Merrill
Deputy Director
Office of Policy Coordination, Bureau of Health Planning and Resource Development
Health Resources Administration

Roger G. Noll
California Institute of Technology

Don K. Price
Kennedy School of Government

Mitchell Rabkin
Beth Israel Hospital, Boston

Marc Roberts
Harvard School of Public Health
Kennedy School of Government

Milton I. Roemer
School of Public Health
University of Southern California at Los Angeles

Ruth Roemer
School of Public Health
University of Southern California at Los Angeles

Colin Rorrie
Deputy Director
Bureau of Health Planning and Resource Development
Health Resources Administration

Eugene Rubel
Special Assistant to the Administrator
Health Care Financing Administration

A. M. Schmidt
Vice Chancellor for Health Services
University of Illinois Medical Center

Paul Schwab
Health Policy Analyst
Health Resources Administration

Herbert Sherman
Harvard School of Public Health

Mitchell Spellman
Harvard Medical School

Jack Stelmach
Director
Family Practice Program
Baptist Memorial Hospital, Kansas

Daniel C. Tosteson
Dean
Harvard Medical School

Peggy Washburn
Grants Management Specialist
Office of Health Manpower
Health Resources Administration

Caspar Weinberger
Vice President
Bechtel Corporation

Milton Weinstein
School of Public Health
Kennedy School of Government

J. Skelly Wright
United States Court of Appeals

Don Young
Chief
Health Services and Health Resources Branch, Office of General Counsel

Dan Zwick
Associate Administrator
Office of Program Evaluation and Legislation
Health Resources Administration

1. Organized by the J. F. Kennedy School of Government, Harvard University and convened in Cambridge, Massachusetts, February 27–28, 1978.

2. Source material on which the discussion was based (see Chs. 5 and 6 *infra*): (1) "The Reform of Economic Regulation," by Stephen Breyer, Harvard Law School: and (2) written "reactor" papers by Berman, Brown, Enthoven, Marmor, and Weinberger.

3. See Ch. 1 *supra*.

4. Source material on which the discussion was based (see Ch. 3 *infra*): "A Structured Framework for Policy Interventions to Improve Health Resource Allocation," by Milton C. Weinstein and Herbert Sherman.

5. Source material on which the discussion was based (see Ch. 2 *infra*): "Magic Bullets or Seven-Card Stud: Understanding Health Care Regulation," by Penny Feldman and Marc Roberts.

Regulation of the Health Care Sector

EDITOR'S NOTE

In his introduction to the Feldman/Roberts chapter, Robert J. Blendon highlights the distinctive service background from which the modern, largely not-for-profit health care institutions have emerged. Because they possess boards of trustees, by-laws, and other accoutrements of corporate structure, it is tempting to consider regulating them by the same methods as used to regulate other corporate bodies in the private sector. However, Blendon suggests that given the tradition of scarce resources for public service and the plethora of third-party payments (i.e., neither by patient nor by institution but by an insurance company or government agency, etc.) for a very large portion of hospital costs, such conventional regulatory approaches will not be productive.

The main discussion in this chapter, by Professors Penny Feldman and Marc Roberts, sets forth a very clear description of the problems that beset the implementation of regulation in general and health care specifically. Their paper is unusual because it treats health care regulation within the context of the American political system. The chapter is important because very often those who propose regulation do so from some concept of public "good" or some particular economic bias, ignoring the realities of the interplay that must take place between all the several classes of regulators and administrators themselves. Two specific "reactor" papers follow the Feldman/Roberts presentation. Harold Cohen comments on the applicability of Feldman and Roberts' ideas to his work with the Maryland Rate Setting Commission. Roger Noll evaluates the Feldman/Roberts propositions in terms of current knowledge concerning political relationships that arise from regulation of institutions that provide professional service to the public.

Comments by John T. Dunlop and Judge J. Skelly Wright conclude this chapter, highlighting the dilemma one faces in working things out between all interested parties so as not to exclude those who might be affected by the bargaining relationship that Feldman/Roberts (and Dunlop) espouse.

THE THIRD SECTOR [1]
IN THE HEALTH FIELD

Robert J. Blendon, *Vice President, Robert Wood Johnson Foundation*

There is an apparent truism that has emerged from the almost never-ending health conference circuit. Discussions of the rival merits of price competition in the medical marketplace versus planning and regulation of health care as if it were a public utility are notable for the production of much controversy and disappointingly little practical consensus about the shape of the health sector in the future. Individuals continue to leave these conferences frustrated by the unwillingness of the public decision-making process to embrace the economic precepts growing from the merits of one side or the other of this contentious debate. I believe the reason for this continuing lack of consensus is often misunderstood.

The current debate revolves around two different policy choices for the future: market orientation or planning and regulation. The debate itself takes no recognition of the fact that for over 100 years, a third set of economic forces has been at play in the health field. As most political figures recognize, health institutions have been subject to a set of economic laws quite different from those seen by either of the two sides of this argument. The economic realities are clearly quite different, possibly calling for a different course of action. Yet many public figures are still reluctant to intervene in the economics of the health world with which they are familiar in order to move in either of the two proposed directions, feeling intuitively that hospital and health care delivery is somehow "different."

I would like to limit my remarks to my perception of the economic forces which have shaped the "third sector" and the nature of the health field. To do this most expediently, I will use the focused question-and-answer format utilized by staffers during congressional hearings.

1. Q. Your name and occupation.

A. Robert J. Blendon; my occupation, Foundation Executive; my job, banker to the third sector.

2. Q. Where does the idea of a third sector in the health come from?

    A. As historian Daniel Boorstin has observed, this country has had a tendency to rely on voluntary nonprofit organizations to pursue community purposes such as health care. Communities often existed before formalized governments or private forms of economic activity were there to provide community services. Thus a third sector of voluntary collaborative community activities resulted. Sometimes government or private enterprise followed later on. Many of these institutions operated under a set of economic laws which would have been considered as highly irrational by many of today's economists.

3. Q. What was this irrational economic behavior?

    A. First, most of these community services were established on an economic basis where they were partially financed by user charges. Given the fact that services were often provided to individuals of low income, these user charges often did not cover the full cost of providing the services. Second, this industry continued to operate with the understanding that the remainder of the costs of these services was to be paid for by sources other than users, though these funds were often provided on an irregular and unpredictable basis. Third, facilities for these services were not paid for by users. Capital for some facilities was often provided by gifts from the community based on some measure of social need. The ability to generate income to repay these gifts or to maintain the operation of the services was usually not a determining criterion.

4. Q. Who owns third-sector institutions? What kinds of individuals are behind them?

    A. If you look at hospitals, which are the largest of the third-sector institutions in the health sector, you see that the overwhelming majority of the institutions are owned by *four* kinds of sponsoring agencies: (1) Religious organizations, (2) universities, (3) nonprofit community associations, and (4) state and local governments (often operating as quasi-independent authorities). For example, one-third of community hospitals are owned by religious organizations. The largest hospitals in terms of budget, staff, etc. tend to be those owned by major universities. Historically, these sponsors have not behaved in ways which have made them models of either functioning market economics or public utilities. For had they been, they clearly would have fled the inner city when most other businesses did, stopped providing service and credit to those who would never pay their bills, and refrained from building new facilities across the street from existing institutions.

5. Q. What kinds of people run these third-sector industries? Who

are the "industrial titans" of this field?

A. Although because of a growing emphasis on professional management in the last decade the norm has changed, for most of the years since World War II, most hospitals have been directed by religious orders, nurses, social workers, public health administrators, and academic physicians. If you were looking for the "giants" in this sector they would often turn out to be religious leaders and physicians with backgrounds in medical research and all with a strong sense of social mission.

6. Q. Are firms in the third sector multinational or conglomerates? Do single firms dominate the market in a particular area or field?

A. There are few multinationals and these are mostly religious organizations. Many of the firms, however, are conglomerates. In addition to hospitals and clinics, many third-sector corporations also operate nursing homes, child care programs, museums, secondary schools, churches, colleges, ambulance systems, and research centers. With 7,000 hospitals and 25,000 clinics, few firms can be said to dominate the industry. The only exception tends to be in downtown areas of large cities where universities often control most of the hospital beds and outpatient services.

7. Q. Has the third sector had a history of restricting market entry to these fields? Take, for example, hospitals.

A. In general, no. In 1876 there were fewer than 200 hospitals. By 1976 there were 7,200 of every type and kind, one-half of which were below 150-beds size. One example to the contrary. Voluntary institutions resisted the growth of proprietary hospitals. The issue was the unwillingness of for-profit institutions to provide care to charitable patients.

On the entry issue, it is important to separate interinstitutional behavior from that of individual hospital behavior of physicians. Physicians on hospital staffs have often considered themselves independent contractors with hospitals. As such there is a long history of efforts to limit other independent contractors from entering communities. But community institutions have behaved quite differently to each other.

8. Q. What is the economic problem in the third sector in the health area?

A. The dramatic increase in user payments has distorted the economic discipline of these institutions. A combination of pent-up labor and professional demands, and rising public expectations about medicine has led to a total loss of control of institutional expenditures. It is worth saying that probably the same phenomenon would occur with colleges, private secondary schools, museums, day care centers, voluntary ambulance squads, etc. if the availability of user payments were to dramatically increase.

9. Q. Does not much of the cost problem relate to the growing power of physicians over hospitals?

A. The answer is clearly yes. Physicians determine individually what happens to each patient. These decisions involve the bulk of health care costs.

Again it is worth pointing out that this growth of professional power is not unique to the health world. University faculty, secondary school teacher unions, and day-care professionals are all exerting significant dominance over their respective institutions to such an extent as to have an enormous economic impact on their sectors of activity.

10. Q. How does third-sector leadership in health think it can solve its cost problems?

A. Most people do not know what to do. For years, the economic problem was that low- and moderate-income patients could not pay for the cost of the services they needed. Now insurance has solved much of this problem, but unexpectedly it has created a whole set of different economic issues. For over 100 years there were only 2 phrases that were dominant in the third sector in health. They were "shortage of professionals and facilities" and "not enough money." Now all the talk is around "surpluses" and "too much money." It will take awhile for the leadership to adjust.

11. Q. What do you think the third sector is going to do about the cost issue?

A. In the short term relatively little. Given a 100-year history, it is very difficult for institutions to adjust to the new economic realities.

Over the long term there will be a good deal of studying of alternatives for resolving these issues. I think the leadership of the third sector will remain relatively cautious. The whole economic climate facing the third sector in health has changed rapidly over the last fifteen years, and unquestionably will continue to change. Yet certain basic functions relating to a special sense of mission that have been characteristic of much or all of third-sector activity still remains. This is regardless of the particular service or health cause involved. There is a sense that these functions are still important today. As a result, there is likely to be a good deal of resistance to any political intervention which would have the effect of destroying the special historical role of third-sector institutions.

NOTES

1. The concept of "third sector" has come into use to describe "not-for-profit" or voluntary agencies and institutions that are community-oriented and bridge the gap between the "for-profit" private institutions and federal and state agencies.

MAGIC BULLETS OR SEVEN-CARD STUD: UNDERSTANDING HEALTH CARE REGULATION

Penny Feldman, *Harvard School\ of Public Health, Kennedy School of Government*
Marc Roberts, *Harvard School of Public Health, Kennedy School of Government*

INTRODUCTION

The growth of third-party payment and the attendant escalation of health care costs have been accompanied by vastly increased regulation of the health sector. The federal and state governments are now engaged in ambitious efforts to control the price, use, and quality of health care resources. Our work examines these efforts and their results. By analyzing past and current experience, we hope to contribute to improved regulatory performance in the future.

The essence of public regulation is the attempt by government to alter the resource allocation decisions of those outside its direct control.[1] This essential characteristic of "action at a distance" underlies our analysis. While many different typologies are possible, at a minimum regulation includes attempts to control prices; attempts to specify what is being produced, how it is produced and by whom; and attempts to use rules and sanctions to elicit changes in behavior.

Several economic and political concerns have traditionally been used to justify regulatory efforts. Much of the classic rationale for government intervention is derived from perceived imperfections on the supply side of some specific economic market. Because of economies of scale (e.g., bigger firms are more efficient) or because of economies of networking (e.g., it only makes sense to have one electric line down any given street), consumers sometimes confront a situation in which there are only a few suppliers or perhaps only one, who therefore can charge a high (monopoly) price. Government responds with price regulation.

On the other hand, some regulatory efforts have been defended by reference to perceived inadequacies on the demand side of the market. That is, for one reason or another, consumers have been deemed unwilling or unable to make informed and appropriate choices. Examples here range from government specification of weights and measures through health inspection and licensure laws to railroad and airline safety standards. All are part of a long series of regulatory interventions typically aimed at setting standards for producers, processes, and products to protect the consumers of those products from possible mistakes in their own judgment. In addition, public intervention has sometimes grown out of the failure of certain markets to avoid spillovers or externalities—situations in which producers do not bear the full burden of costs they impose nor receive compensation for the full value of benefits they might generate. Zoning laws, environmental controls, and vaccination programs are all of this type.

Finally, explicitly or implicitly, many regulatory activities have been aimed at altering the distribution of economic benefits among groups of producers and consumers. Early efforts to control unfair competition, the development of the Robinson-Patman Act to limit discounts to large purchasers, and the development of fair trade laws and the like all have had elements of such redistribution. Indeed, recent economic historians have pointed out that some of the industries subject to early economic regulation—railroads and utilities, for example—perceived potential economic advantages in regulation.[2]

Early regulation of doctors and hospitals consisted primarily of medical licensure proposed as a protection for consumers but carrying significant redistributive effects. Only recently has health care regulation been defended overtly on economic grounds, just at a time when economic regulation is coming under increasing academic and public criticism.[3] At the root of the large number of new health regulatory programs is a complex series of events which we cannot review here. Fundamental, however, has been the rapid increase in health care costs. Rising from less than 5 percent of the GNP in 1950, these costs now constitute 9 percent of the GNP. Certain components of these costs have increased especially dramatically: For example, hospital expenditures increased 15-fold between 1950 and 1976.[4]

There are currently at least four major government initiatives in cost containment. One of these is the attempt by the federal government to use its granting mechanism to encourage new and more efficient provider organizations. Foremost among these are Health Maintenance Organizations (HMOs), which by employing salaried doctors and treating patients for an annual fee are intended to alter management practices, the provision of care, and incentives to providers within the care system.[5] While the federal HMO program is not a traditional regulatory program, it attempts to influence the behavior of providers through rules and penalties as well as through financial inducements.

A second government initiative is the growth of "prospective reimbursement" or rate-setting activities. In many states, Medicare and Medicaid as well as Blue Cross and other insurers have traditionally reimbursed hospitals for whatever costs they incurred. As a way of dealing with the resulting lack of incentives for cost containment, a number of states have developed programs designed to set rates prospectively and then hold hospitals to those rates.[6] While the nature of the process varies greatly from state to state, this is clearly a step in the direction of classic utility price regulation. Closely related are the Economic Stabilization program, in force between 1972 and 1974, which was essentially a national price control effort,[7] and President Carter's proposed Hospital Cost Containment program. In its most recent form, reimbursement regulation tends to focus on revenues as opposed to rates—in the form of "maxicaps" on hospital revenues.

Third, classic product quality regulation is being employed in the service of cost containment. Originally, this involved utilization review activities in which hospitals were asked to review either concurrently (at the time) or retrospectively (after the fact) how long patients stayed in the hospital, with the intent of reducing unnecessary hospitalization.[8] Utilization review has now evolved into a more elaborate activity called Professional Standards Review Organizations (PSROs). PSROs, local bodies mandated by federal law, are intended to control a variety of aspects of professional practice in addition to hospital length of stay. By applying norms and standards of appropriate medical practice, they are supposed to serve the dual and perhaps conflicting purposes of both controlling costs and maintaining minimum acceptable levels of product quality.[9]

Finally, the most innovative aspect of the new medical regulation is the attempt to use entry controls in order to control costs, a purpose for which they have not heretofore been employed. No one, for example, has tried to limit the number of airplanes used in order to limit the size of the nation's expenditure on air transport. However, with regard to health facilities, we now have an elaborate series of regulatory mechanisms (typically called Certificate-of-Need (CON) regulations) intended to constrain costs by controlling the construction of new facilities, the purchase of new equipment, and the provision of new services.[10] In the manpower area, there have been parallel efforts at controlling the flow of foreign medical graduates into the United States. In addition, a series of federal requirements are designed to limit the number of residency positions in certain specialties so as to control the flow of doctors into that kind of practice.[11] Furthermore, there is widespread talk at both the federal and state levels of slowing down or even reversing the growth in numbers of medical school places.

These last efforts reflect an ironic and historic reversal from previous government policy. Earlier, under the Hill-Burton Act, the federal government was a major sponsor of the expansion of the hospital sector.[12] Similarly, in the post-war period, a perceived shortage of doctors (in certain areas, in particular) led to heavy federal investment in the growth and development of new medical schools. However, in recent years, academic opinion has begun to argue that the imperfections of consumer decision making on the one hand and the dynamics of the supply side on the other, lead to a situation in which "supply creates its own demand."[13] That is, hospital beds tend to be filled once they are built and doctors tend to find procedures to perform once they are in practice. Hence, limiting supply becomes a way of limiting costs, since market forces will not act to do so.

In short, health care regulation has moved from a concern with the inability and/or inappropriateness of buyers choosing for themselves to a concern with inappropriateness of relying on competition among suppliers to provide incentives for efficiency and cost control. Not only is classic price regulation in various forms becoming more widespread, but the regulation of product characteristics and the entry of new suppliers into the sector are also being deployed—somewhat novelly—for cost-control purposes.

In subsequent sections of this paper, we describe our general view of the regulatory process and consider how various characteristics of that process are likely to influence its outcome. Then we move to a discussion of the health care sector and explore our general arguments in that context. In particular, we draw on available literature on the effects of health care regulation and attempt to use our general framework to account for observed results. We conclude with some discussion of the implications of our arguments for the way regulatory activities should be structured and managed.

THE REGULATORY PROCESS

The diverse economic, social, and political motives which converge to produce regulation mean that regulatory programs, like others, often embody vague and/or conflicting objectives. Thus the regulatory agency has two major tasks: First it must decide exactly what it is it wants regulatees to do, and then it must decide how to get them to do it. Our aim is to understand what influences those choices and what their consequences are likely to be. The essence of our argument is that the process by which regulatory intent is translated into regulatory outcome is a complex set of bargaining games involving both regulators and regulatees. Therefore the consequences of any particular regulatory effort depend on what the respective parties want and on their relative bargaining power.[14]

Regulatory Choices

In deciding how to define their mission and carry out their operations, the regulators face a complex series of conceptual and procedural questions. While these are not always (ever?) recognized and resolved in logical order in the real world, it is useful to distinguish them as implicit in all regulation. At a fundamental level, regulators have to decide what to regulate. If they are going to set standards with regard to products or processes, then what aspects of those products or processes are they going to control or limit? If they are going to give away grants or limit entry into an industry, what kinds of behavior are they going to reward or discourage? Exactly whose behavior is to be subject to regulation: everyone's or only that of large or important participants? And what activities are to be of interest: all or only the most significant by some standard? Such definitional questions are basic to the more specific questions about what standards to set, which grant applications or petitioners to choose, what prices or fares to allow, and the like.

Having defined their scope of operations, regulators must create procedures and practices for reaching specific decisions. Should they regulate behavior on a case-by-case or a formula basis? If they choose a formula for setting rates or determining the number of competitors or specifying allowable water pollution, then how specific or restrictive will the formula be, and how much flexibility will regulators allow themselves in responding to the particularities of specific instances? If they set standards, will they proceed by specific or by generic hearings? At what points and in what ways will affected parties be involved in standard-setting? If they encounter competing applications, will they consolidate the proceedings or hear them one at a time? Will they organize the process so that applicants can proceed unless they are disapproved, or cannot proceed unless they are approved? Where will the burden of proof be and how heavy a burden will be imposed? Will regulatees be asked to prove that what they propose to do might *possibly* be justified, is *probably* justified, or is almost *certainly* justified?

Along with these questions, regulators must also consider monitoring and enforcement procedures. How will they monitor and measure compliance with their rules and decisions? Under what circumstances will they impose sanctions for noncompliance, and what procedures will be followed in imposing those sanctions? What kinds of sanctions will be applied, and how will their magnitude be determined?

In answering these questions, regulators are faced with a trade-off between their limited resources and their need to accomplish regulatory objectives. Almost by definition, since they are trying to get other actors in the system to change their behavior, they cannot always expect to accomplish their aims simply by announcing them. Instead, they must make some effort to alter the consequences to other actors in the system of behaving in various ways, so that those other actors will in turn alter their behavior. The problem they face is that in doing so, they consume their own scarce resources.

Insofar as the problems regulators have to solve are not easy or well-understood, the institutions they regulate are numerous and disparate, the behavior they monitor is difficult to observe, or the imposition of rewards and penalties is cumbersome, they will find themselves unable to do everything they would like. Hence they have to set priorities, either implicitly or explicitly. Furthermore, insofar as they are personally committed to achieving regulatory goals or are rewarded by the larger political system according to how well they achieve these goals, regulators have reason to pay attention to this priority-setting problem. They have reason to want to solve it well as opposed to poorly, to accomplish more as opposed to accomplishing less.

The priority-setting problem of regulators is complicated by the fact that regulatees, the people on the other side, have some capacity either to complicate or to simplify the life of the regulators at their own discretion. That is, the more regulatees cooperate voluntarily, the easier regulators find it to carry out their mission. On the other hand, since voluntary cooperation means that regulatees are changing their behavior, it is not clear why regulatees should want to cooperate voluntarily. And indeed, by not cooperating, regulatees can impose costs on regulators.

By challenging a single standard or a proposed enforcement action, regulatees can force regulators to devote a substantial proportion of their scarce resources to defend a small portion of their activities. In addition, the possibility of widespread dissent from a regulatory decision, combined with limited agency resources, puts regulators in a position not unlike that confronted by most law enforcement authorities. If everyone broke the law, then law enforcement agencies would not have sufficient resources to catch all the lawbreakers. And, indeed, widespread disobedience will lessen the probability of any one offense being detected, to the point at which enforcement no longer constitutes an effective deterrent. Hence regulation, like law enforcement, can be successful under most resource situations only if the majority of those subject to the rule comply more or less voluntarily. Furthermore, like prosecutors who plea bargain in order to save scarce prosecutorial resources for other cases, regulators have some incentive to reach agreement with those they regulate if, by doing so, they can prevent extensive hearings, appeals, and political battles.

Remember, what regulators would like regulatees to do and what the latter would like to do if left unconstrained typically differ. Otherwise there would be no need for the regulatory authority. Hence, the regulatory process has key elements of bargaining or conflict resolution built into it. In some cases, the bargaining may be perfectly explicit. For example, environmental protection authorities have been known to sit down with a steel plant to agree upon levels of control and a timetable that are mutually acceptable. In other cases, the bargaining is implicit, analogous to what Schelling has called "tacit bargaining" in a slightly different context.[15] People make proposals which they hope others will subscribe to, recognizing the bargaining implications of the discussion.

At each point, the participants have to ask what they might lose by a failure to reach an agreement. On the one hand, regulators risk overburdening their resources if they are too unyielding; on the other, they may fail to achieve their objectives if they are too lax. Regulatees, too, face difficult calculations. Like regulators, they will bear resource costs if they are subject to enforcement actions. On the other hand, modifying their behavior in order to comply is also likely to be costly.

Both regulator and regulatee must calculate their own actions in the face of uncertainty about what the other will do. In brief, regulation is less like a "magic bullet" for solving social problems than a game of seven-card-stud poker. Whoever holds the cards often wins, but the information each side has about the other is imperfect, so that bluff and counterbluff are not unknown. And the process of reaching any given outcome is often time-consuming and nerve-wracking.

The nature of this bargaining process can be illustrated by considering some of the choices that regulators and regulatees must make. Consider the threshold question, the issue of how small a producer or how small an activity must be before it escapes regulatory attention. For example, what size firm should be subject to occupational health and safety inspections? What size capital investment by a hospital should be subject to CON controls?

From the regulator's point of view, the lower it makes the threshold, the more likely it is to review every conceivably relevant source or decision. On the other hand, by doing so it drastically increases the use of its own resources in the review process and runs the risk that it will systematically divert those resources into less important and less interesting cases. Furthermore, low thresholds may be perceived as excessively burdensome by regulatees and provoke them to evade regulatory authority or challenge that authority in the courts or in the legislature. If the threshold is set too high, however, the regulator may miss a set of decisions which, while individually small, are important in the aggregate and likely to affect regulatory success. In addition, high thresholds might be construed by regulatees as a sign of regulatory indifference and signal widespread disregard for the regulatory process.

In deciding, then, what threshold to apply, the regulator is in essence engaged in a bargaining game with regulatees. The choice of a given threshold reflects the regulator's assessment of what resources it can afford to devote to review in light of the cooperation or resistance it expects from regulatees and the relative importance of cooperation to its overall objectives.

Consider next the problem of choosing between a case-by-case versus formula approach to regulation. Under a case-by-case system, rates, licenses, permission to produce a specific product, or the like are determined in a separate review for each regulatee or regulated product. Case-by-case review allows regulators greater flexibility than formulas in reaching decisions and is likely to meet less resistance from regulatees. It does, after all, offer them wider latitude to present the particularities of their individual circumstances. Yet the choice of case-by-case review may be interpreted by regulatees as a sign that the agency has not been able to garner sufficient expert consensus or political support to establish a strong set of general rules to guide specific decisions. To the extent that this is so, regulators will be at disadvantage in keeping the field of negotiations within limits they can manage. The problem may be exacerbated by the necessity of reviewing a multitude of individual cases in a limited time with limited agency resources. If the review process is too lengthy, or negotiations too prolonged, it can logjam the whole system. Moreover, regulators may encounter significant information problems since as outsiders they are

not in an ideal position to judge the validity of the submissions they are
eliciting.

In contrast, formula systems impose their greatest constraints on regulators at the rulemaking phase but reduce pressure on monitoring and on individual case review. The prospect that they will be subject to the comparatively rigid and arbitrary specifications of a formula is likely to stimulate regulatees to try to influence the formula itself. The risk from the point of view of regulators is that implementation will be tied up at the early stages of program development and that the formula which finally emerges will reflect a series of inconsistent and unsatisfactory compromises. The substance of these compromises may have important negative effects on program outcomes. On the other hand, the fact of compromise itself is likely to ease the regulators' burden of applying formulas and making them stick. Moreover, because the ramifications of allowing exceptions to a formula are more serious than granting concessions in case-by-case reviews (where decision criteria are vaguer), regulators will have greater incentive for consistent enforcement under a formula system.

It is possible, however, that regulatees will try "to have their cake and eat it too." That is, they will seek to influence the formula and then, having done so, will appeal the application of the formula to particular institutions on the grounds that they constitute legitimate exceptions. To the extent that such appeals are successful, the relative advantages of a formula system over case by case budget review are reduced. Furthermore, even when appeals are not extensive or successful, a formula may undermine the accomplishment of regulatory goals. This will most likely be the case when the regulated behavior is very complex and the formula overly simple. The choice of how to proceed, then, is an extremely difficult one, involving regulators in multiple estimates of their own limits and resources and those of the regulatees.

Consider finally the situation of an agency which is imposing conditions on grants. Typically, grant-giving agencies are, like other regulatory agencies, seeking to elicit the production of goods and services that would otherwise be unavailable or to modify the kinds of goods and services that are being produced. Insofar as the grant-giving agency is merely trying to increase the quantity of services which producers would supply of their own volition to any willing buyer, its task is relatively straightforward. It can simply dispense money within the limits of fiscal accountability. However, often the grant-giving process is used to modify behavior. In such cases the grantor/regulator faces a difficult choice in deciding how restrictive a set of conditions to put on the grants. The more stringent the conditions, the greater the change they are likely to accomplish in the behavior of any given grant recipient. But if they are too restrictive, the total number of applicants and recipients may decline to the extent that the goals of the program itself are threatened.[16]

Indeed, the same argument applies to any standard-setting process. If standards are too stringent, they will incur the opposition of those at whom they are directed. This may make them extremely difficult to enforce. On the other hand, insofar as those standards are weak, they may not accomplish the manifest purposes of the regulation, regardless of their enforceability. Thus in setting standards, as in most other regulatory transactions, regulators are involved in much implicit bargaining based on the anticipated reactions of those whose behavior they would like to change through the regulatory process.

ACCOUNTING FOR REGULATORY OUTCOMES

Regulators and regulatees do not bargain in a vacuum. Their bargaining strategies, their bargaining power, and their relative success or failure depend on key features of their environment as well as on their internal resources. Our view is that the external environment of the respective parties defines the (uncertain and imperfectly known) consequences of their behavior, while internal factors influence their choices among alternatives offered by the outside world.[17]

In understanding bargaining behavior, we need to see how the incentives and opportunities confronting individuals within regulatory and regulated organizations combine with their own values and beliefs to account for their individual decisions. Then we must see how those individual decisions combine to produce patterns of organizational action which in turn combine into regulatory interactions. We make no presumption that action is always "rational" or "selfish" or "habitual." Rather, we must be prepared to describe and account for whatever kinds of behavior we actually encounter. In accounting for regulatory outcomes, we try intentionally to avoid identifying any one set of consequences as "the effects" of a regulatory program. Instead, we consider to what extent regulators and regulatees will be able to achieve various specified goals and objectives (whether their own or others). We begin with features of the external situation and then move to internal characteristics that shape organizational responses to them.

The Political Context

Political support is important for any regulatory program in several ways. As a routine matter, legislatures affect agency budgets, organization, and policy making. In addition, legislators provide a political court of last resort to disgruntled "victims" of regulation. The possibility that the legislature might override a particular regulatory decision or cut an agency's budget or even alter an entire program enters into the calculations of both sides as they formulate their bargaining positions.[18] Regulators know, for instance, that to the extent they work for stringent controls or impose heavy regulatory costs, they may antagonize their best-organized and most-concerned constituents: Regulatees. After all, those being regulated have the most at stake in regulatory processes, and they find it relatively easy to be informed enough to participate in them. In contrast, given the diffuse nature of many public benefits, public support for vigorous regulation is likely to be less well-organized and less capable of sustaining itself.

Insofar as a program does have widespread public support, however, the costs to regulatees of overt opposition to the program may increase drastically, taking the form of poor public relations, public retaliation elsewhere, a strengthening of regulatory programs, or the like. Public support will also impact the calculations of regulators. The likely costs to them of failing to achieve regulatory objectives will often depend on the extent of that larger support. Political superiors, for example, will be more concerned with agency accomplishments, and distribute rewards and punishments accordingly, in a context of greater political attention. Indeed, the program's importance to key politicians can be critical to the balance of pressures on the agency.

Such political concern can arise in several ways. One is if the program has well-defined beneficiaries, which, however, many regulatory programs are lacking. Broad ideological constituencies—with a public interest embodiment—are another possibility. As James Q. Wilson has noted:

> To the extent that a large political market exists for programs with diffused benefits and to the degree that the interests which must bear the cost of such programs can be defeated through the skillful use of the media, American politics has lost one of its principal characteristics—the capacity of an organized interest to "cast a veto" on policies that affect it powerfully and adversely.[19]

These arguments suggest the following hypothesis:

1. The political process will enhance regulatory power and effectiveness to the extent that:
    a. There are clear beneficiaries of the program.
    b. There are organized interest groups that support regulatory activity.
    c. There are key elected officials or political parties to whom program success is important.
    d. There is broad popular support for the program and consensus as to the importance of program objectives.

The Bureaucratic Context

One of the products of the political process is the bureaucratic environment in which regulation is carried out. Congressional responsiveness to key interest groups, the need to act before sufficient analysis has been performed, limited staff resources, and ad hoc improvisation—all contribute to the multiplication of overlapping federal programs. Similar phenomena also operate at the state level. The result is a fragmented regulatory system in which few agencies have complete control over any one industry or function, while many have partial responsibility for multiple industries or functions. Furthermore, congressional biases toward federalism (given the local political base of Congressmen and Senators) mean that regulation is often not a one-step process. Instead, federal agencies in a wide variety of areas—in health, education, environment, and so on—have to act through state and local governments or through quasi-public organizations to achieve their ends. Not only do they confront the problem of action at a distance, but it becomes action at a distance through one or even two intermediaries who must be remotely and imperfectly controlled.

The bureaucratic environment has important implications for both regulators and regulatees. The regulatory agency has less freedom to bargain with regulatees if its policies clash with those of government agencies or bureaus with overlapping jurisdiction and interest. Conversely, regulatees have greater bargaining leverage if they can play regulators off against each other. Regulators at the Environment Protection Agency may find it difficult to impose stringent emissions standards on the automobile industry if the Department of Transportation has responsibility for setting fuel economy standards. The Federal Trade Commission finds it difficult to enforce antimonopolistic practices in the trucking industry when the Interstate Commerce Commission endorses them. In both cases, the bargaining success of regulators vis-à-vis regulatees depends in part on relationships among the regulators themselves.

Even when regulatory agencies are not in direct conflict with each other, "horizontal fragmentation"—the sharing of regulatory responsibility among multiple agencies—may limit policy coherence and effectiveness. The Civil Aeronautics Board can award airline routes independently of the Federal Aviation Administration, which regulates airline safety, but its decisions might better serve the public interest if they reflected the Federal Aviation Administration's findings. Yet the joint effect of the policies of the two agencies will often escape the explicit consideration of either. The Civil Aeronautics Board, for instance, has provided cross-subsidies for airlines to serve small towns, while the Interstate Commerce Commission has allowed railroads serving those towns to phase out service. The result is a "policy" of replacing rail service with air service without joint evaluation of the economic efficiency or social desirability of the policy.

In theory, the chief executive may have the power to overcome horizontal fragmentation by using his or her authority to require coordination. This is not always the case, of course, given the existence of "independent" regulatory commissions. But even where he or she has formal authority there are practical and political obstacles to exercising that power in a broad range of areas and over multitudes of agencies. Moreover, we would argue, horizontal fragmentation tends to reinforce itself insofar as agencies in such a system have stronger incentives to carve out relatively isolated and insulated areas of operation than to try to overcome the obstacles to coordination. The outcomes that result may be inefficient or undesirable from a global point of view, but agency performance is rarely judged in those terms in the political system.

"Vertical fragmentation"—the degree to which a regulatory agency is dependent on units of government above or below it for clearance and cooperation—is also a critical feature of the bureaucratic environment. Such vertical fragmentation is obvious in many of the new federal regulatory programs. For the federal agencies involved, the process of implementing such regulatory efforts more closely resembles that of typical federal grant-giving and social intervention programs than that of traditional regulation. They must make decisions about conditions for state or local participation, oversight procedures, the circumstances under which participating agencies are to lose funds, etc. The federal agencies are actually a step removed from the regulatory process. To the extent, however, that they try to achieve substantive regulatory outcomes, they have to act through two sets of linkages, compounding the problem of regulatory implementation. In carrying out their tasks, they may confront the kinds of constraints in bargaining with the on-line agencies that those latter agencies face in dealing with target industries.

The on-line agencies themselves face a comparable set of decisions vis-à-vis those institutions they are supposed to regulate. They are directed by law to formulate substantive standards (in some cases, these are called plans rather than standards), to apply them to particular cases, and to enforce them through a combination of influence and negative sanctions. Yet many of their decisions are made in response to federal guidelines and directives and/or are subject to federal review. If they are regulators in relation to certain outside institutions, they are more like regulatees in their relationship to the federal bureaucracy. Their implementation decisions, then, reflect a complex set of calculations about their *own* vulnerability to particular rules and sanctions, as well as the vulnerability of the institutions they regulate. This phenomenon further weakens the bargaining position of regulators while it broadens the scope of opportunities for regulatees to influence the process.

Our discussion of the bureaucratic context of regulation suggests the following set of hypotheses:

2. The bureaucratic context will inhibit regulatory power and effectiveness insofar as:

   a. Regulatory control is fragmented among agencies horizontally and vertically.

   b. Overlapping agencies have a history of independent action and distinct perspectives, missions, or constituencies.

   c. Authoritative mechanisms for coordinating regulatory activities are weak or nonexistent.

   d. The incentives available to indirect regulators for altering the behavior of direct regulators are limited.

Scientific and Technological Context

Even in a congenial political and bureaucratic environment, regulators may face formidable technical obstacles to regulation. We refer here to the available knowledge base and the means of applying that knowledge to regulatory problems. Science and technology influence regulators' capacity to set standards and monitor compliance with them. They also influence the capacity and inclination of regulatees to do what is asked of them.

From the perspective of the regulatory agency, part of the problem of standard-setting is to identify the critical dimensions of regulatees' behavior that are to be regulated. This depends to some extent on the state of knowledge linking behavior and outcomes. Scientific evidence that is clear and widely accepted facilitates the task of reaching agreement within the regulatory agency itself about the nature of appropriate standards. It also strengthens the bargaining position of the agency vis-à-vis regulatees. On the other hand, to the extent that evidence is contradictory, or its validity is called into question, the process of developing standards will tend to be lengthy, controversial, and more heavily political.

The ability of a regulatory authority to acquire and use such information depends on many features of the situation. Since the relevant scientific understanding may take years to develop, agencies will often be quite dependent, at least initially, on whatever prior work happens to have been done in the field. And as Ackerman et al. have pointed out, that in turn can heavily influence the whole focus of regulatory activity, as agencies focus on the known rather than the relevant.[20] Developing convincing analyses will be more difficult, therefore, when technology and methods of production are changing rapidly—if only because of the time lags involved. Furthermore, since evidence will often be ambiguous or proprietary, an agency needs to have access to experts who do not necessarily fully share the perspectives of regulatees and yet also have access to all the latest information—which often is simply not possible.

Technology also exerts an influence on the monitoring capacity of an agency, which, we have suggested, feeds back into the standard-setting process. To some extent the legitimacy and usefulness of standards depend on whether or not conformance to them can be verified. For example, it is much easier to determine whether or not a piece of equipment has been installed than to police how it is operated. Hence, compliance with standards governing capital acquisition will be much easier to police than those aimed at patterns of professional practice. If the state of detection technology is relatively advanced, this will enhance the range of behaviors the agency can choose to regulate. If it is primitive or unreliable, it will limit regulators' options.

Technology also determines the extent to which the monitoring problem may be alleviated by the use of paper records that report on regulated behavior for other purposes. Tax and accounting forms, medical records, and the like which are prepared for nonregulatory purposes, can sometimes be used by the regulatory agency. This can reduce the cost and administrative burdens of monitoring. Such paper records, however, may not be very reliable—depending on how they are created. They also may not report on precisely the dimensions of regulated behavior in which the agency is most interested. In general, some aspects of behavior will be easier to measure than others, some will be more relevant, and these will not necessarily be the same. Thus in employing existing or other mechanisms for monitoring purposes, a regulatory agency may well face the dilemma of trading off the usefulness of such mechanisms against their cost and availability.

Technology has an impact in other ways as well. If regulatees' production technology allows them to vary their behavior in the short run without costly investments in plant or equipment, they will find it easier to evade regulation. Shifting from one machine to another or substituting one procedure or one drug for another are responses that may be relatively easy for a regulatee to adopt and difficult for a regulator to detect or prevent.

We summarize these arguments by the following interrelated series of hypotheses:

3. To the extent that publicly available scientific evidence clearly links regulatory requirements to various possible ends of regulatory activity, those requirements are more likely to be successfully imposed. The availability of such evidence in turn is likely to depend on:

   a. The rate of technical and scientific changes in the area.

   b. The availability of relevant expertise apart from those being regulated.

   c. The amount of prior social and scientific concern with the relevant issues.

4. The ability of the agency to achieve behavior change successfully depends in part on the costs to it of reliably monitoring the behavior in question. Those costs are likely to depend on:

   a. The technical capacity of regulatees to alter the relevant parameters in the short run (i.e., without making major changes in facilities or personnel).

   b. The state of monitoring technology and the reliability of monitoring devices.

   c. The existence of reliable paper records of relevant parameters.

The Regulated Industry

Several characteristics of regulatees themselves affect their capacity to respond to the environment and to influence the regulatory process. Their homogeneity of interests is a key variable relevant to their bargaining power. When regulatees perceive similar economic interests, and existing or proposed regulation imposes relatively uniform costs (or benefits) among them, they are more likely to enter the bargaining arena in unison and more likely to be effective in influencing regulatory outcomes. When the automobile industry as a whole opposed inflatable air bags, it is in a strong position to block regulatory action. On the other hand, when cable systems and UHF channel holders battle among themselves, the Federal Communications Commission may find it easier to impose its own position. To the extent that those who are regulated do have different interests, their bargaining power is likely to suffer.

In general, the capacity of regulatees to influence the regulatory process is likely to depend in part on their ability to mobilize important political resources. Since mobilizing for political action can be costly, groups which already have a communication and coordination structure find it much easier to participate in influencing both the legislative and the implementation process. Preexisting organization is especially important as attention shifts from the relatively highly visible, dramatic early stages of legislative consideration to the more-detailed stages of bill writing, regulation drafting, and on-site enforcement.

The degree to which regulatees possess (and are perceived to possess) special expertise with regard to the subject matter of regulation is another important bargaining chip. Having real expertise and information at their disposal may be critical to influencing both legislative and bureaucratic processes.[21] It enables regulatees to "help" overworked committee staffers or harried bureaucrats. The latter often need to produce and justify proposals on subjects on which they are not expert and for which they have neither the time nor the resources to become expert or to procure such expertise. In addition, having their expertise widely recognized may result in key regulatory decisions being more or less turned over to the regulated—a result that is only tolerated in society when a group plausibly claims to have unique access to technical information, experience, or the like. Finally, well-accepted expertise provides a basis for appeals to other political and legal forums to reverse objectionable regulatory decisions.

Along with homogeneity, organization, and expertise, the economic strength and independence of regulatees affect their bargaining position. Firms that are subject to other forms of public regulation and that sell consumer products are likely to be more sensitive to the public relations implications of compliance because they have more to lose in this regard. For instance, electric utilities and gas companies who rely directly on public utility commissions for rate increases seem more concerned about their public images as "socially responsible" corporate entities than do steel companies. Vulnerability to unfavorable publicity, then, may be a significant deterrent to noncompliance. On the other hand, when compliance is costly—especially in relation to regulatees' ability to raise capital needed for compliance—economic weakness can be used as an effective tool in resisting regulation.

When regulatees face price-sensitive demand—perhaps because they have competitors—it may be difficult to pass the costs of regulation along to consumers without suffering a decline in sales. This is also likely to promote resistance to regulation. Furthermore, the argument that compliance will contribute to general inflation on the one hand or drive a firm out of business on the other, can be a compelling bargaining weapon of regulatees. Note that large firms may find it more

difficult to use this rationale than small firms. Note too that in a rapidly growing market, capital may be in short supply to the firm, but concern about the market effects of price increases to pay for compliance is relatively less important.

All this suggests several characteristics of the target industry which will influence its ability to influence the regulatory process:

5. Regulatees will have more impact on regulatory outcomes when they:

   a. Have similar economic interests.

   b. Have critical political resources.

   c. Have an ongoing organization that could serve as a basis for political action.

   d. Have a real or perceived monopoly of expertise in the area.

   e. Do not sell directly to consumers who might be influenced by the seller's image.

   f. Do not fear other government regulatory action.

   g. Face higher costs of compliance.

   h. Face slower growing, more price sensitive, and more competitive markets.

The Regulatory Agency

So far we have focused on factors external to the regulatory agency which define its range of alternatives. But the likely consequences of the various actions an agency might take, both to itself and its personnel, are seldom unambiguous. Nor are objectives or consequences necessarily the same for all those within the agency. Thus, internal differences of opinion on how to proceed are both possible and likely, and the process of settling them is likely to have both a political as well as a rational dimension. Various groups and individuals attempt both to convince one another and to assemble effective internal coalitions. Of course, in an hierarchical organization, not all members count equally. Different people may have more or less leverage at various phases of the cycle when an agency notices or defines a problem, generates one or more plans, devises a course of action, and then implements that (or perhaps some other) plan.

Within the regulatory agency, individuals with different backgrounds or career objectives can be expected to behave differently. Commissioners ambitious to run for high political office may not decide the same way as those who are effectively retired from electoral politics. Depending on the salience of regulation and the direction of public opinion, political ambitions may either strengthen or weaken the bargaining stance of a regulatory agency head. In general, agency heads drawn from or sympathetic to the regulated industry will be less inclined to ask regulatees to assume heavy regulatory costs. To the extent that the selection process reinforces proindustry biases inherent in the political environment, this may be a significant constraint on regulatory power. Noll, among others, has argued that candidates objectionable to regulatees often are not appointed.[22] As a result, the distribution of views at the top of a regulatory agency is likely to be more limited than the distribution in the broader society, and the resulting decisions are likely to be closer to a proindustry position than they would otherwise.

If legislation specifies representation from various groups (including both regulatees and others), the distribution of views in the regulatory body may be wider than it would be otherwise. And to the extent that public or consumer representatives represent interested and organized constituencies, they may have the incentive and the resources to influence agency outcomes. Where these circumstances do not hold, however, regulatory decisions are likely to be dominated (whatever the numbers) by representatives of those who have the most to lose from regulatory decisions and who have the most expertise, i.e., the regulatees.[23]

The position of the regulatory agency is also influenced by staff selection and staff incentives. In traditional regulatory agencies, civil service works in the direction of greater stability but also greater inflexibility than in those voluntary or quasipublic agencies where civil service does not operate. Staff stability and consistency may strengthen the agency's bargaining powers insofar as experience and persistence contribute to better standards and stronger enforcement. On the other hand, flexible staff recruitment and promotion enable an agency's management to seek special expertise and to reward vigorous regulatory effort. Under some circumstances, particularly when the regulatory mandate is new or when the agency must shift direction, these will contribute more to regulatory effectiveness than staff security or longevity.

In either case, the professional training and values of staff may be a dominant influence on the substance of standards and the application of rules to specific cases.[24] The impact of legal background on the functioning of a number of regulatory agencies has often been noted.[25] Noll has suggested that the effect of lawyers is to make regulatory decisions more sensitive to the potential of judicial and legislative review.[26] Where other professionals—planners, doctors, applied scientists, or the like—are heavily represented in regulatory agencies, we would expect their impact to be significant. This is especially so when they find ideological support and opportunities for career advancement outside of an agency or program. (For example, the increased role of academic economists in the Environmental Protection Agency, we predict, is likely to move that agency further in the direction of using fiscal incentives.) The influence of various professionals, of course, will depend on the resources they control within the agency and/or their capacity to mobilize support from outside.[27]

All this helps explain why regulatory agencies so often seem captured. Agency heads, as well as senior technical staff with extensive industry contact or background, tend to be sensitive to industry perspectives. The industry also has the greatest stake and the most

expertise, and so is often the most forceful participant in regulatory activities.[28] We emphasize the role of senior staff as well as commissioners, since the former often have superior technical expertise and hence have a major impact on decision making.[29]

In addition to its internal composition of perspectives, a regulatory agency is also influenced by the balance between its resources and the tasks it confronts. The more ample those resources and the lower the costs of setting standards, monitoring regulatees, and imposing penalties on them, the easier it is for the agency to take a tough line in the bargaining process. Resource constraints, of course, do not affect all aspects of the regulatory process uniformly.

The use of generic standards, standard operating procedures, or simple decision rules can lessen the costs of standard-setting and case decision making to the agency. They are likely, however, to increase enforcement costs insofar as regulatees perceive such rules as imprecise, arbitrary, or unfair. Civil penalties imposed by administrative procedures—and simplified legal procedures where action is required—can lower enforcement costs, but only if the behavior in question can be monitored. And the simpler the sanctioning procedure, the more reliable the monitoring has to be if the process is to seem acceptably fair. In some cases, both monitoring and imposing sanctions can be done with relative ease. However, if violations are both easy to detect and carry severe penalties, the very effectiveness of such a program is likely to generate increased attempts to overturn it legally and politically. Programs with mandatory strong sanctions and more difficult monitoring lead instead to selective enforcement.

Effectively graduated sanctions may be critical to enable their imposition to withstand judicial scrutiny. Except for "obviously evil" acts, judges are very reluctant to accept "massive retaliation" enforcement strategies especially when it is clear that only a minority of violators have been apprehended. When sanctions can only be imposed through court action as is often the case, this becomes especially important. Indeed, one great virtue of a recent experiment in Connecticut with fines for delays in complying with air pollution regulations is that they were based on an elaborate—and apparently objective—economic calculation which varied in plausible ways with the apparent magnitude of the offense.[30]

Ironically, when regulators elaborate procedures and lengthen the decision-making process in the interest of thorough and fair review, regulatees protest delay greatly. But when regulators seek to lessen delay through simplified procedures so that decisions can be made more easily, equally fervent protests are heard. As is often the case, procedural protests mask substantive interests.

Our final set of hypotheses includes the following:

6. Agency behavior will tend to reflect the values, objectives, personalities, and professional views of top management and senior technical staff, so that:

a. Agencies headed and staffed by those with backgrounds outside of the regulated industry will not as often make decisions that industry prefers.

b. Agencies operating in areas dominated by authoritative professional groups will behave in ways compatible with those professional norms.

c. Agency efficiency and energy will reflect the extent to which its members are subject to performance-oriented rewards and penalties.

7. Agencies will be better able to achieve their goals to the extent that:

a. They have more resources for rulemaking, detection, and enforcement.

b. They face lower costs in carrying out these processes.

c. They have access to a greater variety of and more precise sanctions.

HEALTH CARE REGULATION

When we apply our preceding hypotheses to the health care sector, we find that health care regulators are at a serious disadvantage in bargaining with those they regulate. Political support for specific health regulatory programs is neither widespread nor intense, while industry opposition is vocal. Legislative ambivalence combined with concern for local prerogatives has created a bureaucratic maze of federal, state, and local agencies responsible for implementing regulation. The scientific basis for regulating health care is weak and the technical obstacles are formidable. The medical profession itself is perceived to have a monopoly on relevant expertise, while the state of the art of health regulation is still rather primitive. Finally, the magnitude of health expenditures and the multiplicity of health care providers severely tax the available resources of regulators. It is no wonder then that existing regulation has not produced dramatic results.

Politics

The most significant aspect of current health care regulation is its emphasis on cost containment. This represents a shift from earlier policies aimed at expanding the health care sector and implies far more stringent controls on the supply and composition of medical resources than were typical of earlier public intervention. Such controls generally promise rather diffuse and insubstantial benefits for the public at large, while they imply rather concentrated costs on health care providers and on local communities threatened with service cutbacks. It is primarily politicians concerned with burgeoning public budgets who see potential rewards from health care regulation, and even they may support regulation more in principle than in practice. Popular political support for health care regulation is not widespread nor is it likely to be so in the foreseeable future. Public interest lobbies in the environmental policy area push for more and tougher regulation based on the belief that unregulated industries do not provide enough pollution control. The costs to the public of such measures are embedded in (and hidden by) the overall price of products, while the costs of lax regulation may be evident in dirty smoke plumes and smelly rivers. In contrast, the problem with the health care sector is that the industry is providing *too much* (not too little!) of a good thing. But the typical health care consumer, protected by substantial third-party coverage, still perceives an interest in more and better health care services.

Popular ambivalence toward health care regulation is reflected in the oft-noted observation that public opinion polls show consumers to be skeptical of doctors in general but confident of their own physicians. A 1977 Roper poll found that 65 percent of a representative sample of Americans listed doctors' services and directions as a factor in hospital cost inflation.[31] Only 32 percent of the sample, however, favored cutting services to reduce hospital costs. Sixty percent opposed cuts on the grounds that they would cause inconvenience and hardship. Thus regulators cannot usually draw on broad popular sympathy in their negotiations with health care providers.

While the impact of health care costs at every level of government has persuaded politicians of the need to curtail the growth of the health sector, they too are often ambivalent. For the most part, they have been unwilling to alter the underlying open-ended financing system which fuels the sector's growth. Instead, they have chosen to enact a variety of entry, price, and utilization controls to be superimposed on the financing system. The need for health care regulators to try to constrain the acquisition of facilities and equipment or the growth of intensive services, when retrospective third-party payment rewards providers for their use, exercises a fundamental constraint on regulatory bargaining.

Furthermore, industry and professional groups in the health care sector are highly organized. The American Medical Association, as the largest single contributor to congressional campaigns, wields considerable political influence at the federal level,[32] and the state medical societies can be highly influential in the regulatory arena. The hospital industry, the nursing home industry, the medical schools, the health care foundations, and the prepaid health groups, to mention the most significant, are all organized to a greater or lesser degree and ready to influence or challenge regulatory standards and decisions depending on the stakes involved. Hospital and nursing home associations, in particular, have strong local bases which enhance their political support in state legislatures and in Congress.[33] While these diverse groups do not always take uniform stands on regulation, their relative bargaining power is often greater than that of regulators.[34]

Finally, the impact of health care services on local economies, the intense local concern over convenient access, and traditional loyalties to local doctors and hospitals place regulators at a further disadvantage when they seek to implement regulation. State legislators, for example, may support hospital cost-control efforts in principle, but they will be strongly tempted to sympathize with local constituents who seek excep-

tions from capital expenditure controls. Successful appeals to state legislatures by disgruntled "victims" of CON decisions have been frequent
enough in some states to cast doubt on the capacity of CON agencies to
make their decisions stick.[35]

In sum, analysis of the political environment does not reveal well-
defined beneficiaries of health care regulation, organized interest
groups actively supporting such regulation, or broad popular support
for significant constraint of the health care sector. Even key elected
officials who have supported regulatory solutions to health care cost
inflation are ambivalent in their support of regulators' efforts.

BUREAUCRATIC ENVIRONMENT

Fragmented regulatory authority further lessens regulators' bargaining
power vis-à-vis health care providers. The new health regulatory programs are characterized by a great deal of fragmentation—both vertically and horizontally. When Congress created the PSROs,[36] and the
health planning programs,[37] it invested regulatory responsibilities in
HEW and its various bureaus, in a number of state agencies, as well as
in some 200 PSROs and some 200 Health Systems Agencies (HSAs) at
the local level. Even the federal HMO program, ostensibly administered
by one department (HEW), had its regulatory and development functions separated in different offices.[38] Furthermore, most state health
care regulation is also divided among agencies by function. Thus there
tend to be separate state agencies administering rate-setting, planning,
and CON Programs.

The new federal health regulatory initiatives create complex vertical
relationships and a pattern of vertical fragmentation quite different
from the situation of the classic independent regulatory commissions.
Like the model cities programs and similar initiatives of the 1960s and
early 1970s, PSROs and HSAs exist in addition to and outside of the
federal and state governments, which in turn stand between them and
the Congress and President. Although mandated by Congress, designated and funded by HEW—with state input in designation
decisions—PSROs and HSAs are defined as voluntary organizations.
Yet their receipt of federal funds subjects them to some discipline on
threat of losing their support, and they could not carry out their public
regulatory functions without governmental approval. PSROs, for example, must negotiate memorandums of understanding with state
Medicaid agencies before they can assume binding authority for judging the appropriateness of medical care paid for by Medicaid. Their
control over hospitals and doctors is therefore subject to state as well as
federal restrictions. HSA decisions, to take another example, are subject
to review by the State Health Planning and Development Agency
(SHPDA) and the state CON authority. Thus health care providers may
seek to circumvent or overturn them through direct negotiations with
the state. Furthermore, HSAs' general operations are subject to federal

monitoring, and dissatisfied groups at the local level may appeal to HEW to alter HSA practices or withdraw HSA funding.

Compounding problems of vertical fragmentation are problems of horizontal fragmentation. The "new regulatory agencies" are directed not simply to clear their activities with state and federal governments but to coordinate them with other similarly constituted agencies. For example, HSAs are supposed to take into account the quality of institutional services when they consider applications for investment or expansion, yet information on quality is produced by PSROs which are separate organizations, protective of their data. To the extent that an HSA (or a state CON or licensure agency) needs PSRO input to regulate effectively health care providers and to the extent that PSROs refuse to cooperate (or vice versa), regulatory power is undermined.

Horizontal fragmentation is also a problem among state agencies. For instance, a hospital might go ahead and purchase a piece of equipment despite CON denial if it believed that the rate-setting body would establish a rate and reimburse for the services involved. Conversely, a hospital might attempt to get a higher rate than the Rate Setting Commission (RSC) would like by arguing that the CON agency has found a "need" for a particular piece of equipment or service. Even though rate-setting and CON agencies are mutually dependent on one another if they are to regulate effectively, their separate legislative mandates and bureaucratic structure can make coordination difficult.

In short, the particularly complex bureaucratic environment in which health care regulation is carried out, and the lack of authoritative mechanisms for coordinating regulatory activities hamper the concerted action of regulators and provide regulatees with multiple opportunities for exercising influence.

SCIENCE AND TECHNOLOGY

Virtually all health care regulators are involved in the two-fold attempt to (1) grapple with the difficult problem of establishing standards for what is medically necessary and appropriate and (2) make health resource allocations reflect those standards. CON programs assume planners and regulators have the capacity to determine what capital inputs are necessary for health care delivery on an institutional or an area basis and to make those priorities stick, while manpower controls make comparable assumptions for labor inputs. PSROs are directed to develop and apply appropriate health care standards to local hospitals and doctors. Rate-setting agencies become involved in determining medical appropriateness when they decide which pieces of equipment and which services will be allowable under their predetermined rates. HMO regulators confront the problem when they try to establish a minimum level of acceptable services or criteria for monitoring HMO quality.

Health care standards, however, are extremely difficult to define and apply. Health is a complex phenomenon which is made up of many components, medical care being only one. We are frequently in the situation of being unable to determine what increments in good health are attributable to improved access and quality of medical care and what increments are attributable to changes in lifestyle and a safer environment. For example, the recently reported significant decline in fatal heart disease among Americans is such a phenomenon. Its implications for the allocation of health care resources are still unclear.[39]

Consider the problem of coronary artery bypass surgery. This is a procedure with substantial resource allocations implications. The cost of an average bypass operation in 1977 was $12,500, and roughly 70,000 such operations were estimated to have been performed in the United States in that year alone at a cost of about $1 billion.[40] Bypass surgery requires special and costly open-heart surgery facilities in hospitals and highly trained teams of surgical and medical specialists. The proliferation of the operation has meant the growth of an industry around it: the multiplication of open-heart surgery in community hospitals, the expansion of surgical capacity in large teaching hospitals, the proliferation of angiography and catheterization facilities, as well as the expansion of training opportunities for cardiologists, cardiovascular surgeons, and radiologists.

There also are some data on the efficacy of this procedure. *The New England Journal of Medicine* reported that for patients subject to the surgery, three-year mortality was not reduced as compared to a random sample of medically treated patients. On the other hand, for a small group of patients—those with a difficult-to-define condition labelled "left main equivalent disease"—the procedure does appear to have had life-enhancing effects; for a larger group, it appears to have enhanced *quality*, although not length, of life by reducing pain of otherwise intractable angina pectoris.[41]

How can such findings, reported in perhaps the most prestigious American medical journal, be used by regulatory agencies to improve the performance of the CON process, or PSRO review for medical appropriateness, or manpower projections for surgical specialties? Such information can enhance regulators' capacity to ask difficult and specific questions. Perhaps it can be used to put an increased burden of proof on those defending the proposed expansion of certain facilities. But it cannot provide clear-cut answers. The relevant studies are imperfect and somewhat controversial. To make matters worse, by the time they were published, they were already out-of-date in that the technique had evolved in the interim. As a result, those who defend the general applicability of coronary artery bypass surgery have not been convinced. Further, the information recently developed, however flawed, comes too late to control much of the expansion in facilities the procedure has engendered. A significant problem is that the scientific method of medicine is often not extended to the process of testing new procedures or therapies until long after they have become popular.

Other examples abound of drugs or procedures later found to be of mixed or no benefit that have been widely diffused before outcome data were available. And having been accepted, they then become more or less resistant to later change. Some, like gastric freezing for ulcers, have fallen largely out of fashion. Others, like tonsillectomies, oral substitutes for insulin, and so-called "vaso-dilator" drugs for heart disease, remain in wide use despite negative—although not undisputed—studies.

Surprisingly enough to an outsider, much of medical practice appears not to be either scientifically well-based or consistently carried out. Wide variations in patterns of practice among adjacent small towns[42] and the ability of paramedical personnel, using protocols, to do some diagnosis equal to or better than physicians reflect this situation.[43] With wide differences of opinion in the profession, and often no well-designed body of controlled clinical trials to refer to, the problems of regulators can be severe. We have argued *supra* that even in regulatory programs where there are ample, well-accepted outcome data, the process of developing regulatory standards which are perceived as reasonable and legitimate may involve long and arduous processes of implicit—or explicit—bargaining. Where data are lacking or ambiguous, however—as they generally are in the medical field—regulators are on extremely weak ground.

HEALTH CARE PROVIDERS: THE REGULATEES

Doctors, hospitals, and other health care providers are in a relatively strong position to exploit the weak scientific bases for regulation as well as to take advantage of opportunities provided by other features of the regulatory environment. We have already indicated that the industry is highly organized and that its well-established organizations—the American Medical Association, the American Hospital Association, the state medical societies, state hospitals and nursing home associations, various medical specialty groups, and the like—serve as an ongoing vehicle for political action. Moreover, the resources at their disposal—money, votes, and influence—are substantial.

The political and organizational strength of the industry is reinforced by its perceived monopoly of expertise. That expertise provides a powerful rationale for medical self-regulation and for preserving the professional autonomy of individual doctors. Claims to expertise are compounded with strong traditions of self-regulation and individual autonomy. As a result, regulators rather than providers are often on the defensive when regulation is being proposed or implemented. Health care regulators must usually rely on doctors for expert input in standard-setting, case decision making and even enforcement.

Because the health care industry consists of many small, independent, and highly individualized producers, claims to uniqueness often can be plausibly made. This in turn can seriously hamper the regulatory processes. Suppose a CON agency is trying to decide which, if any, hospitals in a community should be allowed to expand. Each is likely to submit an application which proposes a different set of services in a different facility under the direction of different trustees, administrators, and physicians. Each will make a strong argument that it should be allowed to grow in the public interest, and the decision-making task of the CON authority will be exceedingly difficult.

When regulators move beyond institutional boundaries to intervene in the medical decision of individual doctors for individual patients, providers' claims of uniqueness are even stronger and the problems of regulatory decision making are even more severe. No one patient is identical to any other, and the possibilities for taking exception to general rules are numerous. Moreover, the individual physician-patient relationship is the area of medical activity traditionally most vociferously guarded against outside encroachment. We should expect, then, that utilization review and quality-of-care regulation will be heavily dominated by the doctors involved.

Another implication of the small size and individuality of health care providers is that they are likely to have limited resources for coping with regulations and find compliance onerous. Since the entities are highly varied, regulatory agencies which group providers into broad categories in order to ease the administrative burden of case review are liable to find that some regulatees feel quite victimized, and hence their determinations are subject to frequent—and perhaps successful— appeal.[44] This is even more likely where some providers can claim to be unable to bear the costs of compliance.

HEALTH CARE REGULATORS

If the health care industry generally has internal characteristics which enhance its bargaining power, the same cannot be said for most health regulatory agencies. Their resources are generally modest and their tasks large.

For historical as well as political reasons, health care providers— usually doctors—are often chosen to head health regulatory programs. While their leadership may inspire industry confidence, it is not likely to result in pressure for significant institutional change. State health departments—often headed by doctors—are notable in this regard. While regulatory functions within those departments may be carried out by nonmedical professionals, the ultimate resolution of policy may well depend on the disposition of the individual physician who heads the department or on the composition of the Public Health Council (usually incorporating provider interests) over which he or she presides. At the federal level, the PSRO program provides the best example of physician-dominated leadership, reflecting the explicit expression of the Congress that regulatory responsibilities are the appropriate domain of the regulatees.

As for the new health regulatory agencies, both PSROs and HSAs incorporate health care providers into their formal decision-making apparatus. PSRO governing boards are composed predominantly of doctors, and consumer representation is not required. Majority consumer representation, as well as provider representation, is required for

HSAs, but health care consumers are not nearly as well-organized nor as easily identified as providers. Nor do they often have the technical expertise comparable to provider representatives. The result may be merely to consolidate the influence of industry and professional groups on HSA boards, while creating an illusion of broad representation.[45]

Internal staffing of health regulatory agencies—given the voluntary nature of HSA, PSRO, and often CON or state health department boards—is likely to have an especially heavy impact on regulatory decisions. Aside from the fact that funds for technical staff are not plentiful, the body of skills and the kinds of training appropriate for health care regulators—and, in particular, health planners—are in an incipient stage. Thus there is not a strong professional counterweight to the norms of the medical profession. Nor is there a strong professional consensus to guide the rulemaking, monitoring, and enforcement tasks of health regulatory agencies.

Moreover, those tasks are formidable. The problems of setting standards applicable to numerous, individualized producers and to highly sophisticated services and technologies that are changing rapidly are common to virtually all health care regulators. In addition, some programs require regulators to have in-depth knowledge of medical practice and/or in-depth knowledge of individual providers' internal affairs. Some also embody sanctions which have a negative effect on consumers as well as on providers and hence must be used with extreme restraint.

Our analysis suggests that those programs whose standards rely most heavily on definitions of medical need and whose decision making is most heavily dependent on case-by-case review will be the least effective in constraining the costs or changing the characteristics of medical care delivery. Such conditions can only enhance providers' already considerable bargaining resources at the expense of regulatory agencies. Conversely, those programs whose standards can be formulated without substantial medical input and applied to groups of providers rather than to individuals have the greatest potential impact on medical care costs. This is because judgments about quality and composition of professional services are almost unavoidably the domain of professionals, while judgments about what the public can afford are more likely to be recognized as the appropriate domain of government. Nevertheless, we should expect that any set of controls with the potential to exercise significant constraint on the quantity and quality of health care services offered under our present financing arrangements will encounter the forceful and influential opposition of the affected provider groups.

Strictly speaking, we cannot test our hypotheses in the format of this paper. Some of them grow out of the very programs against which we would be testing them, and clearly that would not provide independent confirmation. Rather, they are intended to focus on what we believe are a number of key conditions which influence regulatory outcomes and to provide a basis for further refinement and elaboration. And so, we shall "test" them by examining what we know about the effects of health regulatory programs to see if they provide a reasonable explanation of those outcomes, recognizing, of course, that definitions of reasonableness will vary among individuals according to their perceptions and experience.

The studies we have surveyed reveal a striking variability of effects. Studies of entry and capital investment controls suggest that CON programs have been relatively effective in reducing growth in the number of hospital beds in some states, but have had varying impacts on nonbed investments and on hospital costs. Studies of direct cost and price controls indicate that they, too, have had mixed results. There is evidence that programs which set reimbursement rates through hospital-by-hospital budget review are relatively ineffective in controlling hospital costs, while programs making use of formulas have had somewhat greater impact on the growth of hospital prices, costs, and inputs. Studies of utilization or product characteristic controls indicate that, in some circumstances, they have constrained hospital admission rates and lengths of stay, but evidently not in all. If we examine the implications of such findings, we believe that they are consistent with our analysis of regulatory implementation.

ENTRY AND INVESTMENT CONTROLS[46]

Outcome studies in this area are relatively comprehensive and plentiful. Their results can be summarized as follows:

1. Overall, CON controls have been significantly associated with declines in growth in hospital beds.[47] However, declines in some states have been far greater than in others.[48]

2. In some states, CON controls have also been associated with declines in growth in hospital equipment and services as measured by plant assets per bed and total plant assets.[49]

3. CON controls do not appear to have had a significant effect—positive or negative—on per capita hospital costs. For the 5 states which have had such controls the longest, however, hospital expenditures may have been somewhat lower (3.4 percent) than they would have been otherwise.[50]

4. There is evidence from at least one state (Massachusetts) that those institutions which are already large and capital-intensive are the ones that are continuing to expand investment with the approval of the CON agency.[51]

5. There is some evidence that hospitals may anticipate CON laws by increasing their levels of plant investment in the period preceding legislative enactment.[52]

Does our analysis of regulatory implementation provide us with a "reasonable" explanation of these findings? The apparent emphasis of CON agencies on bed capacity conforms to our view that regulators will find it easier to apply standards to context areas where there is the greatest consensus and hence where incentives for regulatees to comply are the strongest. The state of the art of determining need for medical facilities and services is primitive. The only methodologies that are in any sense accepted involve setting crude limits on beds in relation to population. The whole question of what technology and services should be offered, in contrast, lacks even this elementary analytical framework. In fact, most available methodologies for establishing bed limits are seriously flawed. They either merely reflect current custom and use, or else are based on forty-year old epidemiological surveys and similarly outdated analyses of what "good care" requires.[53] But that does not mean they will not be used when agencies are under pressure to justify particular decisions by reference to some general criteria. That they have been around for some time, and enshrined in Hill-Burton planning requirements, only increases their bureaucratic value—regardless of their intellectual limits. Thus, a 1975 survey of SHPDAs found that 72 percent of those with developed standards applied the demand-based Hill-Burton formula for review purposes.[54]

Not only are bed-need standards practicable, they are enforceable: (1) Both regulators and providers are accustomed to using them; (2) outcomes are easy to measure; and (3) they have not been controversial in general, since hospitals apparently have been reducing the number of their beds on their own in recent years. Even hospitals in states without CON programs have been reducing their bed investments over the period in which such controls have been developed in other areas.[55] The bargaining position of regulators is obviously enhanced when the standards they are applying push in the same direction in which providers are moving themselves!

The bargaining powers of agencies that might try to develop and apply standards for new investments in equipment or technology are, we believe, far more tenuous. There is no analogy to the Hill-Burton bed-need formula—weak as that might be—in the technology area. Monitoring is much harder, and rules harder to defend. Nor is there evidence that hospitals are moving on their own to limit investment growth in equipment and technology.

In fact, evidence points in the opposite direction. If the "more is better" phenomenon has begun to erode in the beds area, it is still pervasive in the technology area. What Havighurst and Blumstein have called the "quality imperative"—the popular and professional belief that any increment in quality is worth attaining regardless of its marginal cost—is a powerful constraint on any agency that tries to impose controls on investments in new technology.[56] In this area, the burden is apparently on would-be regulators to prove the harm of any investments they might deny rather than on providers to prove the marginal value of any investments they might propose. While some states have attempted to impose limits on a few selected machines (e.g., CAT scanners, radiotherapy machines, and the like), these efforts have been problematic.[57]

While our analysis explains why CON agencies should be inclined to interpret their mandate rather narrowly, it does not preclude the likelihood that some agencies will be more ambitious, more vigorous, or more successful than others. Where the hospital industry is particularly large or well-organized, however, we would expect the effects of CON controls to be weaker than where the hospital industry is smaller or less well-developed. The industry in the former situation will have greater financial, political, and technical resources at its disposal for influencing both the legislative and the standard-setting processes and for appealing unfavorable decisions. Similarly, we would expect CON agencies to have a harder time constraining the behavior of large, sophisticated hospitals than that of others. Not only do such institutions have superior bargaining resources, but the whole rationale for CON controls favors them. The program, after all, is intended to consolidate tertiary care activities in the large medical centers which are believed to perform them best.

Data on both intrastate and interstate variations in CON outcomes are scarce, but they are not inconsistent with this analysis. The Massachusetts study, cited *supra,* found that large urban teaching hospitals were more likely to gain CON approval than others.[58] In addition, there is evidence that of the five states which have had CON controls the longest, the three smallest, in which the hospital sector is smallest and least sophisticated—Rhode Island, Connecticut, and Maryland—have been the most successful. California and New York, on the other hand, have been the least successful.[59] Moreover, the differences in effects have been dramatic in some instances. The *decline* of growth in plant assets per bed (a measure of service intensity) in Connecticut, for example, between the period 1963–1968 (pre-CON) and 1969–1974 (post-CON) was 19.2 percent. In contrast, between the same 2 periods, pre- and post-CON, New York experienced a 66.4 percent *increase,* and California a 60.5 percent *increase* in plant assets per bed.[60] The size and political influence of the industry in the two large states may, indeed, have more severely limited the effectiveness of regulators than in the smaller ones. It is also likely that implementation choices have been affected by other aspects of the financial, political, and organizational environment in the respective states. Both Connecticut and Maryland, for example, have strong rate-setting bodies which, if their decisions were coordinated with the CON agencies, might have provided additional sanctions for investment controls. The fact is, however, that we lack systematic comparative data on those factors which would allow us to make valid inferences about the impact of program operation on program outcomes.

That hospitals may anticipate CON laws and avoid compliance by taking action before they are implemented is consonant with our view that the capacity of regulated industries to vary their behavior in the short run has an important effect on regulatory outcomes. Accelerating investment decisions to avoid new regulation and altering the character of investments from physical plant to equipment, or from ordinary equipment to exotic technology, are actions which, if feasible for providers, can undermine the decisions of regulators. These, then, are some of the obstacles to successful implementation which help account for the insignificant effect of CON controls in the aggregate on overall hospital costs.

RATE-SETTING REGULATION

Outcome studies in this area can be summarized in four points:

1. There is evidence that prospective rates set through hospital-by-hospital budget review are not effective in constraining hospital costs.[61]

2. There is evidence that rates set through formulas are associated with decreased growth in prices and average costs per patient day and admission.[62]

3. Decreased growth in average hospital costs may not be proportionate to decreased growth in prices and charges.[63]

4. Decreased growth in average hospital costs may not be associated with decreased growth in total hospital costs.[64]

The apparent ineffectiveness of hospital-by-hospital budget-review systems is directly explainable, we believe, by our analysis of the bargaining process inherent in implementing regulation. Although in principle budget review systems allow regulators to scrutinize hospital accounts thoroughly and to root out inappropriate or inefficient budget allocations, in practice they may become unwieldy if regulators try to do that. Of necessity, regulators know a lot less about the individual hospitals' financial situation than those who prepare the budget. The former must deal with many institutions, while the latter usually deal with one. Hellinger has observed that "in order to convince an appeals panel that certain expenditures are unnecessary, operating agency staff members must spend a considerable amount of effort researching and investigating the activities of each hospital."[65] Furthermore, in face-to-face encounters, hospital representatives are in a strong position to persuade both regulators and appeals boards to bend what are flexible rules to begin with. Time and resource constraints, then, as well as the probability of losing on appeal, pressure regulators to engage in relatively superficial and uncontentious case-by-case review.

In contrast, formula systems alleviate regulators' time and information problems and reduce the amount of one-to-one bargaining in the rate-setting process. Because formulas specify explicit operational rules that govern individual decisions, rate-setting authorities are loathe to make exceptions and hospitals are less likely to expect them. The clearer effect of formula programs seems attributable to the increased leverage which such rules provide regulators.

If regulators have greater bargaining power under formula rate systems, why have those systems not produced decreases in average and total hospital costs proportionate to their impact on regulated rates? In some instances this occurs in part because the state hospital industry is able to influence the legislation and regulation writing enough to soften the impact of the formula. This may result, as it did initially in New York State, in significant loopholes. For example, the New York formula originally encompassed only routine hospital charges and not charges for costly ancillary services. It also excluded out-patient departments which nevertheless generated (and became a vehicle for shifting) significant hospital expenditures.

Furthermore, when rules are known in advance, hospitals may have an opportunity to exploit the system. For example, in Massachusetts some hospitals have apparently obtained higher daily rates from the RSC by purposely underestimating projected volume, and have collected greater revenues than the rate-setting authority "allowed" by exceeding the estimated patient volume. To take another example from New York, penalties for excess hospital capacity were built into the formula to encourage hospitals to close beds. Combined with per diem reimbursement, however, they evidently had the opposite effect of inducing hospitals to increase occupancy rates as well as lengths of stay.[66]

Moreover, any formula is likely to be imperfect—not only because of political compromise or provider gaming, but because of technical and administrative considerations. Formulas—like all substantive standards—must specify parameters which are observable and administratively feasible, even if they are not necessarily ideal from the viewpoint of program objectives. Per diem hospital rates, for example, may not be the ideal parameter by which to reimburse hospitals because of the incentives they create (as in the New York case, discussed *supra*). Alternatives, however, such as figuring reimbursement on a per capita, per admission, or per case basis, may be both administratively and technically difficult.

Such constraints inherent in regulatory implementation help explain why on the one hand formula systems have been more successful than case-by-case review systems, while on the other, their impact on system costs has not been more substantial.

UTILIZATION AND (QUALITY) CONTROLS

Because of the newness of the PSRO program and the lethargy of federally mandated review activities prior to its passage, most outcome studies in this area are based on private-professional rather than on publically administered programs, which somewhat limits their generalizability. In October 1977, however, HEW's Office of Planning, Evaluation and Legislation (OPEL) released the results of an early evaluation of the PSRO program's impact on Medicare utilization. The results of the OPEL evaluation and of other extant outcome studies indicate the following:

1. On the whole, there is no evidence that utilization review programs have significantly constrained hospital costs.[67]

2. Available evidence suggests that concurrent review programs—those that monitor the necessity and appropriateness of hospital stays while patients are in the hospital—by and large have been no more successful in constraining hospital admission rates or lengths of stay than retrospective review programs.[68]

3. In at least one instance, preadmission screening has demonstrated a constraining effect on hospital admissions rates.[69]

4. In a few instances, retrospective review of specific medical procedures (the use of certain injections, for example) and both retrospective and concurrent review of hospitalization have had constraining effects when closely tied to public reimbursement sanctions.[70]

The relative effectiveness of preadmission, concurrent, and retrospective review programs is, of course, important because one of the implicit assumptions in the PSRO program is that concurrent review will be more effective. The PSRO amendment authorizes but does not require PSROs to review elective hospital admissions before patients enter the hospital, but so far few, if any, have exercised that prerogative. It is really on-site review that is the keystone of the program.[71] Decisions about the necessity and appropriateness of hospitalization are made by reviewers while the patient is in the hospital, and payment cannot be denied retroactively on medical grounds if care has been approved.

How does our analysis of regulatory implementation let us "explain" the rather unimpressive results of on-site review? In some ways, the process by which medical criteria are applied to individual cases in concurrent review activities is analogous to the hospital-by-hospital budget negotiation approach we discussed *supra*, with all its attendant constraints on regulators. The number of patients whose admissions are to be monitored and for whom appropriate lengths of stay are to be assigned is even more numerous than the number of hospital budgets which rate regulators have to scrutinize. To cull too many exceptions would overload the resources of the handfull of reviewers in any one hospital. (There is, of course, the possibility of monitoring only a sample of patients or of targeting review on specific groups of patients, but for the most part "targeted" review has not been widespread.) Obviously, too, the physician knows more about the individual case than can the reviewer. Even if the principal reviewer is a physician (which he or she rarely is), the attending physician will have the advantage of familiarity with the patient. And the variety of justifications for admitting a patient or extending a length of stay are nearly as numerous as the variety of individual patients.

Furthermore, once the patient is in the hospital, the burden is on the reviewer to prove "unnecessary" or "inappropriate" care rather than on the physician to justify his or her decision. A negative decision will not mean merely that a patient is not admitted or that the hospital is not reimbursed, but probably that the patient will have to leave the hospital.[72] The appearance of evicting a patient from the hospital puts the reviewer in an extremely disadvantageous bargaining position. Preadmissions review, on the other hand, should both lessen the pressure on the reviewer to make a positive finding and at the same time provide greater incentive for physicians to propose admission in those cases where hospitalization is most clearly warranted. This may explain why in Sacramento, for example, a preadmission review program evidently produced a significant decline in hospitalization rates for Medicare patients.[73] Retrospective review programs should lessen even further the pressures on reviewers to make positive decisions since they are in essence denying payment to hospitals rather than treatment to patients. That, on the whole, they have not been particularly successful, may have less to do with their retrospective nature than with the problems inherent in making judgments of medical necessity.

There is some evidence that programs which emphasize dollars can have an effect on medical services even if they use concurrent review. Lave and Leinhardt concluded from their study of Western Pennsylvania review mechanisms that hospital lengths of stay, adjusted for case mix, declined more for Medicaid patients than for non-Medicaid patients regardless of whether Medicaid review was concurrent or retrospective.[74] While they do not report specifically on rates of payment denial for Medicaid and non-Medicaid patients, we suggest that the availability of and propensity to use such sanctions—which are generally greater for Medicaid than for non-Medicaid programs—may have been a factor in Medicaid's reduction in lengths of stay. Brook and Williams' study of Medicaid-sponsored review of injections in New Mexico also indicates that a review process closely tied to the reimbursement mechanism can be successful in changing physician behavior, although under highly specialized circumstances.[75] Their study, however, does not allow us to separate out the effects of educational efforts to change injection behavior from the impact of reimbursement denials.

Our understanding of the bargaining relationship inherent in implementation suggests that the preponderance of on-site review activities and the general disinclination of review agencies to make use of reimbursement sanctions have weakened their effectiveness. But these, in turn, reflect a more fundamental set of constraints on implementing product characteristic controls for the purpose of controlling health care costs. Insofar as decisions about "appropriate" or "necessary" utilization entail judgments about the quality and efficacy of medical care itself, rather than about how much the public wants to pay for it, they will inevitably depend on medical expertise and medical judgment. Regulators, then, will either have to employ doctors as consultants or be doctors themselves. Doctors who are employed as consultants, however, and who derive their principal livelihood as well as their professional norms from outside government (and this is surely the case with PSROs, even though the organizations themselves are federally funded)

will not have very strong incentives to impose rigorous constraints on
the practice of medicine. This is especially the case when there is a dearth of data which might link specified standards of practice to desired medical outcomes. Even if regulators were doctors themselves, however, and derived their principal livelihood from government, their capacity to change the practice of medicine would depend at the most basic level on their ability to formulate reasonable and valid substantive standards for medical care.

Yet it is precisely this ability which is lacking in any part of the system. Without it, however, utilization and quality controls are likely to be ineffective. The bases for determining need in CON programs and for establishing rates in rate-setting programs are still at an early stage of development. There are, however, areas of expert and political consensus on these problems. In contrast, in the product characteristic area of health regulation this is not the case. Quality decisions are central to the medical profession. Yet it is most reluctant—as evidenced, by the American Medical Association's opposition to public funding for health technology assessment—to subject those decisions to rigorous scientific scrutiny. This suggests that even incipient consensus is still far off.

IMPLICATIONS FOR REGULATORS

A number of the dimensions of regulatory programs that we have argued influence regulatory outcomes are outside the control of regulators. There may be relatively little regulators can do, for example, about the economic circumstances or the diversity of interests among those whom they regulate. Still other aspects of the situation may be alterable—but only at significant cost in time and resources. And perhaps in part for those reasons, influencing such parameters—as the costs of monitoring or the extent of public support—has not always been part of how regulators approach and define their own jobs. Nevertheless, there are some parameters that are influenced by the design and implementation of regulatory programs. These relate to agency resources, the nature of standards, available sanctions, and so on. We shall begin with the more specific and work up to the more general.

The nature of standards Our analysis suggests that cost-effective, clear, and defensible standards derived from well-established methodologies facilitate the enforcement process. This suggests that agencies should reexamine their requirements in light of the costs they are imposing on regulatees and the evidence they have for the benefits to be derived therefrom.

Obviously, we are not proposing that regulators abandon standards which impose substantial costs on regulatees simply because those standards are costly. We are suggesting, however, that they be able to defend their standard-setting priorities by reference to at least a rough calculation which sets out *both* the costs *and* the benefits of controlling a particular dimension of regulatees' behavior, and which considers the likely consequences of alternative approaches.

Such calculations may provide the regulatory agency with additional cards in its game with regulatees. Of equal or greater importance, however, the process of arriving at such calculations may make *internal* decision-making mechanisms more conscious, more visible, and open to a wider range of perspectives from within the organization. To the extent that complex issues are exposed and analysed, the resultant standard should be a better, more reasonable one.

Second, our analysis implies that regulatory agencies should give high priority to standard-setting efforts in areas where there is relative consensus among experts on both the problem and the likely benefits of regulating a given parameter. Where the methodology and the data appropriate for developing a standard are less well-formed, those activities may most appropriately be carried on at the federal level (or under federal auspices). In such cases, the loss of local control may be more than compensated for by greater expertise, resources, and insulation from local interest groups.

We are aware of the danger that waiting for appropriate data and devising acceptable methodologies may create delays in promulgating standards. There is no easy solution to this problem, but it does suggest that substantial investments of resources for developing a particular standard should reflect some strategic calculation of its likely importance and applicability over time. It also suggests that generic standards may well be preferable to highly specific standards in some cases.

Third, our analysis suggests that where disagreement over substantive standards is likely to be strong, the agency place high priority on creating a standard-setting process which is perceived as open and legitimate. As with the problem of waiting for appropriate methods and data, the problem of relying on good process tends to work against pressures for producing timely and relevant standards. Again, this is a trade-off which regulators will have to make in the context of a particular program and a particular standard or set of them. It seems to us, however, that hastily promulgated standards may eventually backfire and require extensive revision in light of real or threatened protests and appeals, or unworkability, or both. Thus, the gains of speed may be illusory.

It should be noted here that interim guidelines and advisories—as distinct from formal regulations—and temporary moratoria or other simple decision rules may be acceptable to regulated parties, so long as they feel reasonably well-assured that decisions made under them will not be reversed (if those decisions are perceived as favorable) and that the period in which they are in force will be used to foster a participative standard-setting process.

Moreover, in some instances at least, participation of regulatees will not necessarily mean that they dominate the process. In the health care area, for example, hospital and nursing home associations have been keen to participate in setting bed-need standards at the state level, yet rarely have they proposed specific formulas themselves—preferring to leave that to public planners and statisticians. This provides the latter with significant latitude for determining the parameters of debate.

Our conclusions about standard-setting should not be interpreted as an apology for regulatory delay. We have perused the recent Government Accounting Office report which documented innumerable examples of delay in promulgating rules in HEW.[76] We are inclined to place more emphasis, however, on the real problems of ambiguity and conflict which often tie up standard-setting efforts than on the admittedly bothersome aspects of administrative inefficiency.

Monitoring and enforcement Lowering the costs to the agency of detecting violations and imposing rules will probably help. In part this can be done by picking parameters to regulate which can be monitored—provided they are relevant—and by encouraging the development of more reliable and less expensive monitoring technology. Where costs would otherwise be prohibitive, systematic scientific sampling may be the only (best) solution. Wherever possible, records required for other purposes should be used instead of new and untested monitoring mechanisms.

Pooling of information or of monitoring resources, of course, presupposes a modicum of coordination among the multiple agencies to which regulatees often report that may be nonexistent. It is possible, however, that some of the resources devoted to inducing regulatees to comply with new and additional reporting requirements might be better devoted to securing cooperation among regulators. Both the importance and the difficulty of obtaining cooperation among government agencies which possess relevant data are attested to in the health field by the recent battle over the format of and access to information obtained by PSROs.[77] Yet, this is precisely the kind of situation in which, it strikes us, the payoffs in greater availability and uniformity of information are worth the expenditure of fairly considerable political resources on the part of those who stand to benefit.

Further, we would argue that regulators should keep their monitoring tasks as simple and straightforward as relevance allows. This implies that they avoid—to the greatest degree consonant with equity and enforceability—elaborate case-by-case reviewing procedures. As we have argued in our analysis of case-by-case rate review, such procedures entangle agencies in a web of particularities, the implications of which are usually clearer to the regulated party than to the regulator. To the degree that sound and reasonable formulas can be derived, we believe they are far more advantageous to regulators—from the point of view of resource scarcity and bargaining advantage—than more in-depth case review.

At the enforcement level, allowing agencies to impose sanctions without court action (by removing subsidies or imposing civil penalties) should also help. Having small sanctions for small violations may facilitate the enforcement process where monitoring is expensive, since it lowers the incentives for lying and corruption.

We have pointed out, however, that there are no easy or readily apparent solutions to the problem of developing and applying sanctions. The availability of graduated sanctions would seem to be a "must."[78] Yet, often the nature of the sanctions available to an agency is defined in its legislative mandate, leaving relatively little room for maneuver in that area, barring some imaginative use of administrative devices for penalizing violators. If a regulatee is a relatively small, resource-poor institution, for example, calling it in for informal discussions and possible agreement prior to proceeding with a formal hearing may be effective, since for a small provider, the formal process itself may constitute a significant sanction, requiring the institution to hire a lawyer, release its manager for a day, etc.

However, agencies are likely to have far more discretion in applying sanctions than in determining their nature. And here, the particular circumstances of the regulatee, the nature of the violation, its negative impact, and the like will be determinant. It does seem to us, however, that regulators looking for symbolic impact should probably focus on large regulatees' significant violations, while those concerned with the cumulative impact of small violations would be better advised to pursue a sampling strategy in imposing sanctions.

Program management Within the broad confines of a program, better management can make a difference. Having enough people with enough expertise may be critical. Having people who are committed to program goals and/or confront some incentives for vigorous job performance can be very helpful. Since bargaining is inevitable, agency leadership that is knowledgeable and effective internally can have a significant influence on how these processes are conducted. In addition, having a distribution of views and/or expertise within the agency may facilitate internal analysis and strengthen the agency's position when it has to be justified to the public, the legislator, or the courts.

Once these observations are made, it is readily apparent that regulatory agencies are often severely hampered in achieving effective internal management. Both the constraints and the avenues open to key managers who seek to promote responsive and responsible agency performance are all too well-known.

Because large private organizations, however, are heavily bureaucratic in nature—with some important exceptions—it is quite likely that regulatory managers stand to learn from management techniques appropriate to the private sector. This suggests that the use of private consultants and the exposure of key personnel to private management insights may have some benefit. It also suggests that public management research might focus usefully on certain aspects of the regulatory process which create particular management strains. Blau's early study of a federal regulatory agency and the use of internal "consultation" to avoid cooptation by regulatees is an example that comes to mind.[79]

Political support Developing appropriate political support for a program may be critical to long-run effectiveness. This means not only

good public relations for regulators, but more assiduous efforts to
cultivate important political actors and supportive private-interest groups.

The use of advisory task forces that include not only industry or professional groups but a broader spectrum of public opinion may have some role in enhancing the access and prestige of public-interest groups which are inclined to support regulation. The smaller and less formal the task force, the more likely it will be to promote real substantive input by participating groups. Whether or not this is useful to the regulatory agency will depend on how the group is composed and how well the agency can manage the process. Of course, agencies that pursue this course may become captive or unchallengeable, or both. But in many areas of health regulation at least, the risk that regulators will become too powerful is clearly less than the risk that they will not be powerful enough.

Part of the effort to build political support also has to involve communicating what is known about the adverse effects of the practices being regulated—to clarify to both regulatees and the general public that, with risks of harm at stake, imperfect information does not necessarily imply inaction. The agency's success in this regard will depend both on the nature of information available and on the degree to which its staff and leadership believe themselves to be on firm ground in advocating a particular course of action.

Scientific justification   In the longer run, there may be some room for regulators to improve the implementation of their programs by developing a more secure scientific basis for their efforts. We noted previously that in the short run, rules should reflect what in fact is known about the situation being regulated. But clearly, research conducted for purely scientific purposes may not be the most useful method to clarify ambiguities about causality and so on that are critical for designing better modes of intervention. This implies that problem-solving, program-oriented research, in some cases, should be a significant concern to regulatory agencies.

Research on the relationship between the proximate outcomes desired by regulators—reducing inefficacious medical procedures, lowering growth in hospital expenditures, obtaining cleaner air, etc.—and the parameters they might conceivably manipulate—investments in technology, hospital revenues, plant emissions, etc.—will obviously enhance the analytical basis for establishing regulatory standards. In addition, research relating variations in program design and implementation to variations in regulatory outcomes may provide useful feedback to regulators in devising alternate strategies.

Program design   Regulators themselves may have only limited powers to influence program design. Yet, often they do have a substantial contribution to make here: either by initiating legislation or amendments, or by suggesting new administrative arrangements or whatever.

In particular, trying to reduce vertical fragmentation, and hence limiting the number of indirect and imperfectly manipulatable linkages that an agency must utilize, is likely to influence program impact positively. Similarly, efforts should be aimed at providing for increased coordination and a capacity to consider, choose, and impose a coherent regulatory strategy on diverse and horizontally fragmented agencies.

Insofar as regulators can successfully impress on legislatures the usefulness of funding to support program-relevant research and evaluation, of graduated sanctions and administrative appeals mechanisms, and of agency budgets sufficient to sustain breadth and depth of activities mandated in legislation, their impact on program design ought to ease their administrative burdens to at least some degree.

A FINAL WORD

All social choice mechanisms are imperfect—regulation being one of them. The now fashionable attack on "overregulation" of the private sector by the government, however, seems to us to confuse several issues simultaneously: concern about economic inefficiency and cross-subsidy, delays and costs of regulatory processes, and arbitrary or mistaken decisions. In the health regulation area, these costs of regulation, however great, are being incurred by the society because—in the view of some at least—the costs of nonregulation are even greater. And, whether one agrees with the specific answer that the political process has arrived at in each case, at least it is clear that "what is the lesser evil" is the correct question. To find regulation imperfect in some respects is to make, at best, half of the necessary argument.

Many of the problems of health regulation, like regulation in general, reflect the fact that we are asking agencies to resolve intellectual and political problems that no one else in the society has been able to address satisfactorily. With poor data, limited resources, insufficient scientific understanding, substantial social conflict, unrealistic time deadlines set by elected officials eager for results, it is no wonder that regulators are often seen as not performing satisfactorily. But in part, that is because of what we have asked of them.

Nevertheless, we do believe that it is possible for regulators to do better or worse. Despite system constraints and larger circumstances, they do have choices to make, choices that can be made in various ways with various consequences. However much we consider grander arguments for regulatory reform, those choices will continue to be made, and it is worth trying to understand how they might be made more effectively.

NOTES

1. See, for example, C. Schultze, *The Public Use of Private Interest* (The Brookings Inst., 1977).

2. See G. Kolko, *Railroads and Regulation 1877–1916* (Princeton University

Press, 1965) and R. A. Posner, "Theories of Economic Regulation," 52 *Bell Journal of Economics and Management Science,* No. 2 (Autumn 1974).

3. For an example of the attack, on economic regulation, see R. Noll, "The Consequences of Public Utility Regulation of Hospitals," in *Controls on Health Care* (Inst. of Medicine, Nat'l Academy of Sciences, 1975).

4. The growth in health care expenditures is documented in the yearly reports that appear in the *Social Security Bulletin.* See, for example, N. L. Worthington, "National Health Expenditures, 1919–1974," *Social Security Bulletin* 3–20 (Feb. 1975); R. M. Gibson and C. R. Fisher, "National Health Expenditures, Fiscal Year 1977," *Social Security Bulletin* 3–10 (July 1978).

5. C. R. Gaus, B. S. Cooper and C. G. Hirschman, "Contrasts in HMO and Fee-for-Service Performance," *Social Security Bulletin* (May 1976).

6. For a description of such programs, see K. Bauer and P. M. Densen, *Some Issues in the Incentive Reimbursement Approach to Cost Containment: An Overview* (Harvard Center for Community Health & Medical Care, 1974).

7. For a description of the Economic Stabilization program as it applied to health care, see S. Altman and J. Eichenholz, "Inflation in the Health Industry—Causes and Cures," in *Health: A Victim or Cause of Inflation?* (M. Zubkoff, Ed., PRODIST, 1976).

8. Utilization controls are reviewed in B. Stuart and R. Stockton, "Control over the Utilization of Medical Services," *Millbank Memorial Fund Quarterly* (Summer 1973).

9. Conflicts inherent in the PSRO program are analyzed in C. C. Havighurst and J. F. Blumstein, "Coping with Quality/Cost Trade-Offs in Medical Care: The Role of PSROs," *Northwestern University Law Review* (Mar.–Apr. 1975).

10. C. C. Havighurst, Ed., *Regulating Health Facilities Construction* (Am. Enterprise Inst., May 1974).

11. P. L. 94-484, *The Health Professions Educational Assistance Act of 1976.*

12. J. R. Lave and L. Lave, *The Hospital Construction Act: An Evaluation of the Hill-Burton Program, 1948–1973* (Am. Enterprise Inst., May 1974).

13. M. Roemer, "Bed Supply and Hospital Utilization: A Natural Experiment," 35 *Hospitals* (Nov. 1, 1961) is one of the earliest statements of this argument.

14. For discussion of regulation as bargaining, see M. Holden, *Pollution Control as a Bargaining Process: An Essay on Regulatory Decision-Making,* (Cornell Water Resources Center, 1966).

15. T. Schelling, *Strategy of Conflict* (Harvard Univ. Press, 1960).

16. See M. Derthick, *The Influence of Federal Grants: Public Assistance in Massachusetts* (Harvard Univ. Press, 1970). See also H. Ingram, "Policy Implementation Through Bargaining: The Case of Federal Grants in Aid," 25 *Public Policy,* No. 4 (Fall 1977).

17. The internal/external distinction is useful, we think, even though it is complicated by the fact that the *in*ternal characteristics and actions of regulatees constitute part of the regulators' *ex*ternal environment and vice versa.

18. See discussion in R. Noll, *Reforming Regulation* 40–42 (The Brookings Inst., 1971).

19. J. Q. Wilson, "The Politics of Regulation," in *Social Responsibility and the Business Predicament* (J. M. Mckie, Ed., The Brookings Inst., 1974).

20. B. Ackerman, S. Ackerman, J. W. Sawyer and D. W. Henderson, *The Uncertain Search for Environmental Quality* (W. W. Norton, 1974).

21. R. Bauer, I. Poole and L. A. Dexter, *American Business and Public Policy* (Atherton Press, 1963).

22. Noll, n. 18 *supra* at Ch. 4.

23. See Ackerman et al., n. 20 *supra,* for the role of various interest group representatives in the Delaware River Basin study.

24. See H. Kaufman, *The Forest Service* (Johns Hopkins Press, 1960).

25. See, for example, S. Weaver, "Decision-Making in the U.S. Anti-trust Division," Diss. Harvard Univ. (1973).

26. Noll, n. 18 *supra* at Ch. 4.

27. The opportunity to "jump" from an agency to an outside job can free such an individual from the incentive system of that organization. But it can also make one eager to compile an exemplary record, as Weaver has argued in relation to young Antitrust Division lawyers.

28. R. E. Caves, *Air Transport and Its Regulators* (Harvard Univ. Press, 1962).

29. See, for example, R. G. Noll, M. J. Peck and J. J. McGowen, *Economic Aspects of Television Regulation* (The Brookings Inst., 1973).

30. M. J. Roberts and S. Farrell, "The Political Economy of Implementation: The Clean Air Act and Stationary Sources," forthcoming in *Approaches to Controlling Air Pollution* (MIT Press, 1978).

31. *Medical World News,* Oct. 17, 1977.

32. 5 *Health Security News,* No. 6, Sept. 29, 1976 and 6 *Health Security News,* No. 5, Aug. 31, 1977.

33. See, for example, G. F. Feeley and P. H. Feldman, *Certificate-of-Need Regulations,* Case in Health Policy and Management (Harvard School of Pub. Health, 1978).

34. Outside the health care industry, both labor and management have become concerned about health care costs and the impact of financing health insurance on the entire wage bargain. (T. B. Morehart and J. Rue, "The Impact of Rising Health Insurance and Health Care Costs on Business," 24 *Arizona Business* 9–16 (Jan. 1977)). Recent statements by leaders of companies like General Motors that they now pay more for health insurance than steel reflect this concern. Employee resistance to reduced benefit packages and employee demands for sufficient wage increases to keep up with the general rate of inflation have combined to make management extremely concerned about the apparently open-ended commitment it may have to financing health care benefits. To what extent business concerns will reinforce the political resources of regulators, however, is unclear. It appears that management is pursuing for now its own health care cost containment strategies rather than vigorously supporting regulation.

35. The recent flurry of exemptive legislation in Massachusetts is a prime example of industry attempts to override the CON process. See "Doctors, Hospitals and Politics," *Boston Globe,* October 5, 1977, p. 22.

36. P.L. 92-603, *The Professional Standards Review Organization Amendment of 1972.*

37. P.L. 93-641, *The National Health Planning and Resources Development Act of 1974.*

38. D. Alexander, *HMO Implementation*, Chap. 1, n. 33 *supra.*

39. W. Walker, "Changing United States Life-Style and Declining Vascular Mortality: Cause or Coincidence?" *New England Journal of Medicine* (July 2, 1977).

40. E. Braunwald, "Coronary-Artery Surgery at the Crossroads," *New England Journal of Medicine* 661–663 (Sept. 22, 1977) "Special Correspondence: A Debate on Coronary By-Pass," *New England Journal of Medicine* 1464–1470 (Dec. 29, 1977).

41. *Ibid.*

42. J. Wennberg and A. Gittelsohn, "Small Area Variations in Health Care Delivery," 182 *Science* 1102–1108 (Dec. 14, 1973).

43. A. L. Komaroff et al., "Quality, Efficiency and Cost of a Physician-Assistant Protocol System for Management of Diabetes and Hypertension," 25 *Diabetes*, No. 4, p. 297 (1976).

44. This phenomenon is discussed in A. Enthoven and R. Noll, *Regulatory and Nonregulatory Strategies for Controlling Health Care Costs*, Sun Valley Forum (Aug. 1977), and Graduate School of Business, Stanford Univ. (Sept. 1977).

45. For discussion of representation issues, see B. C. Vladeck, "Interest-Group Representation and the HSAs: Health Planning and Political Theory," 67 *American Journal of Public Health*, No. 1, pp. 23–29 (1977).

46. We have not included outcome studies of new manpower controls here, because they do not exist. O'Donoghue et al., provide a review of accreditation controls and their impact, but new federal requirements which seek to restrict entry of foreign medical graduates and to control geographical and specialty distribution are only now being put into place.

47. D. S. Salkever and T. W. Bice, "The Impact of Certificate of Need Controls on Hospital Investment," 54 *Health and Society* 185–214 (1976); D. S. Salkever and T. W. Bice, *Impact of State Certificate of Need Laws on Health Care Costs and Utilization*, Final Report, Contract No. HRA 106-74-57 (Nat'l Center for Health Serv. Research, HEW, Jan. 1976).

48. *Ibid;* see also D. Cohodes, *Certificate of Need Controls and Hospitals: An Outcome Assessment*, Unpublished Paper (Harvard School of Pub. Health, May 1976).

49. *Ibid.*

50. *Expenditures for Health Care: Federal Programs and Their Effects* 33 (Congressional Budget Office, Aug., 1977).

51. C. R. Britton, *Certificate of Need Legislation in Health Care Delivery*, Unpublished M.Sc. Thesis, (Sloan School of Management, MIT, May 1975).

52. F. Hellinger, "The Effect of Certificate of Need Legislation on Hospital Investment," 13 *Inquiry* 187–193 (1976).

53. E. Correia, "Public Certification of Need for Health Facilities," 65 *American Journal of Public Health*, No. 3, pp. 260–265 (Mar. 1975). Also M. J. Roberts

and A. Lawthers-Higgins, *The Concept of Need in Regional Health Care Planning,* unpublished paper (Harvard School of Public Health, 1979).

54. Cohodes, n. 48 *supra* and M. M. Melum, *Assessing the Need for Hospital Beds* (Interstudy Publishing, 1976).

55. Cohodes, n. 48 *supra.*

56. Havighurst and Blumstein, n. 9 *supra.*

57. See, for example, M. Gillick, "The Criteria of Choice in Medical Policy: Radiotherapy in Massachusetts," *Minerva* 15 (Spring 1977).

58. Britton, n. 51 *supra.*

59. Cohodes, n. 48 *supra.*

60. *Ibid.*

61. F. J. Hellinger, "Prospective Reimbursement through Budget Review: New Jersey, Rhode Island and Western Pennsylvania," 13 *Inquiry* 309–320 (Sept. 1976).

62. Altman and Eichenholz, n. 7 *supra*; also R. E. Berry, Jr., "Prospective Rate Reimbursement and Cost Containment: Formula Reimbursement in New York," 13 *Inquiry* 292–301 (Sept. 1976).

63. Altman and Eichenholz, n. 7 *supra.*

64. Berry, n. 62 *supra.*

65. Hellinger, "Prospective Reimbursement," n. 61 *supra.*

66. Berry, n. 62 *supra.*

67. *Assessing Quality in Health Care: An Evaluation* (Inst. of Medicine, Nat'l Academy of Sciences, Nov. 1976); *Expenditures for Health Care,* n. 50 *supra*; see also *Professional Standards Review Organizations: Program Evaluation,* Rep. No. OPEL 77-12 (OPEL, Oct. 1977).

68. P. Bonner, "On-Site Utilization Review: An Evaluation of the Impact of Utilization Patterns and Expenditures," Diss. Harvard School of Pub. Health (Feb. 1976); R. Brook and K. Williams, *An Evaluation of New Mexico Peer Review* (The Rand Corp., Fall 1976); J. R. Lave and S. Leinhardt, "An Evaluation of a Hospital Stay Regulatory Mechanism," *American Journal of Public Health* (Oct. 1976).

69. M. Kolins and D. K. Baugh, "An Evaluation of Medicare Concurrent Utilization Review Project: The Sacramento Certified Hospital Admission Program," Unpublished Paper (Social Sec. Administration, Nov. 1976).

70. Brook and Williams, n. 68 *supra*; and Lave and Leinhardt, n. 68 *supra.*

71. See the Senate Comm. on Fin. on Professional Standards Review, S. Rep. No. 92-1230, pp. 254–269 (Sept. 26, 1972).

72. See Havighurst and Blumstein, n. 9 *supra,* for elaboration of this argument.

73. Kolins and Baugh, n. 69 *supra.*

74. Lave and Leinhardt, n. 68 *supra.*

75. Brook and Williams, n. 68 *supra.*

76. *Report to the Secretary of HEW on Fundamental Improvements Needed for Timely Promulgation of Health Program Regulations* (GAO, May 1977).

77. This issue is highlighted in issues of *PSRO Reports* (formerly *PSRO Update*), 1977 and 1978, and is currently being litigated.

78. See, for example, D. Chapman Walsh and R. Feeley, "Graduated Sanctions to Enforce Nursing Home Standards," *New England Journal of Medicine* (July 22, 1976).

79. P. Blau, *The Dynamics of Bureaucracy* (Univ. of Chicago Press, 1963).

RESPONSE TO "MAGIC BULLETS OR SEVEN-CARD STUD"

Harold A. Cohen, *Executive Director, Health Services Cost Review Commission, Maryland*

Penny Feldman and Marc Roberts have presented an insightful argument on the problems associated with health care regulation. This response will underline those points which I believe are most important, give specific examples of the predicted problems, and discuss some possible solutions. The examples herein are taken from Maryland's regulatory experience. They are not meant to be unbiased. It is at least conceivable that the lack of objectivity on the part of this respondent might explain why most (if not all) examples suggest that rate-setting is more responsive to the types of concerns mentioned in Feldman/Roberts and Breyer (see Chapter 5 *infra*) than is health planning.

The Feldman/Roberts model suggests that both planning and utilization review will encounter more problems in implementation than will rate review. This follows from what Feldman/Roberts and others have described as the ambiguity, tension, and conflict of the legislative mandate coupled with vertical fragmentation in which the incentives available to indirect regulators for altering the behavior of direct regulators are limited, and the data which might link specified standards of practice to desired medical outcomes are lacking.

The legislation creating rate review, planning, and utilization review (PSROs) set up dual mandates for agency concern. These dual concerns are as follows:

Rate review	Cost containment–equity
Planning	Cost containment–access
PSRO	Cost containment–quality

These principal directives of rate review legislation are almost never in conflict. Cost containment relates to "the size of the pie" while equity refers to the "allocation of the pie among classes of payors." The technical problem of designing a rate structure which places the proper incentives upon providers so as to be cost containing and allocates the resultant cost equitably among patients is not trivial, but it is at least readily recognized as possible.

This is not meant to imply that rate reviewers never have clearly incompatible legal mandates. In our case, due in part to the political strength of the Maryland Hospital Association, the Maryland Health Services Cost Review Commission (HSCRC) Enabling Act requires the Commission to approve rates which will permit nonprofit hospitals "to render effective and efficient service on a solvent basis" (Section 568V (2)(a)) while "rates are set equitably among all purchasers or classes of purchasers without undue discrimination or preference (Section 568VU(a)).[1] Further, hospitals may not "charge for services at a rate other than those established in accordance with (this Act)." The Commission is powerless to assure payment by Medicaid and Medicare on the basis of commission rates and so solvency and equity among classes of purchasers are in conflict. The Commission has opted for solvency and, in effect, approves charges to payors other than Medicare and Medicaid at rates which, in the aggregate, are above what equity considerations alone would have generated. (That choice, itself, is clearly predicted by almost every regulatory model. See Breyer, Chapter 5).

The only clear conflict between cost containment and equity is in regard to cost determination of "equitable" hospital cost allocation. The Commission has adopted an economic rather than legal definition of price discrimination.[2] Applying this strictly would require measurement of the cost differential in treating different patients. Generally speaking, the Commission has expressly opted for cost containment when the expected cost of improving equity was perceived as being more costly than the attached benefit.

Thus, room rates do not reflect the differences in nursing or house staff time associated with particular patients. One example in which we were thwarted was a proposed regulation that would require hospitals to bill separately only for medical supplies over fifty dollars (such as pacemakers and prostheses). All less costly items would be averaged out and included in the room rate. We believed the cost saving to the hospital would outweigh the decrease in equity. One Medicare intermediary ruled that unless medical supplies were separately listed on itemized bills, it would not authorize any Medicare payment for medical supplies. (The Medicare intermediary can decide which services must be allocated on the basis of the ratio of Medicare patients' itemized charges to those of other patients). Given that ruling, the Commission decided that the increased equity of having Medicare contribute toward medical supply costs outweighed the cost-containing advantage of the per-patient allocation. Since Medicare can force other payors to pay "their apportioned share" of the cost of that type of decision, it will tend to underweigh the cost containment aspects of increased equity. The possible solutions are to have Medicare pay separately for its compliance costs (and the cost of measuring them)—a step appropriately taken with regard to utilization review—or to have Medicare allow an independent agency to decide the differential to which it is entitled, if any.

COST CONTAINMENT VERSUS ACCESS

The way in which planners are to foster cost containment is through limits to entry and expansion as well as identification of unneeded capacity and services. The closure of existing services clearly reduces access and denying entry impedes the growth of access. Thus, the two principal concerns of health planners—access and cost containment—are in direct conflict. One apparent solution would be to develop an acceptable standard for access and indicate that if the standard is threatened—that is, if access proves too difficult—enhancing access takes priority; otherwise cost containment takes precedence. An example of such a standard would be that there be a .999 probability that obstetrical and related services be available within 30 minutes normal driving time for all females of childbearing age who need them.

Why have planning agencies generally not given operational definitions of access? I believe the Feldman/Roberts model, in conjunction with existing market imperfections, explains this reluctance. Key imperfections in the health market are the separation of benefit from payment responsibility (the academically inclined might review the writings of Anthony Downs and J. M. Clark among others);[3] the incentives associated with the fee-for-service system;[4] the disparity between price and out-of-pocket expenditure due to insurance;[5] and the influence of cost-based reimbursement for hospitals.[6] These lead Feldman/Roberts to suggest that the problem with the health care sector is that the industry is providing *too much* (not too little) of a "good thing." Yet health system agencies (HSAs) institutionalize the separation of benefit from payment. The local planning agencies which decide whether a service is to be provided get the full benefit of the services they approve, but share the burden of paying for them with taxpayers and health insurance purchasers from the rest of the state and country. It is in their best interest to have too much access. The dearth of data linking access to health status makes it easy to justify a system in which access determination can always be used as the binding constraint. Only when the self-interest of existing firms coincides with cost containment efforts (such as retarding entry as opposed to expansion) is there much hope of cost containment dominating access.

This is a good example of vertical fragmentation. The federal agencies may place a high priority on cost containment but are unable to

enforce that priority upon the line agencies responsbile for the decisions. The political strength of the American Medical Association or
American Hospital Association has thus far kept that power out of
federal hands.

The planning agencies' natural desire to maintain both access and
the often excessive current levels of utilization is exemplified by a
current disagreement between the HSCRC and the Central Maryland
Health Systems Agency (CMHSA). (The CMHSA covers over half the
state's population and capacity.) The CMHSA's proposed plan[7] notes
that the inpatient utilization rate in their area is 1,149 bed days per
1,000 population and that the national guidelines for health planning
propose a standard of 1,000. Yet they project needs for 1980 and 1982
based upon the use rate of 1,149 (CMHSA). A Commission staff report
develops the cost of an 1,149 use rate over a 1,000 use rate in 1980 and
1982 at 1977 prices as approximately $66 and $68 million, respectively.[8]
The hospital association is doing all it can to minimize the rate reviewers' influence in CON decisions and in the plan development. One
obvious solution would be to pass something such as Title II of the
President's Cost Containment Act. This says that local planners can
exercise their priorities regarding local access so long as the total cost
does not exceed a particular amount.

The second obvious solution regards federal standard-setting relative
to health plans. In order to get full designation and be named the
planning agency, an HSA must submit a plan giving high priority to
cost containment. Thus far, very few HSAs have submitted satisfactory
plans. It also remains to be seen whether CON decisions will coincide
with plans. It is well known that many planning agencies have approved more beds than they themselves identify as needed.[9] The
CMHSA's draft plan gives top priority to achieving 85 percent occupancy in all hospitals (despite what we tell them about the lessons from
New York), but they recently approved an expansion project in which
the hospital forecasts an 80 percent occupancy in 1982. The CMHSA
draft plan calls for the elimination of all metropolitan obstetrical services with fewer than 1,000 births by 1979, but they just approved a
capital project for one of the two obstetrical services their proposed plan
would eliminate. The reason: It is unfair to apply a *draft* plan to these
hospitals.

COST CONTAINMENT–QUALITY

While cost containment and equity are almost never in conflict, and cost
containment and access are almost always in conflict, the relation between cost containment and quality is not that clear. What is clear is
that when it is inconsistent the physicians with local authority would
be expected to opt for quality for reasons analogous to the discussion
supra on access. Given the inability of anyone to measure quality by
way of patient outcomes and the lack of a proven relationship between
process and health status, there is every reason to believe that almost

any incentive giving more weight to cost containment is socially desirable. Yet faulty rate design and faulty efficiency screens by rate reviewers and Medicare have tended to make cost containment even less attractive to utilization reviewers.[10]

Again, the appropriate federal bureau (the Bureau of Quality Assurance) has proposed guidelines for full designation which give high priority to cost containment. Coupled with the Office of Management and Budget suggestions that the PSRO be scrapped, this may lead to local adoption of federal priorities. I doubt it. One cannot help but wonder what type of pressure will be put on the federal bureaus to approve HSAs and PSROs which do not give priority to cost containment.

The Commission, for its part, has developed a rate design which makes effective utilization review in the hospital's financial interest. Inpatient revenue is based on case-mix adjusted admissions (see Appendix 2-A at the end of this discussion.)

Given this background of the different weights attached to cost containment pursuit by the three agencies, it is not surprising that horizontal fragmentation would lead to "horizontal confrontation." Maryland has, and is witnessing such confrontations. Mercy Hospital's capital project presents an interesting example. Mercy is an inner city Baltimore hospital offering several "outreach" clinics in various parts of the city identified as "primary physician poor." It applied for an $11 million project almost entirely associated with backup facilities for these outreach clinics. The commission recommended against the project on the grounds that plenty of backup facilities were available at Maryland General Hospital—about ten blocks away. The planning agency approved the project as it felt it was not fair to penalize Mercy because of the close proximity and adequate facilities of Maryland General. A series of similar differences led to the following very revealing interview with Richard Staffs of the Comprehensive Health Planning Agency (CHP) staff which appeared in a local newspaper: "The problem with the HCRC, Staffa [sic] says, is that the agency is charged with holding down health costs in Maryland and they must 'look at every project as it affects the whole system. Our agency tempers this a bit by looking at a hospital's specific needs.' "[11] In spite of these continual differences, the Commission and the state's CHP are supporting legislation to formalize relationships. Hopefully, the HSAs and the State Health Coordinating Council (SHCC) will join in support. (A draft agreement—which needs that legislation to be implemented—is attached as Appendix 2-B). The Maryland Hospital Association is lobbying very strongly against the agreement.

"CAPTURE" THEORIES

Feldman/Roberts give various reasons why regulators might make inappropriate decisions. At least one of those reasons—asymmetric appeal costs—deserves more recognition than it has received. If an agency is accountable through the courts if it says "no" but not if it says "yes", then, given the need for all regulators to economize on their own resources, "yes" will be said too frequently. Maryland's early CHP history was rife with this type of asymmetry, the nadir of which was reached in the matter of Gaithersburg Community Hospital. Two applications to build 200-bed hospitals in Gaithersburg, Maryland were filed and reviewed simultaneously. The local planning agency, the state planning agency, and both hospitals agreed that only one hospital was needed. One application was for a proprietary hospital; the other was for a branch hospital operated by the Seventh Day Adventists in conjunction with the hospital they already owned in the same county. Both hospitals submitted capital and operating budgets. The Commission recommended the proprietary hospital be approved as it was less costly. The planning agency approved the other hospital and denied the proprietary hospital's application. The proprietary hospital appealed to the Board of Review which handles all CHP appeals before they reach the courts. When asked the basis for its decision, the lawyer for the planning agency stated that both applicants were equally good, only one was needed and so they "flipped a coin." (They obviously could not say they picked the more costly among equals.) The Board of Review decided: (1) Flipping a coin is arbitrary, and (2) if the appellant was equally good as the hospital which was approved, it too must be approved. It thereupon directed CHP to approve the proprietary hospital so that both were finally approved. Sometime later I had reason to review the transcript of the hearing before the Board of Review and was told that the record had never been transcribed because the board had approved the hospital's appeal and no one could appeal its approval. Both Blue Cross plans in Maryland have attempted and failed to attain standing to appeal CHP decisions. Maryland's legislature corrected this problem and gave payors standing to appeal CHP decisions effective July 1, 1977. The Commission, by regulation, made all major payors "designated interested parties" in all rate cases.

Feldman/Roberts discuss theories of capture associated with preponderance of participation and with a monopoly on data. If regulators see themselves as reviewing line items on wish-list budgets, they are doomed to failure. As Feldman/Roberts indicate, they could never sustain the burden of proof. Systems can be developed which eliminate that problem. Further, payor input not only can help maintain the long-run integrity of regulators, their data base often exceeds the industry's. For example, in a case in which University Hospital's wage rates were being challenged, the hospital claimed that high productivity could explain its wages. Blue Cross submitted testimony which, utilizing statewide bills for their patients, developed a case-mix complexity index. It showed University Hospital's length of stay was significantly higher than its complexity explained. Peninsula General Hospital's inhalation therapy budget was challenged. Blue Cross used their data base to show that for sixteen diagnoses which generated most use of inhalation therapy, per-case use at Peninsula General Hospital far exceeded the average.

While such reviews of base costs can occasionally be successful, Feldman/Roberts make an important point in suggesting that regulation not be based on case-by-case review but on generally applied parameters.

THRESHOLDS FOR REVIEW

Feldman/Roberts discuss the importance of threshold setting as it relates to the utilization of the regulatory agency's resources. Threshold setting can be used as an incentive in the system, as well as a recognition of regulatory priorities. The Commission has developed an inflation-adjustment system. This is an extremely formulaic method of adjusting approved base-year costs and rates, and using a modified order granting new rates for the next year. The process is painless to the hospital and takes less than a month to complete. Hospitals which are not willing to accept that "threshold of reasonableness" review, undergo a lengthy and often embarrassing public hearing. In all likelihood, hearings will be held on only five to eight of Maryland's fifty hospitals this year.

In determining issues for a public hearing on the original base budgets, the threshold for presumptive unreasonableness was the 80th percentile of hospitals in the same class. That screen was applied departmentally. We often did not raise an issue if the amount challenged was less than $20,000. Agency capacity was a consideration in setting the screen.

Threshold setting can also apply to jurisdictional questions. The same "resource consuming" analysis as advanced by Feldman/Roberts is appropriate. Thus, while CON could conserve resources by raising the threshold from $150,000 to $300,000, a more intelligent economization of its resources might result from the elimination of its jurisdiction over HMOs, home health agencies, nursing homes, etc. An argument can be made that some early planning agencies deliberately extended their jurisdiction to consume their resources and give themselves an excuse for not developing an operational plan for acute hospital facilities.

One question that Feldman/Roberts raise is just how simple should thresholds of reasonableness formulation be. This, too, relates to the incentives the rate-setter wants to build into the system. If all dollars are treated equally, the hospital is equally at risk for all aspects of its business and the public is at risk for all projections made at the time of rate approval. The Commission's inflation-adjustment system is quite complicated mathematically. (It is less complex for hospitals on the Guaranteed Inpatient Review Program (GIR) as discussed in Appendix 2-A, as the GIR contains the incentives more directly.) Base-period approved costs (we want a long regulatory lag) are adjusted by commission-specified inflation indices. The hospitals know these indices in time to avoid incurring costs beyond the threshold. (See Appendix 2-C for a memorandum on computing prospective rate adjustments

which was sent two months before union contracts had to be re-
negotiated.) These costs are adjusted departmentally for changes in
volume on the basis of each department's specific estimates of the
proportions of fixed and variable costs. Hospitals not on the GIR are not
at risk for volume changes. In developing rates from the newly approved costs several further adjustments are made. Some adjustments
apply to estimates made in developing earlier rates from approved costs
where the hospital is not meant to be at risk, i.e., it should be neutral as
to the accuracy of the prediction. For example, if the percentage of
payors receiving a differential varies, an adjustment is made. This is
because the differential is not based solely on cost savings to the
hospital but also on estimated cost savings to the system. If any approved cross-subsidies are over- or under-realized due to differences in
departmental volume change, adjustments are made. The above prospective adjustments represent a "doubling," i.e., there is an adjustment
for previous results as well as one for the future period. The inflation-
adjustment system also includes a compliance system. If hospitals fail to
charge the approved rates, those adjustments are also made departmentally. The Commission has recently published regulations which specify
the penalty in the case of an overcharge. Undercharges are not in
violation of the approved rates but a 2 percent or more undercharge
would be recoverable.

Hospitals are currently at risk for the approved proportion of uncol-
lectible accounts built into their rate structure. The commission believes
that hospitals should be at risk for bad debts but not for charity care.
The Commission has published a proposed regulation to distinguish
operationally between these two types of nonpaying patients. The
inflation-adjustment system will then see that the hospital is neither
penalized nor rewarded if it serves more (or less) charity patients than
projected at the time of rate approval.

An example of what can happen when cost review systems are
complex—as opposed to simple like those based upon an 80 percent
occupancy rate—was revealed to the commission in the *Franklin Square
Case* (Franklin Square Hospital et al.).[12] We prepared a document
meant to describe how the staff reviews hospital budgets. Twenty-five
hospitals in a declaratory judgment suit claimed the document was an
illegally approved regulation. The document had been badly written
and the judge correctly noted that there were many statements which
appeared to be regulations. He went on to describe some aspects of the
document as "the largest chunk of gobbledygook it has been my dis-
pleasure to read during forty-two years at the bar and on the bench." The
four examples he gave of "gobbledygook" were all mathematical
standards—they included references to Laspeyre's index, to information theory, to regression techniques, to the 80th percentile, to the
median, and to square roots. It is easy to sympathize with those who
would use simple occupancy rate standards to define excess capacity
when a judge can levy such extreme criticism against the use of a
Poisson distribution.

Feldman/Roberts give an excellent discussion of the problems associated with service and process standards for medical care. This is appropriately a recurrent theme throughout their article. My feelings could not be better expressed than by the following quotation from a speech made by Alvin M. Powers, Chairman of the HSCRC:

> As much as possible, health care standards should be patient oriented, they should not be input or paper compliance oriented. Setting a standard such as a 3 percent hospital induced infection rate makes sense. (It may be unenforceable, though). Requiring X numbers of nurses per patient day makes no sense. Its being enforceable cannot be allowed to overcome its basic irrelevance.
>
> Standards must avoid any implication that more inputs are better. Without better patient outcome, more inputs are simply inefficient. This goes for such self-serving measures of quality as asset to bed ratios, number of "services" offered, employees per occupied bed, etc. Hospitals and physicians should have to show that "more" leads to "better" patient outcomes and how much better. The rate reviewers might still decide the better outcome is not worth the additional money, but at least the decision will be made on appropriate estimates. In many cases, follow-up review will be needed to see if the forecasted improvements did occur. (How many previously undetected operable tumors did your scanner find last year?).
>
> Thus, the only approach to health care standards I would endorse has to do with the way health care is provided—length-of-stay, error rates in drugs, infection rates, lab test per admission, etc. And minimum standards should not be set only maximum ones. This flies in the face of what many PSROs are doing, but I trust physicians to not do too few lab tests or X-rays.
>
> My proscription of input standards includes most emphatically "credential" standards. I would never require a hospital administrator to have a masters degree in hospital administration or a laboratory administrator to be a physician of any ilk. Infection rates, error rates, death rates and other patient care measures are infinitely superior.
>
> Thus, using outcome measure standards for evaluating patient care will not get in the way of using industrial engineering standards for approving inputs."[13]

Rate monitoring is rather easy. Every hospital reports quarterly volumes and revenues by department. The revenue and unit collection systems are subject to spot audit by the Commission. We are considering requiring some additional verification (other than that usually performed) by the hospital's independent CPA.

The major monitoring and enforcement problems in rate review relate to reporting requirements and to policing "fraud and deception" which are generated by the incentives to link reported costs to rates. An important current example relates to nursing home rate determination for Medicaid. The New Jersey Health Department and the HSCRC decided to share consultants and work jointly on a reasonable cost

system for nursing home rate review. We began by deciding that we would not become police agencies reviewing the various financial arrangements by which homes are owned and financed. After all, when we buy an apple do we care if the farmer leased the farm from his mother or has a 99:1 debt/equity ratio? We developed a "capital facilities allowance" based on age and location of the facility. It recognized, up to some screen (a maximum standard), actual building square feet and land acreage.

Apparently the federal government will not accept this allowance but will require that reimbursement be based upon book cost, interest payments, and lease payments. It appears to insist on developing a system which requires that every building transaction be closely examined and every existing contract be scrutinized. This type of review mechanism is exactly the kind of standard Feldman/Roberts correctly warn against.

CONCLUSION

The Feldman/Roberts paper contains many insights regarding problems a rate reviewer is likely to encounter. The major policy question regards whether prospective hospital rate setting is a necessary or sufficient condition for securing an effective and efficient hospital delivery system. In a world of high coinsurance and great HMO penetration, it might not be necessary. Without an attack on the fee-for-service system, it is clearly not sufficient. Without either of the above two criteria it is almost certainly better than retrospective reimbursement.

The "biggest ticket item" is probably the utilization rate. Rate setting may help contain it but cannot generate the wholesale reductions that are possible. The second biggest ticket item, at least on the East Coast, is labor—both quantity and wage rate. No system can work unless the public and the relevant government agencies are willing to see several people lose their jobs. In a recent television program, NBC suggested that Denver could save a lot of money by closing 1,500 beds. The program suggested that money could be saved without causing major disruption to a lot of lives by closing beds and buying fewer machines like CAT scanners. Closing 1,500 beds will not cause much saving unless the (approximately) 4,000 people who staff them are laid off. Unless the government is willing to accept this consequence (and use other policies as necessary), no rate-setting agency (or planning body) will operate with the support it needs.

NOTES

1. Art. 43, Ann. Code of Md.

2. E. Singer, *Antitrust Economics* 225–226 (Prentice-Hall, 1968).

3. See A. Downs, *An Economic Theory of Democracy* (Harpers, 1957); and J. M. Clark, *Studies in the Economics of Overhead Costs* (Chicago, 1923).

4. See J. S. Cook, "A Discussion of the Causes of Hospital Cost Inflation," Staff Paper (Health Serv. Cost Review Comm'n, Oct. 5, 1977); and H. Cohen and J. S. Cook, "Hospital Reimbursement and Utilization Incentives, A Maryland Experiment," in *Profile of Medical Practice, 1978* (J. C. Gaffney, Ed., AMA, 1978). See also M. Pauly and M. Redisch, "The Not-for-Profit Hospital as a Physicians' Cooperative," *American Economic Review* (Mar. 1973).

5. See H. Cohen, "The Rationing Ability of Price in the Market for Hospital Services," in *Compendium on the Development of Human Resources* (Joint Economic Comm., U.S.C., Mar. 1968); see also Cohen and Cook, *ibid.*

6. H. Klarman, "Reimbursing the Hospital—The Differences the Third Party Makes," *Journal of Risk and Insurance* (Dec. 1969).

7. *Draft: Health Systems Plan and Annual Implementation Plan, 1978,* Central Maryland HSA.

8. Cohen, "Projected Cost of Excess Beds and Excessively Used Beds in the Central Maryland Health Systems Area." Unpublished Report to the HSCRC (1978).

9. See D. Salkever and T. Bice, "The Impact of Certificate of Need Controls on Hospital Investment," in *Milbank Memorial Fund Quarterly/Health and Society* (Spring, 1976); and C. Havighurst, "Regulation of Health Facilities and Services by Certificate of Need," *Virginia Law Review* (1973).

10. Cohen and Cook, n. 4 *supra.*

11. J. Price, "State Orders Carroll Hospital Probe," *Baltimore News American,* Jan. 13, 1978.

12. Franklin Square Hosp., et al. v. Health Serv. Cost Review Comm'n, in the Circuit Court for Baltimore County, Docket 104, Folio 293, File 82047.

13. A. Powers, "The Government as a Regulator," Unpublished Speech (Methuen, Mass., Nov. 17, 1977).

APPENDIX 2-A: MEMO FROM THE HEALTH SERVICES COST REVIEW COMMISSION OF THE STATE OF MARYLAND

TO: All Hospitals–Chief Financial Officers
        –Chief Executive Officers

FROM: Harold A. Cohen

DATE: October 18, 1976

SUBJECT: Inflation Adjustments to Hospital Rates

Inflation adjustments to rates will continue to be available to all hospitals. For those hospitals not yet on Commission-approved rates, general inflation orders will be issued periodically. Hospitals which are charging Commission approved rates are not covered by the General Inflation Orders, but may apply after notice by the Commission for an inflation adjustment. The information required in order to calculate an inflation adjustment is given in the attached paper. Requests for inflation adjustments should be addressed to Mr. Robert Vovak.

The main purpose of this memorandum is to indicate to hospital management the amount that will be included for average salary inflation in these adjustments. For hospitals in the Baltimore metropolitan area, the factor for salary inflation will be the increase in the Baltimore Consumer Price Index (CPI) for the period September 1975 to September 1976. This is expected to be about 5.5 percent. For hospitals in the Washington metropolitan area the Washington CPI for the period November 1975 to November 1976 will be used (this is expected to be about 5.9 percent). For other hospitals, the National CPI for the period October 1975 to October 1976 will be used (about 5.6 percent). These percentages will apply to the total bill for salaries, wages, and fringe benefits.

We are informing you of these figures so that you are aware of future revenue increases available without a thorough budget review. As soon as the Bureau of Labor Statistics publishes the precise figures we will send a note of them to all hospitals.

You should recognize that the Commission's emphasis is upon allowed

121

increases in rates. Thus, in a metropolitan Baltimore hospital for which the labor and fringe package represents 70 percent of its cost, we currently expect to approve a 3.85 percent (.70 × 5.5) increase in rates as the labor induced factor included in the forthcoming inflation adjustment.

APPENDIX 2-B: AGREEMENT BETWEEN ST. AGNES HOSPITAL AND THE HEALTH SERVICES COST REVIEW COMMISSION REGARDING THE ADOPTION OF THE GUARANTEED INPATIENT REVENUE PROGRAM

INTRODUCTION

The Guaranteed Inpatient Revenue (GIR) Program has been developed by the Maryland Health Services Cost Review Commission to provide hospitals with financial incentives to moderate the increase in the amount of resources used per-patient admission in order to slow the rise in the cost of health care. This approach recognizes that the cost of health care is dependent not only on the amounts spent for individual personnel, supplies, and services, but is also dependent on the quantity of tests and examinations ordered for patients and on their average length of stay.

The GIR is applicable to inpatient service only and is being implemented on an experimental basis, initially for an eighteen-month period. Hospitals selected for this program are those with relatively well-developed information systems and with the capacity for detailed utilization review. Hospitals participating in this experiment will be provided with normal periodic rate increases as prescribed in the Commission's rate-adjustment system. The eighteen-month period during which St. Agnes Hospital will be subject to the GIR is the period ending March 31, 1979.

COMPUTATION AND APPLICATION OF THE GIR

The first step in the computation of the GIR is to specify the base period. The base period for St. Agnes Hospital will be October 1, 1976 through March 31, 1977.

For the base period the Hospital shall develop certain charge data applicable to live discharges other than newborns. Specifically, the Hospital shall first classify each patient (other than deaths and newborns) served in the base period according to their discharge diagnosis and whether or not the patient was under age sixty-five. Within each classification the Hospital will then compute the average billed charge. These statistics will be referred to as the base-period charges.

The Hospital shall adjust the base-period charges so as to bring them to the level they would have been throughout the experimental period, thereby taking into account all rate adjustments subsequent to the first day of the base period but prior to the last day of the experimental period. The resulting charges will be called the adjusted base-period charges.

The adjusted base-period charges represent the guaranteed average revenue per diagnostic-age classification for each live discharge other than newborns during the period of the experiment. The computation of the GIR for the experimental period is then carried out as follows:

1. For each diagnostic age classification, the adjusted base-period charge is recorded along with the number of live discharges.

2. The product of the base-period charge and the number of live discharges is then summed over all applicable discharges.

The Hospital shall receive a prospective rate adjustment at the end of the experimental period or as often as monthly during the experimental period if the Hospital so chooses, equal to the difference between the actual revenue and the GIR during the experimental period. This adjustment will be modified so as to account for changes in the number and severity of illness of patients served according to the method outlined in the "Methodology Of Computing Prospective Rate Adjustments Under the Guaranteed Inpatient Revenue Program" which is attached to this agreement as Exhibit B (Appendix 2-C).

ADDITIONAL COMMENTS

The Commission recognizes the experimental nature of this program and will consider adjustments to the Hospital's GIR based upon documented and quantifiable changes in the burden of illness faced by the Hospital.

At the end of the experimental period the Hospital may choose any alternative rate structure then applied in any hospital within their bed-size category. The bed-size categories will include those hospitals with 400 beds or more and those hospitals with less than 400 beds.

St. Agnes Hospital shall receive, in addition to normal periodic rate increases, a provision of $100,000 in order to monitor and analyze actively the Hospital's case-mix patterns. In the event that the Hospital increases preadmission testing or other outpatient services as a result of this program, funds will be provided in rates to offset increases in bad debt losses and charity allowances created by such efforts. It shall be the responsibility of the Hospital to report to the Commission changes in revenue associated with increased outpatient services.

APPENDIX 2-C: METHODOLOGY OF COMPUTING PROSPECTIVE RATE ADJUSTMENTS UNDER THE GUARANTEED INPATIENT REVENUE PROGRAM

The purpose of the following paragraphs is to explain the method used to adjust the Hospital's inpatient revenue for variations between the number and severity of illness of discharges used to establish the GIR, and the number and severity of illness of discharges actually realized during the period that the GIR is in effect. This method begins by determining whether or not the total projected inpatient revenue of the Hospital exceeds the inpatient revenue actually realized. Because inpatient charges approved by the Commission are cost-based—i.e., one department does not subsidize another—it follows that if the Hospital's actual revenue exceeds its projected revenue, then the Hospital's income will have exceeded its projected cost (assuming no change in the proportion of patients in the various payor categories). Moreover, it is reasonable to assume that the Hospital's income exceeded its actual cost. This follows because the additional services provided admit of economies of scale; each additional service unit can be produced at a marginal cost which is less than the average cost of producing the budgeted number of service units.

Since charges are cost-based, the average income per unit of service equals the average approved cost and hence exceeds the marginal cost of additional units. Thus, total income exceeds total cost when actual revenue exceeds projected revenue in a cost-based pricing system. The Commission is currently carrying out a study to determine the marginal cost of the daily patient care services and of the major ancillary departments in a number of hospitals. A result of this study will be a precise method for determining the reasonable variation in cost associated with changes in the volumes of service provided. In the interim, the Commission is assuming that 60 percent of the cost of the daily patient care services and 40 percent of the cost of ancillary services vary with increasing volume. In most hospitals these assumptions imply that on average about 50 percent of a Hospital's inpatient cost is variable, and hence, that 50 percent is fixed. This percentage of fixed cost is applied to any increase in actual and budgeted revenue and is used as a rate offset in subsequent periods.

During a period when hospital volumes are declining, the Hospital's short-term fixed cost will, however, exceed 50 percent. The pattern of declining volumes must first be established, followed by personnel reductions made through attrition or lay-offs. Such reductions frequently involve payment for back pay, accrued leave, severance pay, and increased unemployment insurance compensation. Thus, short-term fixed cost clearly exceeds 50 percent. To encourage the elimination of marginal and unnecessary admissions, the Commission has established 80 percent as the fixed-cost factor for unrealized admissions of less than 5 percent and a 50 percent fixed-cost factor for any additional unrealized admissions.

To illustrate the formulas implied by these concepts, let us assume that 50 percent of a Hospital's cost varies with volume. Then, if the Hospital's actual revenue (R_a) exceeds its projected revenue (R_p), 50 percent of the increased revenue should be subsequently recovered:

$$R_a > R_p \text{ implies } .5(R_a - R_p) \text{ to be recovered}$$

If the Hospital experiences less than a 5 percent decline in admissions and its actual revenue is less than its projected revenue, then 80 percent of the lost revenue should be subsequently included in rates. Letting A_p denote the projected number of admissions and A_a the actual number, we have:

$$.95 < \frac{A_a}{A_p}$$

and $R_a < R_p$ implies

$$.8(R_p - R_a) \qquad \text{to be included in subsequent rates}$$

Finally, if the Hospital experiences a decline in admissions of more than 5 percent (and a loss in revenue), then the Hospital shall recover in subsequent rates 80 percent of the revenue lost as the result of the first 5 percent drop in admissions and 50 percent of all additional lost revenue. Of the lost revenue, $R_p - R_a$, the proportion lost as a result of the first 5 percent drop in admissions is the ratio of 5 percent of projected admissions, $.05\, A_p$, to the total drop in admissions, $A_p - A_a$. The proportion of the lost revenue attributable to the additional drop in admission is the quotient of the total drop in admissions less the 5 percent of projected admissions already accounted for, $(A_p - A_a) - .05\, A_p$ and the total drop in admissions $A_a - A_p$. Hence:

$$\frac{A_a}{A_p} < .95$$

and $R_a < R_p$ implies

$$\left[.8\left(\frac{.05 A_p}{A_p - A_a} \right) + .5 \left(\frac{A_p - A_a - .05 A_p}{A_p - A_a} \right) \right](R_p - R_a)$$

is to be recovered.

The adjustments outlined above will allow a Hospital sufficient income to offset its reasonable cost. The GIR program, however, adjusts income in accordance with the Hospital's performance. To explain the adjustments associated with the GIR, it will be useful to introduce some notation:

R_a = actual billed revenue $\left.\vphantom{\begin{array}{c}a\\a\end{array}}\right\}$ As before
A_a = actual discharges and deaths

A_d = number of deaths or discharges with diagnoses not occurring in the base period

A_L = number of discharges

R_d = revenue attributable to patients who died or with diagnoses not
occurring in the base period

R_L = revenue attributable to discharges

The following identities hold:

$$R_a = R_d + R_L$$
$$A_a = A_d + A_L$$

Also, let us denote by G_A the guaranteed inpatient revenue per admission, during the period of the GIR. Since the GIR only applies to discharges (not deaths), the GRA has only been exceeded if $G_L = (R_L/A_L)$ exceeds G_A.

There are six possible adjustments depending on which of the three revenue adjustments applies and on whether or not the GRA has been exceeded.

Case I

The GRA has not been exceeded, $G_A > G_L$ and the Hospital's actual revenue exceeds the budgeted revenue, $R_a > R_p$. We have already determined that the Hospital's income has exceeded its reasonable cost by $.5(R_a - R_p)$ (assuming 50 percent variable costs). Thus, the Hospital's rates will be adjusted in subsequent periods by

$$- .5(R_a - R_p)$$

On the other hand, the Hospital has not exceeded the GIR limit. Since the GRA applies to live discharges the difference between the total revenue guaranteed under the GIR and the total revenue actually received is:

$$A_L(G_A - G_L)$$

The cost saving attributable to not exceeding the GIR is this amount of revenue multiplied by the proportion of variable cost (.5). Thus, the Hospital will have added to its rates

$$.5[A_L(G_A - G_L)]$$

The total adjustment is, therefore

$$-.5(R_a - R_p)$$
$$+.5[A_L(G_A - G_L)]$$

Example Hospital X had budgeted $1,500,000 in inpatient revenue and realized $1,760,000. The Hospital had 1,100 discharges who were charged on average $1,600. The GRA was $1,700. The Hospital's adjustments would be as follows:

$R_a = 1,760,000$	$-.5(1,760,000 - 1,500,000)$
$R_p = 1,500,000$	$+.5(1,100)(1,700 - 1,600)$
$A_L = 1,100$	$= -130,000$
$G_A = 1,700$	$+ 55,000$
$G_L = 1,600$	$= - 75,000$

Proof of Example Assuming charges equal cost equal income:

Approved cost R_p	$1,500,000	(1)
Expected cost $R_p + .5(R_a - R_p)$	1,630,000	(2)
Allowance for beating GIR $.5A_L(G_A - G_L)$	55,000	(3)
Total approved income (2) + (3)	$1,685,000	(4)
Realized revenue R_a	$1,760,000	(5)
Adjustment	−75,000	(6)
Income	$1,685,000	

Case II

The GIR has been exceeded, $G_L > G_A$ and the Hospital's actual revenue exceeds the budgeted revenue. The reasoning and adjustment formula are exactly as in Case I.

$$-.5(R_a - R_p)$$
$$+.5A_L(G_A - G_L)$$

Example Hospital X had budgeted $1,700,000 in inpatient revenue and realized $1,760,000. The Hospital had 1,100 discharges who were charged on average 1,600. The GRA was $1,500. The Hospital's adjustment would be as follows:

$R_a = 1,760,000$	$-.5(60,000)$
$R_p = 1,700,000$	$+.5(1,100)(-100)$
$A_L = 1,100$	$= -85,000$
$G_A = 1,500$	
$G_L = 1,600$	

Proof of Example Assuming charges equal cost equal income:

Approved cost R_p	$1,700,000	(1)
Expected cost $R_p + .5(R_A - R_p)$	1,730,000	(2)
Disallowance GIR $.5A_L(G_A - G_L)$	−55,000	(3)
Total approved income	$1,675,000	(4)
Realized revenue R_p	$1,760,000	(5)
Adjustment	−85,000	(6)
Income	$1,675,000	(7)

Case III

The GIR has not been exceeded, $G_A > G_L$, the Hospital's actual revenue is less than budgeted revenue and admissions have dropped by less than 5 per cent.

We have already determined that the Hospital's income has been insufficient to cover $.8(R_p - R_a)$ of its reasonable cost. Therefore, this amount must be added to the Hospital's subsequent revenue. In addition, the Hospital has not exceeded the GIR. As before, the total revenue reduction associated with this reduction in unnecessary or marginal services is

$$A_L(G_A - G_L)$$

The cost savings attributable to not exceeding the GIR is this amount of revenue multiplied by the proportion of (short-term) variable cost (.2). Thus, the Hospital will have added to its rates.

$$.2A_L(G_A - G_L)$$

The Total adjustment is, therefore

$$.8(R_p - R_a)$$
$$+.2A_L(G_A - G_L)$$

Example

$R_a = 1,680,000$	$.8(25,000)$
$R_p = 1,705,000$	$+ .2(1,050)(1,700 - 1,600)$
$A_L = 1,050$	$= \$41,000$
$G_A = 1,700$	
$G_L = 1,600$	

Proof of Example   Assuming costs equal charges equal income:

Approved cost (R_p)	$1,705,000	(1)
Expected cost $R_p - .2(R_p - R_a)$	1,700,000	(2)
GRA allowance $.2A_L (G_A - G_L)$	21,000	(3)
Total approved income (2) + (3)	$1,721,000	(4)
Actual income (R_a)	1,680,000	(5)
Adjustment	41,000	(6)
Total income	$1,721,000	(7)

Case IV

The GIR has been exceeded, $G_L G_A$, the Hospital's actual revenue is less than the budgeted revenue and admissions have dropped by less than 5 percent.
    In this case, the adjustment formula is precisely the same as in Case III.

$$.8(R_p - R_a)$$
$$-.2A_L(G_A - G_L)$$

Example   Hospital X had budgeted \$1,800,000 in inpatient revenue and realized \$1,750,000. The Hospital had 1,750 discharges, an average charge of \$1,000 per discharge and a GIR of \$950. The adjustment is then

$R_a = 1,750,000$	$.8(1,800,000 - 1,750,000)$
$R_p = 1,8000,000$	$+ 2(1,000)(950 - 1,000)$
$A_1 = 1,000$	$= 40,000$
$G_A = 950$	$- 10,000$
$G_L = 1,000$	$= 30,000$

Approved cost R_p	\$1,800,000	(1)
Expected cost $R_p - .2(R_p - R_a)$	1,790,000	(2)
GRA disallowance $.2A_L(G_A - G_L)$	$-10,000$	(3)
Approved cost	\$1,780,000	(4)
Actual income	\$1,750,000	(5)
Adjustment	30,000	(6)
Total income	\$1,780,000	(7)

Case V

The GIR has not been exceeded, $G_A > G_l$, the Hospital's actual revenue is less than budgeted and admissions have dropped by more than 5 percent. We have already seen that the Hospital's expected cost exceed its income by

$$\left[.8\left(\frac{.05A_p}{A_p - A_a}\right) + .5\left(\frac{A_p - A_a - .05A_p}{A_p - A_a}\right)\right](R_p - R_a)$$

The quantity in brackets [F] is the average percentage of fixed cost not reimbursed during the period of the GIR. If A_L denotes the number of live discharges during the GIR period, then the amount of unbilled allowable charges is:

$$A_L(G_A - G_L)$$

The cost savings associated with this reduction in charges is:

$$(1 - F)A_L(G_A - G_L)$$

Thus, the formula for this case is:

$$F(R_p - R_a) + (1 - F)A_L(G_A - G_L)$$

Case VI

The GIR has been exceeded, $G_L > G_A$, the actual revenue is less than budgeted, and admissions have dropped by more than 5 percent. In this case, the formula and reasoning are precisely the same as in Case V.

THE GAME OF HEALTH CARE REGULATION: COMMENTS ON FELDMAN/ROBERTS

Roger G. Noll, *California Institute of Technology*

INTRODUCTION

The system for delivering and financing health care in the United States is complex. It demands that the approach to health care policy be sophisticated enough to avoid causing unintended, undesirable social consequences of well-intentioned public policy interventions.

Judging from the actions of individuals in making decisions about health care and insurance, and of government in enacting numerous laws pertaining to health care since the mid–1960s, the purpose of any legislated change in the medical care system would be:

1. To improve the health status of the population generally and of certain target groups (i.e., the poor, the young, the elderly, members of racial minorities, and residents of rural areas) in particular.

2. To assure that all citizens can receive adequate health care in case of catastrophic illness without suffering financial ruin.

3. To promote the development of more effective methods and technologies for providing medical care.

4. To achieve all of the above at a reasonable cost.

The last objective has become more pressing in recent years because of the rapid rate of increase in medical expenditures. Part of this increase is due to inflation as medical care prices have risen more rapidly than have prices generally. Part is also due to the fact that more of society's resources are being devoted to medical services. The alarming feature of rapidly rising medical expenditures is that they do not seem to be achieving very much in terms of their primary objective, the improvement of the health status of citizens.

Public Policy Instruments in the Health Sector

Nearly every type of public policy instrument available to government has been used to some degree in the health care sector.

- Tax incentives promote private insurance, defray part of major medical expenditures above insurance reimbursement, and encourage capital investment and drug research in for-profit enterprises that operate in the sector.

- Direct governmental expenditures pay for most of the health care for the poor and the elderly, finance construction of medical schools and hospitals, and underwrite extensive research to develop new methods of treatment.

- Licensing authorities control entry into most medical care professions, the hospital industry, and the drug market.

- The quality of medical care is influenced by the courts, through medical malpractice litigation, by professional review groups, and by reimbursement policies of Medicare and Medicaid.

- Prices are influenced by reimbursement policies, and in about one-half the states hospital rates are directly regulated.

- Insurance companies are subjected to regulation of financial practices and profit rates, and employers who provide medical insurance as part of fringe benefits for workers are required to offer access to a "qualified" local prepaid health plan (HMO) if one exists.

The last policy is the only one that is explicitly procompetitive in that it seeks to use the forces of consumer choice to further public objectives in the health care sector. Even in this case the procompetitive thrust of the policy is blunted by regulation (i.e., "qualifying" a plan, permitting an HMO to obtain hospital facilities to begin operation). Moreover, the result—a choice between one conventional insurance package and one HMO (there is usually only one in an area)—is short of any definition of robust competition.

If anything, the trend of policy during the past ten years has been away from reliance on the use of incentives and competition, despite the limited growth (with some limited encouragement from government) of HMOs. Instead, the trend has been to establish formal regulatory processes to control more and more of the decision making of medical care professionals. With each wave of increase in medical care expenditures, a new "cause" is identified: overbedding, inflation, or expensive new technology. Each cause is attacked with a new regulatory authority to control the culprit, such as by licensing hospital capacity, controlling fees or total expenditures, overseeing treatment decisions, and limiting the diffusion of new technology.

The importance of the Feldman/Roberts study is that it sheds light on where this trend—if it continues—will take society in terms of the quality and cost of medical care delivery. Feldman/Roberts are telling us by a painstaking, detailed chain of arguments not just that regulation is an imperfect instrument of public policy (regardless of our opinions on what ought to be done, we all know that), but that social scientists who have studied regulation now provide important insights about the likely success of regulation in various economic environments. They are able to point to ways in which the nature of the technology and market structure affects the outcome of regulation in terms of meeting the kinds of policy objectives that were set forth *supra* in this essay.

This approach is especially useful. It avoids a fruitless, dichotomized debate on the totally irrelevant question of whether the medical care sector ought to be regulated. Obviously, regulation of certain aspects of medical care delivery and finances is here to stay. The relevant debate is about the proper combination of policies, including actions that facilitate competition in certain parts of the medical care sector as well as regulatory, expenditure, and taxation policies.

THE FELDMAN/ROBERTS POSITION

The theme of the Feldman/Roberts study is that regulation ought to be regarded as a complicated game involving numerous agents and including regulated entities, regulatory officials, executive and congressional political overseers, bureaucrats with related responsibilities, and various groups who are customers of the regulated sector.

While most of these players may well subscribe to the idea that regulation should work to make the regulated market operate more efficiently with more equitable outcomes, each is also motivated by personal objectives that may be irrelevant or even antithetical to these ends. And each player, given these objectives and the environment in which regulation takes place, pursues these objectives by selecting a set of informational, legal, and political strategies to influence regulatory policy. Regulatory outcomes depend upon the interaction of these strategies, the nature of the regulatory problem, the procedures, the authority and enforcement capability of the regulatory agency, and other important features of the regulatory environment that are likely to vary from case to case.

The objectives of the Feldman/Roberts study are to develop the detailed structures of the regulation game in a fashion that enables it to identify situations in which regulation is likely to be passably effective, and to examine regulatory programs in the medical care sector to see whether the conditions for relatively effective regulation are present.

Players in the Game of Regulation

At the risk of making generalizations that do not do justice to the many subtleties of the argument, the following is offered as a summary of how Feldman/Roberts roughly characterize the players and environment of the regulation game.

Political overseers are motivated by the quest for reelection, and in a media-rich, informed contemporary America, their public policy positions have an important impact on their electoral fortunes. Thus, they advocate the objectives listed at the beginning of this essay. But politicians, being technically limited, overworked generalists, tend to provide only vague guidelines to agencies, leaving much discretion in developing policy to the latter. Hence direct political controls over the regulatory process tend to be weak.

Regulators, facing a relatively vague mandate, imperfect information, and limited resources, must rely upon other players for information and program proposals in carrying out policy. The regulatory authority must work out the details of defining what to regulate (specific actors and activities), the procedures for gathering information and making decisions, and the sanctions and enforcement mechanisms for assuring compliance with regulatory rules. The strategy of regulation, given limited resources for the regulator, involves trying to have an impact without incurring unsupportable expenses in making and enforcing decisions, including fighting legal and political battles with recalcitrant regulated entities.

Regulated entities, in turn, presumably do not want to behave as the regulators wish, or else there would be no point to regulation. They, too, have limited resources for participating in the regulatory process, fighting decisions of the regulators, complying with rules, and paying fines for noncompliance. Their strategy will depend on the behavior of other regulated entities (massive noncompliance makes the risk of noncompliance minimal for any regulatee); the degree to which they are well-organized for effective collective participation in the regulatory, legal, and political processes; and the relative costs of influencing the outcome and either complying with the rules or failing to do so.

Customers of regulated entities may be organized for collective action, in which case one strategy is to confront regulated interests directly in the regulatory process and subsequent legal and political appeals. More likely, at most a few customer groups will be organized, in which case the principal strategy for influencing policy must be issue voting in elections.

The regulatory environment can vary in several important ways. Authority can be more or less fragmented among different agencies, giving regulators more or less ability to control the performance of the regulated sector. The technical basis of regulation—that is, the knowledge of cause-and-effect relations pertaining to the problems that first gave rise to regulation—may be more or less perfectly known, which affects the confidence regulators have in the consequences of their actions, the costs of achieving a given degree of perfection in policy decisions, and the extent to which, with limited budgets, regulators must rely on outsiders for information in making policies. The number of actors in the regulated sector can be more or less numerous and heterogeneous, with greater numbers and heterogeneity raising the costs of monitoring and enforcing a regulatory rule, and with greater homogeneity making it easier for any group to organize for effective collective action to influence policy.

In examining the various forms of regulation that have been applied to health care, Feldman/Roberts discover that the nature of the health care sector and of the problems regulators are mandated to solve are not compatible with effective regulation.

Politicians play especially weak roles in overseeing aspects of health care policy that deal with cost containment because it is not a very salient political issue. Third-party reimbursement dilutes the impact of rising medical expenditures so that consumers do not cast votes on the basis of cost containment policies. Regulation of medical care is fragmented among numerous federal, state, and local authorities, none of which is clearly responsible for the overall performance of the sector. Moreover, health care is provided by a very large number of independent actors who are also well-organized in homogeneous professional organizations. The latter maximizes their political threat to regulators, and the former maximizes the cost of enforcement of regulatory rules. In addition, regulators face considerable uncertainty with regard to pertinent technical issues.

Medical science is complex and imperfect, as is knowledge about the likely response of institutions who provide service to changes in their economic and organizational environment. Consequently, effective regulation requires substantial technical input and inevitably leads to imprecise decisions. Thus, for these and other reasons, regulation is likely to be expensive, ineffective, and especially sensitive to the interests of regulated groups in the health care sector unless its purpose is limited to a few issues with great, general political salience or to achieving objectives that impose relatively minor compliance costs on regulated entities.

Feldman/Roberts affirm this conclusion by summarizing recent research on the effects of various types of medical care regulation. Most of this research concludes that regulation has had only a marginal effect on the quality and costs of medical care.

Feldman/Roberts rightly conclude that the appropriate inference to be drawn from their largely pessimistic analysis of the prospects for effective regulation is not necessarily that society ought to abandon its objectives in health care policy, nor even that it should abandon rather extensive reliance on regulation. The appropriate conclusions are: (1) Regulation can be done more or less well, depending upon how it is set up; (2) the appropriate frame of reference for judging whether regulation should be used is a comparison of an imperfect, unregulated world with an imperfect, regulated one; and (3) the efficacy of regulatory interventions is sufficiently predictable that such a comparative evaluation before the fact is feasible.

THE FELDMAN/ROBERTS POSITION: RIGHT OR WRONG?

Feldman/Roberts have played a dangerous game by trying to write a scholarly discussion in sufficiently general language that it can be understood by virtually any intelligent person. The advantage of their approach is obvious: The way to affect policy is to communicate with those who make it. The danger is that elements of the analysis that have sound analytical or empirical foundations will be mistakenly regarded as ex cathedra pronouncements, having no more weight than personal opinions.

For the most part, the arguments in the Feldman/Roberts paper are syntheses or natural, logical extensions of the results of solid theoretical and empirical examinations of various public decision-making processes.[1] The essential part of the Feldman/Roberts model of regulation is their description of the interactions among regulators, regulated entities, and the general public that presumably is intended to be the beneficiary of regulation.

Two observations by Feldman/Roberts are consistent with all scholarly research on regulation in the past two decades: (1) Regulation systematically tends to redound to the benefit of groups that are well-represented in the regulatory process, and (2) regulators generally have too few resources to find good solutions to technically difficult public policy problems and to force compliance with extensive and complicated regulations.

These two observations are related. The tendency of regulators to be less than vigorous in constraining the behavior of regulated entities reflects the need for regulators, in the face of inadequate resources, to rely on regulated entities for information and to adopt largely consensual rules that keep enforcement requirements within the agency's limits.

On somewhat less secure footing are the arguments by Feldman/ Roberts pertaining to the effects of regulated entities. Theoretically, their argument is sound, in that it is a logical extension of received doctrine in the area of applied game theory that deals with mechanisms for making collective decisions. Empirically, however, very little work has been done to confirm the theory. Most of the evidence is anecdotal. Nevertheless, in the words of a leading political scientist, Raymond Wolfinger, the plural of anecdote is data, and the data seem to be consistent with the theory.

The least secure component of the Feldman/Roberts argument is their characterization of the strategies of legislators with respect to regulatory policy. Their model here seems to combine issue voting in competitive elections with symbolic politics in creating institutions for carrying out public policy. Both points of view are controversial, and each is one among several competitors for explaining the behavior of congressmen.

The Incumbent Advantage

Until relatively recently, the dominant theory about voting decisions was that traditional party loyalties explained voting, that the pattern of these loyalties in the population was stable and could be explained by a host of socioeconomic variables, and that what actually was said in an election or was done by incumbents had little effect on election out-

comes. The key empirical results of the 1960s and 1970s that have
eroded confidence in this theory are the simultaneous declines in party loyalty and the competitiveness of congressional elections. Moreover, since the late 1950s, if survey data are to be believed (a big if), the degree of satisfaction of the electorate with the performance of representatives has also declined.

If voters are paying more attention to issues, giving less attention to traditional loyalties, and feeling less satisfied with public policy, the unanswered question is why are they also reelecting virtually all representatives who stand for reelection? Several explanations of these phenomena have been advanced and found wanting for lack of empirical support.[2]

One is the idea that gerrymandering followed the Supreme Court requirement that districts have approximately equal populations. Another is the proposition that incumbents, by their greater access to free communications channels to constituents, capture important advantages in terms of name-recognition and salesmanship. Still another is that incumbents have an easier time raising money for campaigns. Unfortunately, none of these or other factors thus-far measured explains the rising incumbency advantage.

After taking account of the influences on voting that have been advanced, incumbents still get about 5 percent more of the vote than can be explained—an amount that is sufficient to convert their reelection possibilities from slightly better than a toss-up to a virtual certainty.

The Ombudsman Theory

One explanation for the rising incumbency advantage has received some weak empirical confirmation, and has important implications for the prosecution of regulatory policy. It is that contemporary representatives are not elected as makers of policy (and hence on the basis of issue positions), but as ombudsmen and sources of favors. The argument runs as follows.[3] A single representative is unlikely to have much effect on public policy. A representative is only 1 of 535 relevant votes on legislation, and in any event the President, by virtue of the national mandate behind the office and the natural role of the Chief Executive, is more influential in shaping policy than is the legislature. But a single legislator can be effective in providing favors to constituents: He or she is a source of information about where to approach the bureaucracy to receive the benefits of a particular program, a person who might be able to speed up a grant application or a social security check with a few well-placed phone calls, and a provider of specific program favors to constituents seeking a "fair share" of a program or perhaps "fair treatment" by a regulator.

The weak confirmation thus far available for this view of Congress is explained in three ways. First, the theory does a good job of explaining "pork barrel" programs—that is, programs that have widespread legislative support; that distribute funds on the basis of specific project grants, each of which is approved separately by Congress; and that provide negative net economic benefits. Second, while the incumbency advantage has risen, the allocation of congressional staff between policy-related work and constituency service has shifted dramatically toward the latter; meanwhile, agencies have responded to growth in inquiries from Congress by establishing legislative liaison offices for dealing systematically with requests from the Hill. Third, one in-depth study of two congressional districts that traced their competitiveness through the 1960s and 1970s found that county chairpersons of both parties attributed the decline of competition to the election of representatives who downplayed their policy positions and emphasized their ombudsman activities.

The importance of the preceding argument to the Feldman/Roberts study is that it established a congressional connection to the tendency of agencies to work for compromises with the well-organized groups that are affected by their policies. First, these groups are as able to request help from their representatives as they are to participate in the regulatory process. Second, if agencies are provided with too few resources to regulate effectively, perhaps it is because their congressional overseers want to encourage consensual regulation and the dependence of regulators on outsiders for information and assistance in assuring compliance.

What this specifically means with respect to health care is that Congress would be expected to make regulators dependent on medical professionals for providing the information on which regulations are based and for bearing some of the load of enforcement, either through private enforcement mechanisms or through voluntary compliance (presumably because requirements are not onerous enough to fight).

By Any Theory, A Tough Problem

Of course, the general conclusions of Feldman/Roberts do not depend upon the validity of either view of Congress—their own or the ombudsman theory. For whatever political and institutional reasons, their observations about how the regulatory process works and the kinds of outcomes it produces are, as remarked *supra*, sound.

Perhaps all that is required to drive home the validity of their dire prediction about the problems of regulation in the health care sector is simply to state concisely the problem of regulators in this area. The benefit of tight regulation is to lower cost of care. Arrayed against the regulator's attempt to impose tight regulation are providers of care who see costs as income and who warn of the possibility that tighter controls may kill people by denying them possibly efficacious treatment.

Moreover, patients tend to like their doctors; indeed confidence in a doctor has therapeutic value. Insulated from the financial consequences of personal medical care by third-party payment and tax rules, these patients are not likely to apply political pressure to reduce the care they

receive. In this milieu, and faced with uncertainty about the efficacy of
alternative treatment strategies, regulators cannot reasonably be expected to accept the subjective risk of a medical disaster to achieve cost
containment objectives.

POLICY CONCLUSIONS: A CRITIQUE

Feldman/Roberts state in their conclusion that regulation can be made
to work better or worse, but they do not provide a concrete, detailed
development of this theme for the case of health policy. In order to
provide greater detail in policy conclusions, more concreteness must
be added at certain points in the development of their argument.

First, a better definition is needed of the policy alternatives that are
available for changing the performance of the medical care sector. Perhaps Feldman and Roberts too readily dismiss the seemingly "sterile"
and "academic" exercise of careful definition, for their characterization
of regulation—any attempt to change the behavior of some sector of the
economy—is too broad. Their discussion of regulatory environments,
procedures, and strategies really applies only to a class of policy instruments that is far narrower, e.g., in no significant procedural way are tax
incentives or National Science Foundation grants equivalent to regulation. This vagueness thereby suggests the unwarranted conclusion that
if regulation is found too ineffective the only recourse is to abandon the
attempt to make things work better.

Second, as Feldman/Roberts argue, the details of an acceptably effective policy instrument can not be specified unless the nature of the
problem that the policy is intended to solve is also described in detail.
Feldman/Roberts leave as an exercise for the interested student the task
of making explicit exactly what are the most important things to change
about the American medical care system, and why these particular
problems have arisen in the first place.

Suppose that the problem is as stated at the outset of these comments: Medical care expenditures are rising rapidly whereas the health
status of the population does not appear to be improving commensu-
rately. What explanations could lie at the root of this problem?

First, maybe Americans receive care of substantially lower quality
than could be provided at the same total cost. If so, the problem is that a
substantial number of providers are either poorly informed or charlatans. This happens to be one problem that regulation can probably deal
with fairly effectively. As long as most medical professionals are not
charlatans, the medical profession has an interest in helping to solve the
problem, particularly if government will pay part of the cost of educating the uninformed and ferreting out the frauds. Just as most police
departments do not try to protect criminals, and the Food and Drug
Administration acts swiftly to take soup off the market if it causes
botulism, so, too, can regulators deal with equivalent problems in the
medical care sector.

Second, maybe the nature of the health problems that are prevalent in the population is such that gains in health status can be accomplished only at very high cost. If so, society really has no choice but to continue footing the bill or to rethink whether it really wants to spend so much money on obtaining small gains in health status.

Third, maybe society has created institutions for providing and financing care that generate powerful, perverse incentives that favor expensive treatment of extremely—even hopelessly—ill patients in comparison to treating more mundane but curable illness; to providing better preventative and early diagnostic care; and to dealing directly with important potential causes of illness, such as environmental chemicals, smoking, and occupational hazards. If so, regulation is at best a palliative. It is unlikely to be very effective because it is working against more powerful institutions that push the system in the opposite direction from that which the regulators would like to move. Effective policy in this instance requires changing the institutions that create perverse incentives. Obviously, one such change is to promote plans for financing and providing care that do not involve third-party, fee-for-service payment.

If the last is the case, regulation still has a role. If open panel health insurance that covers virtually all major medical expenditures can somehow be subjected to real competition from plans that have incentives for more efficiency, regulators can be free to focus on those areas they can do better than controlling costs and specifying acceptable treatment strategies. Examples are nondiscriminatory enrollment policies; information requirements in standard formats for insurors and providers; minimum-service requirements for plans receiving federal financial assistance; and standards of financial soundness, perhaps coupled with government coinsurance in case of financial failure.[4]

Regulatory responsibilities such as these can be relatively effectively carried out because they do not attempt major, unnatural changes in the behavior of most members of the groups being regulated. Consequently, these regulatory policies are not likely to be challenged seriously, and regulated entities are likely to be relatively cooperative in helping the regulators do their job. Even if a particular regulated entity dislikes a policy, as long as the policy has general acceptance, the incentive will be to go along. Sympathetic political ears will be hard to find, professional organizations will not be supportive (and may even help catch cheaters should they fail to comply), and in any case compliance will not cost much.

By the same token, the generosity and fairness of health care policy bears no direct relation to the choice of the policy instruments that are used to achieve policy objectives. The government can pay for as much of the bill for any group as it would like, relying on the rules for payment to a provider to assure that care be available to particular target groups. Of course, very generous support for medical expenditures blunts the incentive of the patient to consider costs in deciding whether to undergo a particular treatment. The advantage of HMOs is that they permit generosity, but preserve an incentive to consider cost in the decisions of the physician. The physician is in the best position to have the information necessary for making difficult trade-offs between costs and potential gains from treatment, by virtue of a knowledge of the personal needs of the patient, the patient's health status, and the technical options available. Consequently, HMOs that operate in a competitive environment, combined with informational requirements, peer review, financial regulations, and the like, can be both generous and efficient.

NOTES

1. For a survey of this literature, see P. Joskow and R. G. Noll, *Regulation in Theory and Practice: An Overview*, Social Science Working Paper, No. 213 (Calif. Inst. of Technology, 1978).

2. J. A. Ferejohn, "On the Decline of Competition in Congressional Elections," *American Political Science Review* (Mar. 1977).

3. M. P. Fiorina and R. G. Noll, "Voters, Legislators and Bureaucrats: Choice of Technology in the Public Sector," *American Economic Review* (May 1978).

4. See more generally, A. Enthoven and R. G. Noll, *Regulatory and Nonregulatory Strategies for Controlling Health Care Costs*, Social Science Working Paper, No. 185 (Calif. Inst. of Technology, 1978).

EDITOR'S NOTE

At intervals during the conference, overview papers were delivered by Professor John Dunlop and by the Honorable J. Skelly Wright, United States Court of Appeals, District of Columbia Circuit.

In view of the ideas advanced by Feldman/Roberts, Dunlop and Wright's papers are included here. Professor Dunlop reinforces the idea of consensus building in order to achieve effective regulation whilst Judge Wright deals with the need to observe due process and fairness in developing any regulatory position that will eventually be officially promulgated.

THE ROLE OF CONSENSUS IN REGULATION WRITING

John T. Dunlop, *Lamont University Professor, Harvard University*

Regulation should be viewed in the broad context of the whole regulatory process. Regulations arise in different settings. First, whenever government gives money away or subsidizes a program, regulations necessarily follow. Second, regulation is pervasive in that new systems of regulation are placed on top of old systems, as in the case of agriculture and inflation controls (which may account for conflicting incentives). Third, regulation in health care is intertwined with a variety of other social, political, and economic problems. OSHA, welfare, and inflation control policies, for example, all have impacts on the health care system. Fourth, economic regulation of price rates and entry is the earliest form of regulative activity of governmental agencies.

There is a need for the formation of a policy group on health to bring together persons from different policy fields and disciplines to deal with the problems of health care regulation is an integrated manner. The problems which deserve the most attention are: (1) cost-constraints, (2) delivery and financing systems of care, (3) the regulatory process, (4) the distribution of care, (5) the minimum standards of care, and (6) the organizational management of health care institutions.

The only way to escape the present state of defensive regulation writing and overlitigiousness is to work to develop a concensus on health issues before regulatory decisions on these issues are made. Regulations that cannot be promulgated and updated in a fast, efficient manner without undue politicization, cause problems. *First,* the necessary coordination between business and government does not take place. *Second,* academics are not remaining neutral (to criticize and evaluate alternative forms of regulating health care problems); instead they are taking sides, as paid expert witnesses during the drawn-out litigation and hearings which precede the final promulgation of regulations. *Third,* regulations which become obsolete—as they quickly do in a rapidly developing field like health care—cannot be replaced, but

143

instead are counteracted by new layers of regulation. *Fourth,* regulation easily becomes overpoliticized, thereby discouraging the study of worthwhile subjects of regulation because the potential to influence decisions on how to regulate appears limited.

Thus, consensus on regulations improves the chances of compliance by regulatees and of active encouragement of programs by regulators. In addition, negotiating a policy consensus prevents having to deal with issues in a crisis, when they are so easily dealt with inappropriately in attempts to meet political pressures. And, in spite of the need to think broadly about regulation before a crisis occurs, we must realize that Congress rarely appropriates the necessary money or provides required staff for a successful regulatory program. Congress needs input and study from outside of government to be able to take any long-range view on health care regulation.

NEGOTIATIONS AND EX PARTE
CONTRACTS IN REGULATION WRITING

Judge J. Skelly Wright, *United States Court of Appeals, District of Columbia*

The issue of federal judicial review of rulemaking often involves questions of due process associated with public participation and adequate notice. Such notice in the form of a public comment period assures public dialogue through hearings and the entry into the public record of studies, data, and comment which affect the regulation in its final form. The record is crucial to the due process requirements of a reasoned and substantiated decision by the agency. In the *Overton Park* case, the Supreme Court required lower courts "to make a searching review of the public record," to assure that the agency or department did not act arbitrarily or capriciously in promulgating a regulation. A regulation which fails to meet this standard obligates a court to overturn the regulation or remand the issue to the agency for further clarification or specification.

The question was raised whether this decision meant that informal negotiations, undisclosed to all the parties and to the public, which take place after the issuance of a notice of proposed rulemaking in the informal rulemaking process under Title 5, U.S. Code, Section 553, may be seen by the courts as unwarranted *ex parte* contacts violative of due process. Because such negotiations take place "off the record," they preclude comment by nonparticipating interested parties on them and judicial review of them, yet they may affect the substance of the regulation issued at the end of the rulemaking.

It was asked how can agency personnel, trying to formulate rules in highly complex and technologically dependent areas, develop enough information to generate sound regulation if they are not allowed to consult widely and informally at initial stages of the process with experienced persons who are knowledgeable in the field?

The response given was that putative rulemakers should educate themselves before publishing the notice of rulemaking and place in the public rulemaking file the information obtained, and its source, while

145

being educated so that interested persons not consulted during their education can comment during rulemaking on the information, and the reviewing court can consider the information as well as the comment thereon in determining the legality of the regulation.

CHAPTER THREE

A Structured Framework for Policy Intervention to Improve Health Resource Allocation

EDITOR'S NOTE

There is little published work which indicates that health regulatory agencies or legislative bodies concerned with health care issues truly consider all alternatives open to them. Yet to do so without a framework to identify *relevant* dimensions of choice in the design and implementation of government intervention in health is a task of considerable magnitude. One normally would have to start de novo each time an issue was considered. While Chapter 5 *infra* by Breyer sets forth a generalized "road map" or framework with which to analyze regulatory options, the diversity of health care and the many agencies involved at federal, state, and local levels seem to require that a specialized framework be built for the health care system.

Fortuitously, a working group at Harvard's School of Public Health has undertaken such an effort, the result of which is this chapter by Professors Milton Weinstein and Herbert Sherman. Weinstein and Sherman set forth an analytic structure useful in examining key variables in designing and operating regulatory schemes. A typology or framework should highlight potential consequences for program implementation and effectiveness resulting from choices made along different dimensions (selecting different variables). Here are some examples:

- For a given policy objective, there may be several alternative stages in the "production" of health care which are suitable targets for intervention (e.g., manpower legislation affecting supply of labor, CON regulations affecting capital, state regulation of nursing home eligibility affecting entry into the process, and state court malpractice rules affecting the substance of practice and the permissible outcomes of treatment).

- There may be important options in deciding what level of government should wield regulatory authority at each stage of the process (if the regulator is indeed a public entity rather than, for example, an insurance company).

- There may be choices available in dividing the role of regulators among the three branches of government.

The usefulness of the Weinstein/Sherman framework in pressing consideration of the role of all three branches of government is particularly helpful in view of what some believe to be an increasing reliance on the courts to resolve regulatory issues. Many features may be at work in this trend. Laws or regulations may be vague or inconsistent. Agency or legislative procedures and records may be deficient. Or there may simply be more litigation due to broadening conceptions of due process or heightened political sensibilities and power. The analysis helps focus on the issues of appropriate roles for the three branches, and emphasizes how program design and implementation choices will affect those roles. In particular, this suggests that legislation and regulations must be drawn in the future with concern for the proper scope of judicial review as well as citizen input.

It should be pointed out that the Weinstein/Sherman study is essentially descriptive rather than substantive or normative. It attempts to remind us of available options, but leaves to others the analysis of the effects of alternative choices, or determination of which choices are better in what environment. In short, the analysis does not attempt to explain how the world actually behaves, only to get one to consider what must be done.

THE FRAMEWORK[1]

Milton C. Weinstein, *Associate Professor, Kennedy School of Government; member, Center for Analysis of Health Practices, Harvard School of Public Health*
Herbert Sherman, *Associate Director for Technology, Center for the Analysis of Health Practices, Harvard School of Public Health*

CURRENT TRENDS IN HEALTH REGULATION

Government intervention in the health care sector has increased dramatically in the past decade. Broadly speaking, most of this intervention has been directed toward the goal of improving the production and allocation of health care resources by improving access to health care, by improving the quality of care, and by controlling the costs of care. In a sense, we as a nation are still experimenting with the use of a variety of interventions—usually described by laws and regulations—to accomplish these objectives. Each intervention that has been applied has been fashioned out of a complex process: Its general nature defined broadly by a piece of legislation, its precise form specified by administrative agencies that draft and implement regulations, and its use reviewed by the courts to be sure that its implementation is consistent with such legal principles as due process.

We learn from experience that the chosen interventions often have consequences that are quite different from what might have been anticipated. Moreover, new and creative policy options are needed where traditional forms of regulation have failed. The need to design future interventions in the health care sector both creatively and carefully is clear, and this process of policy design and evaluation must begin with a structured set of options. Toward that end we offer a working framework, or classification scheme, for policy interventions to improve health resource utilization.

Rationales for Health Regulation

The tradition of medicine in this country as a private, "sacred" profession and the political culture of our free-enterprise system both have tended to reinforce a general preference for a limited governmental role

149

in health care. Over the years, however, public concern that the unconstrained health care sector was inadequately responding to certain basic societal interests has led to increasing governmental intervention. Historically, the goals of such intervention have been, broadly speaking, to ensure the quality of health care, to control the prices and costs of health services, and to provide increased access to health care.

Government intervention to achieve these goals can be justified by the failure of the private health care system to achieve them. For example, the Food and Drug Administration was given responsibility for assuring the safety of drugs because of the perceived failure of the industry to do so. Federal and state governments have taken on the responsibility for underwriting the costs of health care for segments of the population for whom economic barriers inhibit access to adequate health care (the aged, the poor) and for others to whom society feels indebted (the disabled veteran).

Generally, these justifications for governmental involvement exemplify the need for intervention to achieve the goals of efficiency and equity when the private market cannot. Efficiency, or allocation of available resources in a way that achieves the greatest benefit, is a basis for intervention when a competitive market with fully informed consumers and producers does not exist. In health care, such market failures provide a rationale for regulating drugs, accrediting hospitals, and controlling hospital prices. Equity, or the concern for a socially acceptable distribution of benefits, cannot be guaranteed by even the most perfect of economic markets because of differences in the economic means of members of society. Hence, we have government intervention to guarantee access to health care, for example, by paying the costs of health care for the disadvantaged under Medicaid and for the aged under Medicare.

Market failure and concerns for social justice have not been the only reasons for government intervention in health care. Sometimes intervention is needed to compensate for the unanticipated consequences of a previous regulatory action. For example, the move toward regulation to control escalating health care costs in the 1970s can be traced directly to the increase in third-party coverage for medical care, including the emergence of the federal government as the nation's leading third-party payer.

Traditional Regulatory Tools and Their Shortcomings

Whatever the rationales and reasons, regulation in health care appears to be here to stay. That is, as long as we are concerned with efficiency and equity in health care, intervention from outside the unrestricted medical care delivery system will be necessary. This does not mean, however, that intervention must always take the form of centralized, command-and-control regulation. Other alternatives, including education and information mechanisms, economic and other incentives, and administrative measures, need to be explored more carefully and tested.

In health care, we see many examples of the traditional regulatory approach. Hospital rate-setting, licensure of hospitals and nursing homes, and certification-of-need for new capital investments are examples, respectively, of three major types of traditional regulatory tools: economic controls, standard setting, and allocation mechanisms. The most common response of the federal government as regulator, when an objective is articulated by Congress, the Executive Branch, or the courts, has been to choose a command-and-control type of intervention. Concerns for the need for health planning and for limits on the proliferation of facilities and equipment have led to the Certificate-of-Need (CON) program. Concern for quality of care under federal reimbursement programs has led to utilization review. Even federal funding for Health Maintenance Organizations (HMOs), one of the prime non-regulatory approaches to cost containment, has been linked to an involved and cumbersome set of regulations governing the operation of such organizations, including specification of what medical services must be offered and what measures must be taken to ensure the quality of care. (See Chapter 1.)

The answer to the question of why the government almost always chooses a command-and-control type of intervention is complicated. Perhaps, the sheer force of habit is partly responsible. The government has lots of experience with traditional regulation and not much experience with alternative interventions; despite the lackluster record of performance with the old methods, a risk-avoiding government may be reluctant to try new approaches. Another possible explanation might be the single-minded drive of legislators and bureaucrats toward policy objectives; sometimes, it seems most straightforward to prescribe in detail the desired behaviors to achieve a social objective rather than to try more subtle approaches. And yet, this type of approach invariably leads to the discovery of loopholes by the regulated parties, followed by more and more regulations in an attempt to bring their behavior back under control. Often it appears easier in the short run to try to salvage the failing regulatory apparatus than to try to restructure the interventions.

The Need for New Interventions in Health Care

Whatever the explanation for government actions in the past, it is clear that creative approaches are needed in confronting the major task that lies ahead in health care: ensuring the cost-effective and equitable allocation of health care resources. Clearly, neither the government nor a quasigovernmental body can (or should) prescribe in detail what medical procedures, devices, and facilities are appropriate to which patients under what circumstances. And yet, further intervention is going to be needed. The challenge is to discover new and creative approaches to steering the course of our health care system into socially desirable directions.

A few examples of creative approaches can be found in the United States and abroad. Reimbursement for second medical opinions is one way to try to eliminate unnecessary operations; some states have considered making second opinions for surgery mandatory for reimbursement under Medicaid. Under the health plan of the United Mine Workers prior to the most recent contract settlement, the district manager was required to approve all tonsillectomies, thus providing some impedance to the use of this generally overutilized procedure. In Vermont and Saskatchewan, the feedback of data on physicians' frequency of use of various common procedures led to dramatic changes in behavior, with many of the high-utilization doctors reducing their use of the procedure in question.[2] In the United Kingdom, the waiting time for elective surgery is a policy variable that exerts substantial influence. More generally, placing limits on the availability of reimbursement, as in Canada and the United Kingdom or on real as opposed to budgetary inputs to health care, as in Sweden, are effective ways of forcing explicit consideration of priorities in medical resource allocation. The British system is further augmented by a professional process of reaching consensus on the appropriate use of certain procedures (e.g., breast cancer screening, kidney dialysis, and coronary artery surgery). Prospective reimbursement and various forms of prepaid health care plans are other, less radical ways of restructuring economic incentives; several such approaches are being tested in various parts of this country.

Searching for Regulatory Alternatives: An Example

The examples just given are only illustrative of the range of intervention alternatives that could be conceived. One purpose of this article is to explore systematically the range of options that might exist by first identifying the dimensions, or attributes, of an intervention and then exploring the range of possibilities along each dimension. To illustrate our approach before getting into the formal, structured framework, let us consider CON as a regulatory approach and explore, along a number of dimensions, the range of possible alternatives (cf. Chapter 1).

For now, we consider only six dimensions of an intervention and use these to explore systematically the alternatives to CON. The purpose of this approach, illustrated in Figure 3-1, is to provide an aid in disciplining one's thoughts in thinking through what various combinations of regulatory alternatives might accomplish. In many cases, the very performance of a piece of legislation or agency regulation depends on how skillfully legislators and administrators work their way through the maze of options available.

The first dimension or attribute of CON that we consider is its objective. We presume that cost control is the major objective of concern, although others, such as quality of care, cost-effectiveness, and access to care may be involved.

Second, consider the party being regulated, the *regulatee*. CON is

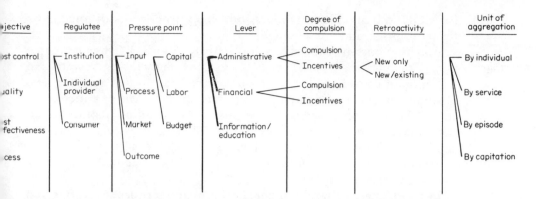

jective	Regulatee	Pressure point		Lever	Degree of compulsion	Retroactivity	Unit of aggregation
st control	Institution	Input	Capital	Administrative	Compulsion / Incentives	New only / New/existing	By individual
ality	Individual provider	Process	Labor	Financial	Compulsion / Incentives		By service
st fectiveness	Consumer	Market	Budget	Information/ education			By episode
cess		Outcome					By capitation

FIGURE 3-1   Regulatory Options (Levers) Available for Use in the CON Process.

directed at health care institutions, although intervention might also be aimed at individual providers or consumers.

Third, the "pressure point" of CON is clearly capital inputs to health care. Labor is not controlled by CON nor are the clinical procedures in which the capital inputs get used nor the mechanism by which services are paid for.

Fourth, we observe that CON is an administrative "lever" not a financial one (e.g., withholding reimbursement for the use of certain facilities), and certainly not an educational nor informational one.

Fifth, we note that CON is fundamentally a command-and-control type of instrument, using compulsion and not incentives. Finally, we note that CON affects only new facilities not existing ones.

With this framework in mind, we can begin to explore alternatives to CON. At least three problems with CON emerge from the very consideration of alternatives: (1) Limits on capital expenditures can lead to the substitution of labor for capital, resulting in diminished cost savings and economic inefficiencies; (2) regulation of proposed expenditures only has no impact on the inappropriate distribution of existing facilities; and (3) by focusing on institutions and not on individual providers, the CON process leaves open the possibility of shifting capital equipment, such as expensive diagnostic instruments, from the hospital to the physician's office, thus escaping control.

The first problem can be addressed by exploring alternatives along the "pressure point" dimension. An expenditure lid on the total budget, rather than restrictions on capital only, can avoid the distortions in the use of labor and capital.

The second problem is more problematic; any gains obtained by limiting new equipment may be lost by failure to address existing overcapitalization. Although closing excess hospital beds is difficult, especially if an expenditure cap is imminent, such a bed reduction might save more money in the long run than would be saved by preventing an institution from purchasing new equipment.

The third problem—evasion of the regulation by transferring equipment to doctors' offices—has been addressed in some states by extending CON to individual providers, but this introduces additional costs for monitoring and enforcement.

Allowing ourselves to explore more freely, Figure 3-1 suggests some more fanciful cost-control alternatives to CON: Franchising hospitals on the basis of cost effectiveness, requiring certification of need for new hospital personnel, and paying physicians on the basis of patient outcomes. Less fancifully, it might be possible to redefine institutions in the market or to replace administrative rulemaking with financial incentives such as taxes or subsidies. After viewing all the options for intervention, the legislator or administrator must remember that doing nothing is also an option.

In short, there certainly appear to be many approaches to hospital cost-control other than controlling new capital expenditures, and some of these are bound to be more effective and to have fewer undesirable consequences. The challenge will be to learn to identify which options are likely to be the most successful at achieving the objective at hand.

RATIONALE FOR A STRUCTURED FRAMEWORK

Our structured framework seeks to define interventions in terms of their essential properties. Each property of interest represents one dimension in the description of an intervention. A well-known example of such a structured framework is a restaurant menu offering a *prix fixe* meal to be selected from among 6 appetizers, 3 soups, 5 entrees, and 4 desserts. There are $6 \times 3 \times 5 \times 4 = 360$ possible meals, but each one can be described in terms of 4 characteristics or dimensions. We offer a "menu" of interventions for health care.

A less frivolous example of such a framework arises in the architectural design of a building. Any building can be described in terms of its materials (exterior and interior), floor plan, energy plant, physical orientation, windows and doors, and several other attributes. An architect takes this array of options and, by selecting a combination of attributes, assembles the design of a building that "works." Through our framework, the component parts of a policy intervention are specified and the various forms each can take are identified.

The purposes of any such framework are modest. It tells us what are the parts that constitute the whole and how they might be combined. It stops short of telling us how the parts combine to work (or fail to work) the way they are supposed to. The "architectural design" of a regulation—based on an understanding of which parts work in what combinations—is a matter beyond the scope of this effort. What we offer is a structured set of options for health regulation. We describe the defining characteristics of a health policy intervention and give names to the important dimensions that determine a particular intervention.

Previous Efforts at Classifying Health Care Regulations

This is by no means the first attempt to impose structure on the spectrum of health regulations and policies. In many fields, including health, the distinction is sometimes made between *economic* and *social* regulation, but this dichotomy surely fails to do justice to the range of goals and policy interventions present in the health field. A somewhat more focused trichotomy for regulations in general is suggested by Breyer in Chapter 5 *infra*. In that chapter, regulations are classified by their broad purpose: price or cost regulation (e.g., rate setting), standard setting (e.g., quality assurance), and allocation of a scarce resource (e.g., CON, licensure to practice medicine). That simple, one-dimensional typology serves well in reviewing the limits of traditional forms of regulation; here, however, we aim to explore more broadly the range of intervention alternatives.

Roemer, focusing on health care specifically, classifies regulations by goal.[3] He categorizes the possible goals of health regulations as: (1) resource production (e.g., licensure, medical education), (2) economic support (e.g., reimbursement under Medicaid and Medicare, direct provision of services under the Veterans Administration), (3) improving access to care (e.g., Hill-Burton, National Health Service Corps), and (4) quality and cost control (e.g., Professional Standards Review Organizations (PSRO), rate-setting). Others, instead of organizing regulatory policies by goal or purpose, organize them by the point of intervention or by regulated party. Bishop, for example, distinguishes regulation directed at hospitals, at insurers, at physicians, and at consumers.[4]

It is our view that these one-dimensional classification schemes (i.e., by goal or by target of regulation) are useful starting points for broad policy discussions, but are not rich enough to develop substantial insights into the diversity of possible approaches to regulation in health care at the level of detail required in actual policy formulation and implementation. Our purpose is to offer a multidimensional framework that encourages focused but creative thinking about regulatory policy options, and which highlights often overlooked distinctions that may have important consequences from the point of view of the legislator conceiving or drafting a bill, or the administrator drawing up or implementing regulations.

The Attributes of an Intervention

Our framework, to be described in more detail *infra*, is intended to describe an intervention in terms of seven groups, or "clusters," of attributes. These are as follows:

1. The context of the intervention What is its objective? Who supported it? Who stands to gain or lose from it?

2. The actors Who is doing the regulating? Who is being regulated? Are they individuals or groups? Is the regulator a public or private entity? Was the regulatory agency established for this purpose, or does it have other missions?

3. The lever Does the intervention seek to change behavior by financial, administrative, social, or educational means? Is the response voluntary, influenced by incentives, or forced?

4. The pressure point Does the intervention apply to inputs to health care (capital, labor, or other), the process of health care, or its outputs? Does it involve a change in institutional or market structure? Is the substance of the regulatee's actions being influenced, or the financial aspects, or other aspects? Does it apply retroactively? Does it apply to each unit of action or to aggregates?

5. The monitoring system What aspect of the regulatee's action is monitored? How often? By what process? How selectively? Which regulatees are monitored, all or just a sample?

6. The performance measures On what basis are the regulators to make decisions? By what criteria will the regulatee's response be judged for purposes of monitoring and enforcement? How will the success of the intervention be evaluated?

7. Basis for actions Under what authority does the regulator act? What assumptions are being made about the way in which the regulatees are expected to respond? What assumptions are being made about their decision-making procedures? How are the regulators expected to implement the intervention?

We expand upon each of these, with examples, in the remainder of this chapter. The categories that are drawn do not constitute an exhaustive set, nor are the boundaries neat. Moreover, many interventions are composites of several elements, each representing a distinct combination of regulator and regulatee, lever, pressure point, and other attributes. Despite these limitations, we submit that this road-map provides a useful guide through the landscape of alternatives, and should make interpolations, extrapolations, and combinations easier to identify.

Aims of the Structured Framework

The framework we present has, in our view, two principal aims. The first purpose is to provide a basis for discussions of the consequences of alternative elements of program design: What specific attributes of a policy intervention are most likely to be associated with (a) successful implementation; or (b) accomplishment of intended goals?[5] By defining the attributes, their separate and interactive influences can be analyzed. For example, one policy dimension relates to whether the controls are targeted at the inputs, processes, or outcomes of health care. Are there general principles to be learned about the problems of implementation associated with each of these (possibly based on experience with CON, PSRO, and medical malpractice, respectively)? Or, must one perhaps probe more deeply into the framework to gain useful insights? What are the enforcement problems presented by different monitoring systems or by the application of different measures or standards of performance?

As another example, when one considers denial of third-party reimbursement as a policy lever, what general principles about the possibilities of adverse consequences can be advanced? The increased use
of hospital services to substitute for outpatient services which are not
reimbursable under Medicare suggests the general problem of substitution when one considers a setting-by-setting or procedure-by-
procedure approach to reimbursement.

The second major purpose of this framework is to provide a systematic basis for suggesting interesting combinations of attributes that may
otherwise be overlooked; in short, to stimulate open-mindedness and
creativity in the formulation of health regulation and policy. For example, has the policy maker considered the use of incentives rather than
direct control? Or leverage on inputs to the production of health care
rather than process? (CON procedures are an example of input-based
interventions, but what about measures to influence the mix of labor
inputs?) Has one considered the possibility of educational measures
directed at the consumer rather than financial measures directed at the
provider? Or the reimbursement on a more aggregated basis rather than
item-by-item (e.g., episode-based rather than procedure-based)? Or
regulation to correct failures of the existing market (e.g., subsidies to
physicians for practicing in needy areas, coinsurance and deductibles,
consumer education) rather than wholesale abandonment of natural
market incentives? Each dimension of the framework suggests alternatives that should be considered, by way of a checklist, at each stage of
policy formation from the broad formulation of policy in the drafting of
legislation to the fine detail of writing and implementing rules and
regulations.

The framework, describing "who does what to whom, how, when,
and why," is meant to organize one's way of discussing the elements of
a health policy intervention, to suggest questions of system response to
these elements that need to be studied, and to stimulate broad thinking in policy design so, at the least, to generate some new approaches
and some creative modifications of existing ones. The user, or peruser,
of the framework will quickly note that its scope is broader than "regulation" in the restricted sense, in that it includes several distinctly
nonregulatory alternatives. This is consistent with one of our main
arguments: that it is essential at all stages of the policy and rulemaking
process to keep an open mind and avoid the pitfalls of conventional
thinking.

SELECTED DIMENSIONS OF THE FRAMEWORK

Our framework consists of a set of dimensions along which a policy
intervention may be characterized. If there were only two dimensions
(e.g., pressure point and lever), we could represent the framework as a
matrix, as shown in Figure 3-2. For example, CON falls into the cell
corresponding to an administrative mechanism for controlling capital

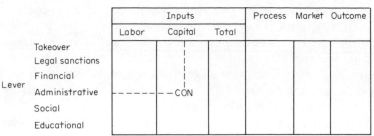

FIGURE 3-2   **Two-Dimensional Cross-Section of the Framework of Interventions.**

inputs. We may think of this two-dimensional display as representing only a cross-section of a much more complex matrix consisting of many more dimensions. Since we cannot visually display such a multidimensional array, we use the terms "matrix" and "cell" as conceptual ways of referring, respectively, to the array of possible combinations of characteristics and to any particular combination of characteristics. Each policy option, if well specified, corresponds to a particular cell in the matrix; conversely, each cell suggests a policy option, although some may be infeasible or, occasionally, nonsensical. There may also be policy options which occupy more than one cell, either because they are actually composites of several regulator-regulatee interactions, or because they involve the simultaneous use of several levers (e.g., carrot-and-stick combinations). More about these composite options later.

We have selected twenty-six dimensions, set out below, which we group into the seven clusters named above. For example, the cluster describing the monitoring mechanism contains seven dimensions.

It is clear that no single classification scheme, especially one of just a few dimensions, can serve all purposes. One might focus on one set of dimensions for exploratory purposes in program design, another for purposes of analyzing implementation, and yet another for purposes of predicting how likely it is that the intervention will achieve its goal. This particular scheme is meant to be suggestive of the important dimensions that seem to be essential to all purposes. Other dimensions can and should be added for specific uses, and some examples of additional dimensions are suggested in Appendix 3-A *infra*. The reader or user can surely think of several more that have been omitted, but which are of particular importance from his or her unique perspective.

The importance of each dimension is illustrated by examples (i.e., existing or proposed policies that differ according to this dimension). An example of the use of the framework to classify an existing regulatory policy follows. Then, we use the framework to explore broadly the range of policy options that might be applied toward the goal of achieving a reduction in the amount of inappropriate surgery.

Cluster 1: The Context

This first group of dimensions describes the motivation behind the proposal for regulation or intervention, which may be an important factor in determining its successful implementation. The exercise of trying to describe the background of a proposed policy measure may be helpful in identifying potential ambiguities and conflicts surrounding its interpretation as well as in predicting who its natural constituency is likely to be.

We cite three dimensions in this group: The purpose (or objective) of the intervention, the source of impetus for the intervention, and the principal beneficiary of the intervention.

Dimension 1-1: Purpose What was the perceived purpose of the intervention?
- a. Cost control
- b. Quality control
- c. Cost-effectiveness
- d. Access or equity
- e. Administrative convenience

This dimension identifies the proximate rationale for the policy, although legislative, administrative, or judicial language on the subject is often ambiguous. For example, rate-setting, price controls, and enforcement against Medicaid fraud are intended primarily for cost control. Nursing home licensing and medical audits are primarily aimed at quality control. New drug or device restrictions are primarily for purposes of assuring efficacy or cost-effectiveness, and Hill-Burton and Medicaid are primarily to ensure access. This dimension parallels the typology of Roemer described *supra*.[6] Its importance lies in assessing the "success" of the intervention in meeting its central goals, and in exploring how the perceived purpose of a regulation may change considerably from its inception to its implementation. An additional motivation for an intervention worth noting is administrative convenience, a major consideration in the proposals for a no-fault malpractice system and for the consolidation of categories of eligibility under Medicaid.

Dimension 1-2: Impetus Who provided the impetus for the intervention?
- a. Consumer
- b. Provider
- c. Labor union (e.g., nurses, allied health personnel, hospital workers)
- d. Delivery institution
- e. Fiscal intermediary
- f. Educational institution
- g. Medical industry
- h. Government (internal impetus)

(1) Executive
(2) Legislative
(3) Judicial

This dimension identifies the locus of initial support for the intervention (compared and contrasted with the identities of the regulatee and regulator [Cluster 2: The Actors]). Within each category may be organized interest groups such as the American Medical Association (providers), the American Hospital Association (institutions), or consumer or employee groups. The role of internal governmental motivation for regulation (e.g., to rectify ambiguities or administrative problems with existing laws and regulations) should not be overlooked. An agency such as the Health Care Financing Administration (including Medicare and Medicaid) falls simultaneously into the categories of fiscal intermediary and government regulatory agency.

Dimension 1-3: Beneficiary Who are the intended beneficiaries of the intervention?
    a. Consumer
    b. Provider
    c. Delivery institution
    d. Fiscal intermediary
    e. Educational institution
    f. Medical industry
    g. Government
        (1) Federal
        (2) State
        (3) Local

This dimension identifies the party or parties who are the intended prime beneficiaries of the policy intervention. This may or may not be the same as the source of impetus identified in Dimension 1-2. Under the rubric of consumers may be special groups such as employee groups, low-income families, or rural families. Among providers may be groups of subspecialists, family practitioners, or nonphysician health personnel. Sometimes the bureaucracy itself is the principal beneficiary, as would be the case with a simplification of administrative procedures. Note that the source of impetus and the actual beneficiaries may, in many instances, differ.

Cluster 2: The Actors (Regulatee and Regulator)

The characterization of the substance of a regulation or other intervention must start with the identification of the principal actors: those who regulate and those who are regulated. In some cases, the relationship is not so straightforward, as is the case when the proximate regulatee is in turn the regulator of the party whose ultimate behavior is of concern. We return to this issue of composite (or "chained") regulations subsequently.

Two dimensions are used to describe the party who is the proximate target of the intervention: Two others describe the actor who affects the target.

Dimension 2-1: Regulatee Whose behavior is being affected?
   a. Consumer of health care
   b. Provider of health care
      (1) In private practice
      (2) In health care delivery institutions
      (3) In occupational setting
   c. Health care delivery institution
   d. Fiscal intermediary
   e. Educational institution
   f. Medical industry
   g. Government (lower level)

This dimension identifies the target party. For example, mandatory deductibles under insurance and health education are aimed at consumers. PSROs and physician fee rate-setting are aimed at providers. Hill-Burton and CON are aimed at delivery institutions. Insurance premium regulation is aimed at fiscal intermediaries. Health manpower laws are aimed at educational institutions. New devices regulation is aimed at industry. Federal cost-sharing under Medicaid is aimed at a lower level of government.

Dimension 2-2: Aggregation of Regulatee What is the level of aggregation of the regulatee?
   a. Individuals
   b. Groups
      (1) Institutional
      (2) Geographical
      (3) Voluntary

This dimension describes the grouping of regulatees for purposes of establishing the intervention. For example, regulation of group health care options is aimed at institutional or voluntary groups of consumers (e.g., labor unions and industrial employee groups); PSRO legislation is aimed at individual providers; and HMO legislation is aimed at voluntary groups of providers. Policies aimed at groups often invite, or require, some kind of collaboration or accommodation among the members of the group (e.g., a CON requirement that at most two hospitals in a region may have a CAT scanner).

Dimension 2-3: Regulator What type of institution is doing the regulating?
   a. Government
      (1) Federal   (x) Executive
      (2) State   (y) Legislative

       (3) Local   (z) Judicial
b. Quasigovernmental body
c. Fiscal intermediary
d. Delivery institution
e. Accrediting group
f. Profession (self-regulation)
g. Laissez faire (no regulation)

This dimension describes the party who is doing the regulating, persuading, or whatever mode of intervention is involved. In any given policy, there may be hierarchies of regulators. For example, the federal government administers the PSRO program, targeted at provider groups which then become professional regulators of their membership.

Within the category of government, the roles of state and local government should not be overlooked. Nor should the ever-increasing role of the judiciary. Indeed, the procedure of judicial review is itself a regulatory policy that carries with it unique implications as to the importance of process in implementing laws and regulations. Note also the roles of fiscal accrediting groups such as the Joint Commission on the Accreditation of Hospitals, and of self-regulation by the medical profession through licensure. Quasigovernmental bodies such as Health System Agencies (HSAs) are assuming an ever-increasing role as planners and, in the broad sense used here, regulators in health care.

Dimension 2-4: Age of Regulator Is the regulating agency:
a. New?
b. Previously existing?

This dimension recognizes that the administrative, legal, and political implications of setting up a new regulatory body or agency must not be overlooked. Can existing machinery be used to implement the intervention?

Cluster 3: The Lever

This cluster of dimensions describes the central attributes of the intervention: What instruments are being used, and with what degree of compulsion are they being applied.

Dimension 3-1: Instrument What is the nature of the instrument being used to affect behavior?
a. Direct takeover
b. Intimidation/legal sanctions
c. Financial
    (1) Fines
    (2) Reimbursement mechanism
    (3) Taxes and subsidies
    (4) Resource ceilings

(5) Alteration of market structure
   d. Administrative
      (1) Explicit
      (2) Implicit
   e. Social
      (1) Peer pressure
      (2) Consumer pressure
      (3) Industry pressure
   f. Information/education

This dimension identifies the instrument that the regulator/intervenor applies to obtain the desired effect. For example, the actual delivery of health services by government (as in the military and Veterans Administration, or state and city hospitals) or production of health manpower and facilities (as by state medical schools or, in times of crises, by control of industrial production) would represent direct takeover. The use of strong Presidential jawboning or stiff penalties for non-compliance represent varying degrees of intimidation and legal sanctions. The use of fines, tax incentives or subsidies (e.g., Hill-Burton), denial of reimbursement, imposed ceilings on hospital revenues, and mandatory deductibles are illustrative of the use of financial levers. HMO laws or a switch to British-style capitation payment would represent financial levers in which the basic market structure is altered. Licensure, permits, second opinion requirements, delayed processing of invoices, and general impediment to action represent explicit administrative levers. Implicit administrative levers include the threat of using other levers in other contexts if the regulatee does not "play the game" (e.g., by shutting down another program at a future date). Reliance upon professional peer pressure under PSROs, consumer pressure on providers to maintain quality, or intraindustry pressure to adhere to the ethics and standards of the hospital or insurance industries represent social levers. Public or professional education campaigns represent attempts to affect behavior by providing information to decision makers.

Dimension 3-2: Compulsion With what degree of compulsion are these instruments being applied?
   a. Strong compulsion or control (e.g., criminal sanctions, direct takeover)
   b. Strong incentives
      (1) Negative (big sticks: e.g., shutdown, severe penalties)
      (2) Positive (big carrots: e.g., large subsidies)
   c. Incentives
      (1) Negative (sticks)
      (2) Positive (carrots)
      (3) Neutral
   d. Voluntary

This dimension describes the extent to which the regulatee is either compelled or merely encouraged to take action. The issue is: How drastically are the payoffs to the regulatee altered as a result of pulling the lever? Strong compulsion or control is usually associated with the use of force, but may refer to criminal sanctions (e.g., for fraud) as well. Strong incentives include large fines for noncompliance with quality standards, and may be viewed as a weaker form of compulsion than the previous category. These may be either positive (irresistible bribes) or negative (intolerable penalties). Incentives may be positive, negative, or neutral: Hill-Burton is a positive incentive program. A policy of restricted (but not denied) reimbursement for inefficacious procedures would be a negative incentive. Prospective reimbursement provides a neutral incentive to control costs in the sense that excess costs must be absorbed but cost saving may become a reward for efficiency. Educational and social levers are usually associated with voluntary changes in behavior on the part of the regulated party.

Cluster 4: The Pressure Point

These dimensions identify the point in the production process where the leverage is exerted and the level of aggregation of the production units with respect to which leverage is applied.

Dimension 4-1: Locus of Pressure Point   Where is the production process?
  a. Inputs to production
     (1) Labor
     (2) Capital
     (3) Operating budget
     (4) Research and development
  b. Process of production
     (1) Entry into process
     (2) During process
  c. Market for services
  d. Outcome of process

This dimension locates the point of leverage as either input, process, market, or outcome. Medical manpower regulations apply to labor inputs, CON requirements to capital inputs, revenue ceilings to budget inputs, and new drug and device regulation to R&D inputs. Preadmission certification in hospitals and nursing homes impacts upon entry into the process, while procedure-specific delimitation and length-of-stay requirements refer to the process itself. Process-directed interventions are usually considered to be the most intrusive into decision making. One such experiment with process-based (b. 2) intervention was recently reported in which the physicians were exposed to an educational intervention in which the lack of difference in complication rates between short and long coronary care unit stay was presented to

them with the additional option of visiting nurse supervision of the
discharged patient.[7] The result was that the average length of stay was
reduced from seventeen to either eleven or seven days. Policies that act
upon the insurance mechanism or the pricing of health services (e.g.,
rate-setting, insurance options such as deductibles and coinsurance) are
examples of leverage on the market, as are antitrust actions or modifications of patent laws to ensure competition in the medical equipment or pharmaceutical industries. Malpractice liability, and possibly
even outcome-based reimbursement (not an outrageous possibility if
the degree of aggregation described by Dimension 4-2 below is broad
enough) represent leverage through outcomes.

Dimension 4-2: Aggregation at Pressure Point How are production
units aggregated for purpose of setting the regulatory policy?
  a. Per individual unit
  b. Per episode (e.g., of illness, of hospitalization)
  c. Per unit of time
      (1) Day
      (2) Year
      (3) Lifetime of a consumer

This dimension describes the degree of aggregation of the units of
production (inputs, processes, or outcomes) for purposes of rulemaking
and rule interpretation. Consider, for example, the use of reimbursement policy. Reimbursement may be linked to each procedure (the
current system); to each episode of illness (the New Jersey Blue Cross
experiment); or to each day, year, or patient's lifetime (the latter being
the capitation approach in the United Kingdom).

Dimension 4-3: Aspect Affected What aspect of the production process is being affected?
  a. Substance
  b. Financial/costs
  c. Other

This dimension describes whether it is the substantive or financial
aspects of the production process at the pressure point that is of prime
concern. Quality audits and financial audits are examples of these two
possibilities, respectively.

Dimension 4-4: Retroactivity
  a. Applies to new procedures, practices, providers, or facilities
     only
  b. Covers existing and new procedures, practices, providers, or
     facilities

This dimension indicates whether the intervention applies retroactively
(e.g., to existing facilities, procedures, physicians, etc.) or only to new

procedures, practices, or providers. CON is an example of the former; utilization review is an example of the latter.

Cluster 5: The Monitoring System

This cluster describes the method used by the regulation to monitor the behavior of the regulatee for purposes of triggering the appropriate levers. Some interventions require no monitoring for purposes of implementation or enforcement (as in educational programs), and this possibility is considered in Dimension 5.1. By consideration of this cluster at the earliest stages of policy design, administrative costs and bureaucratic nightmares may sometimes be foreseen, if not avoided.

Dimension 5-1: Aspect Monitored   What aspect of the regulatee's behavior is monitored?
> a. Substance
> b. Financial
> c. None

Dimension 5-2: Point Monitored   At what point in the production process does monitoring occur?
> a. Inputs
>> (1) Labor
>> (2) Capital
>> (3) Operating budget
>> (4) Research and development
> b. Process
>> (1) Entry into process
>> (2) During process
> c. Market
> d. Outcome
> e. Not applicable

Dimension 5-3: Timing of Monitoring   When does the monitoring occur?
> a. In advance of the regulatee's action (prospective)
> b. At the time of the regulatee's action (concurrent)
> c. After the regulatee's action (retrospective)
> d. Not applicable

Dimension 5-4: Process of Monitoring   What is the process of monitoring?
> a. Inspections
> b. Record review, audits
> c. Invoices
> d. Special reports
> e. Judicial proceedings
> f. Honor system
> g. Not applicable

Dimension 5-5: Selectivity of Monitoring   How selective is the monitoring?
   a. Universal
   b. Sampling
   c. None

Dimension 5-6: Aggregation of Monitored Party   How are the monitored parties aggregated for purposes of monitoring?
   a. Individuals
   b. Groups
      (1) Institutional
      (2) Geographical
      (3) Voluntary
   c. Not applicable

Dimension 5-7: Aggregation of Monitored Item   How are the units of
production aggregated for purposes of monitoring?
   a. Per individual unit
   b. Per episode (e.g., of illness)
   c. Per unit of time
      (1) Day
      (2) Year
      (3) Lifetime of a consumer
   d. Not applicable

It should be noted that the aspect monitored (Dimension 5-1) need not
be the same as the aspect that is the target of regulation (Dimension
4-3); medical invoices may be audited for purposes of quality assurance, for example. Similarly, the monitored point in the production
process (Dimension 5-2) may differ from the ultimate target of the
intervention (Dimension 4-1), as would be the case if purchases of
supplies (inputs) were monitored for purposes of detecting possible
monopolistic practices (market). Under Dimension 5-3, monitoring may
be prospective (e.g., prospective admission certification under utilization review, licensure of physicians); concurrent (e.g., inspections or
peer observation); or retrospective (e.g., tissue committees), and may
be done by sampling or universally (Dimension 5-5). The actual process
of monitoring (Dimension 5-4) may involve inspections, audits, invoices, special reports, or even judicial proceedings and fact-finding
hearings. The aggregation of regulatees (Dimension 5-6) and of production units (Dimension 5-7) for purposes of monitoring need not be
the same as for purposes of administering the regulations. Thus, the
regulation may require that physicians use a particular procedure only
under specified conditions (individual providers, individual processes), but the monitoring may be with respect to records of the aggregate
practices of a group of physicians over the course of a year to identify
likely violators (as is done by some PSROs), rather than with respect to
procedure-by-procedure records review.

Cluster 6: Measures of Performance

This cluster describes the measure of performance by which rules are set and decisions are made, which is monitored for purposes of enforcement or evaluation. Specifically, the measures of performance may be applied to the following three purposes.

Dimension 6-1: Performance/Criteria This purpose concerns rulemaking or establishing criteria for decision making.

Dimension 6-2: Performance/Monitoring This purpose concerns monitoring and enforcement.

Dimension 6-3: Performance/Evaluation This purpose concerns evaluating the effect of the policy.

Within each of these three dimensions, the following kinds of performance measures are possible:

   a. Legality/legitimacy (nonabuse, nonfraud)
   b. Effectiveness/harm
      (1) Mortality only considered
      (2) Mortality and quality of life considered
   c. Cost-effectiveness
      (1) Mortality only considered
      (2) Mortality and quality of life considered
   d. Cost
   e. Quality of service, irrespective of effectiveness
   f. Appropriateness of service, irrespective of effectiveness, cost, or quality
   g. Equity, access, or availability
   h. Other criterion
   i. None necessary

Legality and legitimacy apply, for example, in regulating Medicaid abuses. Effectiveness and harm apply in the regulation of new drugs and devices, and in reimbursement policies linked to efficacy. Cost-effectiveness underlies the HMO approach, and may be linked to reimbursement and planning policies in the future. Cost is the criterion for rate-setting and budgetary ceilings. Quality is the criterion for licensure and in medical malpractice. Appropriateness, as defined here, is exemplified by the decision not to cover cosmetic surgery (or abortion) under Medicaid. The performance measure for purposes of evaluation may be different from that for purposes of decision making or monitoring: For example, outcome-based criteria such as efficacy may not be monitorable in the immediate run, but may be observable in the long run as the policy is being evaluated.

Dimension 6-4: Burden of Proof
  a. Regulatee
  b. Regulator
  c. Independent party
  d. None necessary

This dimension locates the burden of proof in applying the performance measure for enforcement, an important issue in setting regulatory policy. For example, the Federal Drug Administration requires that a new drug be shown to be safe and effective before it is marketed, but if a fiscal intermediary wants to deny reimbursement for an existing medical procedure on the basis of lack of efficacy, the burden may well be upon the regulator. Often, the locus of burden of proof is unclear, and the courts must decide.

Cluster 7: Basis of Actors' Actions

This cluster of two dimensions describes the proximate authority for the regulator's actions, and the behavioral assumptions made about the regulatee's response. The former is an objective assessment of the source of legal authority; the latter is a subjective assessment of the regulatee's anticipated behavior.

Dimension 7-1: Basis of Regulator Action   Under what authority does the regulator regulate?
  a. Constitution
  b. Statute
  c. Executive order
  d. Court order, judicial decisions
  e. Regulation by higher level of government
  f. Consensus of regulatees
  g. No specific authority needed (e.g., free market)

The source of the regulator's authority to regulate has implications for the likelihood of successful implementation and, where relevant, compliance by the regulatee.

Dimension 7-2: Basis of Regulatee Action   What is the basis of the regulatee's response?
  a. Rational optimizing behavior
  b. Satisficing (minimal response necessary)
  c. Antagonism
  d. Confusion
  e. Lethargy
  f. Support/enthusiasm

Many regulations and interventions are designed under the assumption that the regulated parties will respond rationally. In fact, their behavior may be characterized by "satisficing" behavior, or the minimal deviation from present behavior necessary. Other bases for response may include antagonism or animosity—trying to subvert the system, possible confusion about the meaning of the regulations, or even just plain lethargy. Sometimes, the regulatee may even respond with enthusiastic support as, for example, in complying with health measures that are believed to be correct morally or, possibly, out of political allegiance to the regulator. The likelihood of each possible response may depend, in part, on the lever used (Dimension 3-1) and the strength with which it is applied (Dimension 3-2) as well as the identity of the regulatee (Dimension 2-1) and the nature of the monitoring system (Cluster 5). The regulator should pause to assess the basis for response rather than to assume what may appear on the surface to be rational behavior.

To summarize for future reference, the suggested dimensions of the classification scheme are listed in Appendix 3-A *infra*. Additional dimensions are suggested in Appendix 3-B *infra*; the reader or user is encouraged to think of even more.

COMPOSITE INTERVENTIONS

We have pointed out the possibility that a regulatory intervention will overlap more than one category. That is, an intervention may be a composite system made up of a number of components. Two important classes of composite regulatory systems are of special importance: multiple, or "chained" regulators, and combinations of levers and degrees of compulsion.

Multiple regulators In many instances, one regulator regulates another regulator, which regulates either itself or yet another regulatee. Federal-state-local interactions are an example; mandatory peer review, internal quality audits, or certification comprise another class of examples. In addition, there may be different regulators for purposes of planning, rulemaking, monitoring, and enforcement, even though these may all be facets of the same regulatory policy. Thus, the legislature may design the policy, the department head may set the rules, the bureau chief may do the monitoring, and the courts may be involved in the litigation.

Combinations of levers and degrees of compulsion An example of this kind of combined action is a grant program. Matching grants are incentives, but they may have as preconditions strict rules about resource utilization or employment. Hill-Burton is a case in point. Conditions for receiving federal support for an HMO is another. In other words, the regulator offers a carrot, but if the carrot is accepted, sticks are wielded if the regulatee fails to comply with rules on some specified substantive issues such as access or quality assurance.

Another example of this combined use of levers occurs when a regulatee decides voluntarily to be regulated, either by itself or by some

external regulator. The medical profession has done so with respect to
licensure, and now must comply with state laws and federal provisions
governing licensure.

ILLUSTRATIVE USE OF THE FRAMEWORK TO CLASSIFY AN EXISTING POLICY

The usefulness of the framework can best be tested by attempting to classify existing policy measures from this country and elsewhere. We illustrate this use of the framework with respect to the Medicare policy of denying reimbursement for medical procedures generally established to be inefficacious. Although this intervention is rarely applied—because few medical procedures in use are so clearly and universally inefficacious—it does illustrate the use of the framework.

The *purpose* of the policy is primarily to reduce cost and, secondarily, to improve efficacy. The *impetus* came largely from within the agency (then part of the Social Security Administration), although in response to general pressure from Congress for cost control. The *beneficiaries* would be consumers at large (as taxpayers, as patients), and the agency itself.

The *regulatees* are individual providers; the *regulator* is the Health Care Financing Administration, an existing governmental fiscal intermediary.

The *lever* is the reimbursement mechanism; it is used to generate a "big stick" (strong negative incentive), in that a physician will not be reimbursed for procedures on "the list."

The *pressure point* is the process of care, not inputs or outcomes. Procedures are considered on an individual basis, and the provider's practice is affected substantively. Both new and existing procedures may, in principle, be on "the list."

Compliance is *monitored* through the billing or financial system. The process of care in the patient encounter is the point monitored, and monitoring is done retrospectively from invoices. All bills of every Medicare provider are screened for inadmissible procedures.

The *criterion* for triggering the regulator's action is efficacy (of the procedures). At the monitoring stage, however, the criterion is "appropriateness," given the preexistence of "the list;" that is, the judgment of efficacy need not be made each time. The performance of the measure will (or should) be judged in terms of its cost-effectiveness, and not just cost. The burden of proof for determining the efficacy of procedures is on the regulator, with the implicit or explicit concurrence of the medical profession.

The *basis of regulatory action* is statute; the *basis of the provider's response* is assumed to be a combination of financial interest and professional judgment as to what is best for the patient.

We have not attempted here to explore perturbations along any of the dimensions to generate new policy options. The next section, however, demonstrates the use of the framework in a creative mode—to generate policy alternatives aimed at discouraging the use of cost-ineffective, inefficacious, or unnecessary surgery.

AN EXAMPLE OF EXPLORATORY USE OF THE STRUCTURED FRAMEWORK: REGULATING OVERUTILIZATION OF SURGERY

We have claimed that a framework such as this may be especially useful in generating alternatives to standard regulatory approaches: That is, in encouraging open-mindedness in formulating a regulatory intervention. We illustrate this mode of creative use by exploring how variations along several dimensions can suggest a wide range of regulatory options. The example we have chosen is the control of excessive surgery, as typified by the often alleged overuse of such procedures as tonsillectomy. It is not our intent to argue for or against the validity of the claim that such procedures are being done "inappropriately" on a widespread basis. We start with the supposition that the "problem" has been identified, and that a decision has been made to do something about it. (In the following discussion, numbers in parentheses refer to dimensions of the typology as listed in Appendix 3-A *infra*.) What are the options?

One possibility is simply to deny reimbursement for the procedures identified as "unnecessary" on a procedure-by-procedure basis. But what is the criterion to be used to define "unnecessary" (6-1)? Is it proven efficacy, cost-effectiveness, or some unspecified notion of "appropriateness?" And where is the burden of proof (6-4), both at the level of placing a procedure on the list (6-1) and in judging the merits in an individual case (6-2)? Should existing procedures be affected, or only new procedures (4-4)?

Instead of denying reimbursement on a procedure-by-procedure basis, we may want to consider reimbursement by episode of illness (4-2). Thus, the incentive (3-2) to do additional procedures will be diminished. Or, instead of monitoring individual cases, we may prefer to monitor the profiles of a provider's practice over the course of a year (5-7), with reimbursement linked to performance relative to the norm among other providers (another variant of "appropriateness" under 6-2, but at an aggregate level).

Financial levers (3-1) are not the only ones available. Slowed reimbursement is an administrative device that may dissuade the physician from prescribing certain procedures. Second-opinion requirements have been tried in some states under Medicaid, with mixed success. Peer or social pressure may also be generated by the publication of a physician's tendency to do excessive surgery, e.g., five or six times as many tonsillectomies as his peers.

Still more radical departures involve moving the pressure point from process to inputs, markets, or outcomes (4-1). Input-directed interventions may include limits on hospital beds, equipment, operating budgets, or surgical manpower. These rely on incentives (3-2) to allocate the newly constrained resources cost-effectively.

Market-based interventions may involve imposing deductibles or copayments on certain procedures, thereby relying on consumer incentives (2-1, the consumer; 3-2, incentives). Or, possibly, apply positive incentives to the provider or consumer *not* to undergo surgery (i.e., by subsidizing alternative medical therapies). Or, instead of giving the consumer the incentive at the time of medical need, give him or her the choice when it is time to select an insurance policy by offering lower premiums for coverage packages that exclude certain procedures.

Outcome-based interventions can even be conceived, whereby surgeons are reimbursed according to their success in treating a class of illness relative to the norm. If monitoring on an individual basis is impossible, then consider setting reimbursement rates for a procedure on the basis of aggregate outcome data for that procedure. While these outcome-based ideas are perhaps futuristic at best, liability (or denial or reimbursement) for surgical mortality is not.

Further consideration of Dimension 3-2 suggests the use of information to motivate voluntary changes in behavior by both the provider and by the consumer. Feedback to physicians of their profiles of practice relative to others in the community may inspire desirable practices, even without social or peer pressure. Consumer knowledge that tonsillectomies are usually unnecessary may, at least, result in more careful probing of the physician's reasons for the recommendation. Thus, we may want to focus on the consumer and not on the provider (2-1).

The list of possible variations in these and other policy options could go on and on, simply by varying one or two dimensions at a time. While some of the options generated by this fishing expedition may seem infeasible, others are not, and still others are descriptive of existing policies such as PSRO and CON. The point is that before designing or implementing a new regulatory policy, it is often advisable not to do anything standard until having at least considered a few nonstandard variations, either in the monitoring system, the degree of compulsion used, the pooling of regulatees for purposes of monitoring, or whatever the exploration of the dimensions of policy space suggests.

CONCLUDING OBSERVATIONS

Since this effort is no more than a structural framework within which to conduct discussions about regulatory alternatives in the health area, there are really very few substantive conclusions to offer. One, which is really less of a conclusion than a hypothesis to be tested, is that a systematic framework of this kind can in fact be helpful in stimulating creative thinking, and also in separating out the elements of a regulatory policy that are either conducive or antagonistic to successful implementation and achievement of program goals. The latter, the study of the "architectural design" of health policy interventions, is the subject of later chapters of this book (see Chapters Four, Five and Six *infra*).

A second observation is that while this framework was developed with health care in mind, some aspects of it may generalize to other fields. Environmental regulation, for example, involves issues of levers (taxes versus fines versus shutdown versus public relations), pressure point (inputs versus process versus outputs), monitoring systems, and criteria. The development of a similar classification scheme for other areas of regulation and, ultimately, a generalized framework, would be a worthwhile enterprise.

Next, we offer an insight obtained upon consideration of our seventh cluster of attributes, particularly the anticipated response of the regulatee. Perhaps not so many well-meant policies would go awry if the regulator thought out the consequences of different modes of response by the regulatee. At the least, regulators should consider what sort of response they, the clever, harassed regulators might conjure up were they the clever, harassed regulatees instead.

Finally, a note of optimism. In some circles it is fashionable to profess despair at the prospects of alleviating the problems in our health care system: spiralling costs, limited access to quality care for the disadvantaged (or, more significantly in some respects, the working poor); proliferation of expensive but only marginally useful technologies; maldistribution of physicians among specialties and regions; and so forth. At least a few health care analysts of our acquaintance (not physicians) have left the health arena in part, at least, because of the sense that "we've tried almost everything, and nothing seems to work." Our optimism stems from the observation that, of all the thousands of possible interventions suggested by the framework, our nation has actually tried hardly any of them at all! Slight modifications of a basically sound idea (increased sanctions, increased incentives, etc.) might dramatically affect its chances of successful implementation. Of course, one can never try all the possibilities (heaven forbid!), but if we try a few more, we may learn which attributes in what combinations work and which do not, which result in unmanageable bureaucratic tangles and which do not. In any case, there is no cause for despair. Government is just beginning to face the challenge of steering the health care system onto a favorable course, and there is no shortage of options available.

NOTES

1. The authors are indebted for valuable suggestions to many participants in the Harvard-HEW Project on Health Regulation, but especially to Graham T. Allison, Christopher F. Edley, Howard S. Frazier, and Richard S. Gordon, as well as to many members of the Harvard Regulatory Reform Seminar and of the Harvard School of Public Health's Seminar on Analysis of Health and Medical Practices.

2. See J. Wennberg, L. Blowers, R. Parker, and A. Gittlesohn, "Changes in Tonsillectomy Rate Associated with Feedback and Review," 59 *Pediatrics* 821–826 (1977). See also F. Dyck et al., "Effect of Surveillance on the Number of Hysterectomies in the Province of Saskatchewan," 296 *The New England Journal of Medicine* 1326–1328 (1977).

3. M. I. Roemer, "The Expanding Scope of Governmental Regulation of Health Care Delivery," 6 *The University of Toledo Law Review* 591–616 (1975).

4. C. E. Bishop, "Public Regulation of Hospitals: Summary of a Conference," Health Care Policy Discussion Paper, No. 4 (Harvard Center for Community Health & Medical Care, 1973).

5. The remaining chapters of this book are directed in large part, at this question.

6. Roemer, n.3 *supra*.

7. J. F. McNeer, J. S. Wagner, C. B. Ginsburg, A. G. Wallace, C. B. McCants, M. J. Conley, and R. A. Rosati, "Hospital Discharge One Week After Acute Myocardial Infarction," 298 *The New England Journal of Medicine* 229–232 (1978).

APPENDIX 3-A: SUMMARY OF THE BASIC DIMENSIONS OF THE TYPOLOGY

1. The Context of the Intervention

    1.1 Purpose
    1.2 Impetus
    1.3 Beneficiary

2. The Actors

    2.1 Regulatee
    2.2 Aggregation of Regulatee
    2.3 Regulator
    2.4 Age of Regulator

3. The Lever

    3.1 Instrument
    3.2 Compulsion

4. The Pressure Point

    4.1 Locus of Pressure Point
    4.2 Aggregation at Pressure Point
    4.3 Aspect Affected
    4.4 Retroactivity

5. The Monitoring System

    5.1 Aspect Monitored
    5.2 Point Monitored
    5.3 Timing of Monitoring
    5.4 Process of Monitoring
    5.5 Selectivity of Monitoring
    5.6 Aggregation of Monitored Party
    5.7 Aggregation of Monitored Item

6. The Performance Measure

APPENDIX 3-B: EXAMPLES OF ADDITIONAL DIMENSIONS FOR THE FRAMEWORK OF INTERVENTION

The following are examples of additional dimensions that might be of interest in certain applications of the framework. Many more are possible.

Dimension A-1: Benefactor

In Cluster 1, parallel to "beneficiary" (who benefits?) as described by Dimension 1-3, one might want to characterize the "benefactor" (who pays?). Is it the providers, a particular specialty of provider, hospitals or nursing homes, a particular region or income group, an industry, or just the government personnel who have to implement the regulation?

Dimension A-2: Age of Monitoring System

In Cluster 5, there might be a dimension similar to Dimension 2-4 (age of regulator), indicating whether the required monitoring system is already in place or must be developed. With PSRO, the system had to be developed; but it may often be possible to piggyback upon an existing capability.

Dimension A-3: Basis for Estimating Performance Measure

In Cluster 6, it might be useful to specify whether the performance measure used (in enforcement, say) has an objective or subjective basis. When the measure is objective, enforcement problems are usually less difficult than when discretion is permitted. The potential involvement of the courts to resolve disputes over subjective measures and criteria must be considered. The sources of measurements may range from mechanistic manipulation of hard data to quantitative analysis involving softer data to professional judgment.

PART TWO

Economic Regulation and Health Care

Regulation as an Instrument of Public Administration

EDITOR'S NOTE

REGULATION AS AN INSTRUMENT OF PUBLIC ADMINISTRATION[1]

Part One of this book outlined some possible interactions between government and health care systems. With cost escalation currently triggering demand for more regulation, one senior HEW official sees the situation this way:[2]

> The delivery of health care in the United States is replete with problems: The cost of health care is high and growing with disturbing rapidity; the character of health care is frequently inappropriate; the supply of some facilities (e.g., hospital beds) and some skills (e.g., nurses) is excessive, but some areas and groups are badly underserved; the third-party fee-for-service reimbursement system lies at the root of many of these problems.

> To make matters worse, the health care industry adjusts slowly to imbalances because it relies heavily on long-lived structures owned and supported substantially through the not-for-profit sector and because the labor force is a product of very lengthy and very costly training.

> All of this amounts to two basic facts: (1) There are serious problems, [and] (2) they cannot be solved quickly, even if institutions and incentives are quickly set aright. In these circumstances, it is fatuous to expect political figures not to regulate. They see the problems and so do their constituents. Market forces are not working to improve the situation, and even if the market forces are corrected—for example by giving HMOs a better chance to compete—they will not solve the problems quickly and may not completely solve them ever. Politicians simply will not ignore a policy instrument that offers some chance, comprehensible by even the unsophisticated, of speeding the solution of problems. The fact that regulation may not work over the long haul will cut little ice.

> Therefore, the task of lawyers and economists is to identify modes of regulation that offer the best chance of helping the situation and create the

fewest long term threats. Their efforts will be far more fruitful if they try to make systems of regulation work better than if they try to convince an unreceptive political and lay audience that regulation should be scrapped.

In this context, it is vital that scholars view systems of regulations rather than individual regulations taken in isolation. Furthermore, regulations are important in large part because of the way they alter other decision making incentives and the context within which a consensus is reached.

This appeal to lawyers and economists to focus on ways to improve the operation of regulation is not motivated by a belief that regulation will suffice. As long as the financial incentives in the health care industry remain as perverse as they are today, regulatory approaches alone are bound to fail. The growth of HMOs, community health centers, and clinics financed on a capitation basis, and other changes offer unlimited promise.

But, even if successful, they will take time to work. In the meantime regulation *will* occur. Political imperatives guarantee it. Can we make it do more good or less harm than it does today:

The key point is that the issue is not "should we alter cost based reimbursement or regulate?" We *should* do the former; we will do the latter.

If the growth of governmental activity and intervention in health care has led to problems, are such problems similar to those observed in other sectors of society subjected to "traditional" regulation? Or has what has emerged led to problems which are new and distinct, unique to health care? How similar are problems encountered in route allocation and licensing for transportation industries, rate-setting for public utilities, and standard setting for occupational health to difficulties and costs associated with analogous activities in health care?

The work contained in Part Two examines two propositions:

1. Improvement in the regulation of health care can be made if one could understand the basis for success and failure of regulation in other areas; and

2. A framework for thinking about regulation in general can be applied to regulation of health care so as to be helpful to those who must draft legislation for and plan and administer regulation of health care over the next decades.

It is only in recent years that a significant proportion of the United States population has become wary of "big" government and of the increasing involvement of government with private citizens and their employers in places of work and recreation. Generic examination of regulation therefore is a relatively new phenomenon, particularly when conducted independently of a specific societal "problem" or agenda. In fact, some of the contributors to this volume are among the leaders in developing a more systematic view of regulation. One of the prime movers in developing an overview of the regulatory process has been Professor John T. Dunlop. A position paper, drafted during his tenure as Secretary of Labor, is widely regarded as a seminal document. Since

it has never been printed in its entirety, it appears in the following
pages in substantially its original form. It represents one of the first
modern analyses of the regulatory "malaise" gripping the United
States.

NOTES

1. This chapter is derived from documents developed preparatory to the conference organized by the Kennedy School of Government, Harvard University, pursuant to Contract No. HRA 230-77-0037 with the Health Resources Administration of HEW and additional support from ADAMHA and the Commonwealth Fund. It incorporates material developed by Lamont University Professor John T. Dunlop of Harvard University for the Visiting Committee of the Kennedy School.

2. From notes developed during conference discussion sessions, *ibid.*, as written by Henry Aaron, then Assistant Secretary for Planning and Evaluation, HEW.

THE LIMITS OF LEGAL COMPULSION[1]

John T. Dunlop, *Lamont University Professor, Harvard University*

In recent years, a rapid expansion of government controls has been associated at the same time with a growing dissatisfaction with the effects of regulation. Scholarly books and journals have offered detailed criticisms of specific regulatory policies, but these analyses have neither slowed the growth of formal regulation nor encouraged the development of alternative approaches to problems.

The issue confronts those involved in public policy generally. The Department of Labor, however, is an unusual vantage point from which to survey different types of regulatory programs and the arguments about their usefulness. The Department emerged from some of the same social, economic, and political concerns which were involved in the development of private collective bargaining as the predominant means of establishing the network of rules which governs behavior in the work place and work environment. As such, its ties to industrial relations are strong. In recent years, however, the Department has been assigned one of the most extensive set of regulatory programs in the federal government. In 1940, the Department administered 18 regulatory programs; by 1960, the number had expanded to 40; in 1975, the number stood at 134. At present the Department has responsibility for promulgating and administering complex regulations under the Occupational Safety and Health Act, the Urban Mass Transportation Act, the Civil Rights Act of 1964, the Equal Pay Act, the Employee Retirement Income Security Act, and many others. All of these regulatory programs establish substantive—and in many cases quantitative—definitions of acceptable conduct for employers, employees, and third parties.

The Department thus provides examples for a broader comparison between essentially private methods for rule making within a broad and general governmental context—exemplified by collective bargaining—and the more intensive approach of governmental promulgation of mandatory regulations.

184

At the onset a distinction also needs to be drawn between economic regulation of prices, rates or fees, and related conditions of entry to a market on the one hand, and social regulation on the other, affecting conditions of work such as discrimination, health and safety, and the like. In the case of economic regulation it may often be appropriate to raise the question of whether the interests of a sector and the public may not better be served by deregulation. In the field of social regulation, while some deregulation may be appropriate, the major areas of review are likely to be concerned with methods of regulation, involvement of those affected, enforcement, compliance approaches, and communication to those affected. Regulation to achieve a public purpose continues, but the central concern is the methods, approaches, and mutual attitudes of the regulators and the regulatees.

PROBLEMS WITH REGULATION

Over the years, regulation has proved to be a practical and effective approach to some social and economic problems. The inspection of meat and poultry is an obvious example and suggests the sort of concerns that prompted the development of regulation in the late eighteenth century. In the words of a foremost student of administrative law, Kenneth Culp Davis, "Practical men were seeking practical answers to immediate problems. . . . What was needed was a governmental authority having power not merely to adjudicate, but to initiate proceedings, to investigate, to prosecute, to issue regulations having force of law, to supervise." From these perceived needs developed the structure of modern regulation, an approach which is now used without significant modification as our principal policy tool for dealing with occupational disease, discrimination, dangerous toys, and pollution.

A major reason for the attraction of regulation over the years has been the belief that it is a speedy, simple, and cheap procedure. Yet it should be apparent that the administrative procedure is by no means fast or inexpensive, but the prevailing belief is that it is. This misconception in large part is due to the fact that the constraints on the rule-making and adjudicating activities of regulatory agencies are not widely perceived or appreciated. Perhaps, too, because the majority of congressmen are lawyers and not business executives, labor leaders, economists, or labor mediators, they are apt to think of social and economic problems in legal terms. For these and other reasons, when a problem acquires national attention—as pollution, inflation, and occupational disease have in recent years—the natural reaction has been to create a new regulatory agency to deal with it. There are a variety of problems with this approach.

The *first* problem with regulation is that it encourages simplistic thinking about complicated issues. To get regulatory legislation passed in pluralistic society often requires the evocation of horror stories and the mobilization of broad political support. To quote Professor James Q.

Wilson: "Political inertia is not easily overcome, and when it is over-come, it is often at the price of exaggerating the virtue of those who are to benefit (a defrauded debtor, a sick industry) or the wickedness of those who are to bear the burden (a smog-belching car, a polluting factory, a grasping creditor)."

Second, designing and administering a regulatory program is an incredibly complicated task. How successfully and efficiently occupational disease or discrimination in hiring practices will be reduced depends not just on the kind of goals set by Congress or a few key decisions by civil servants in Washington, but upon tens of thousands of individual actions taken by business firms and private citizens across the country. Ensuring compliance with a regulation is far more difficult than promulgating it, though that too can be a complicated and lengthy process. There are, for example, 5 million workplaces and 1,200 Occupational Safety and Health Administration (OSHA) inspectors. All affected parties can never be notified of a new rule's existence and thus reasonably be expected to comply—and the means of informing regulatees of new rules (mainly through publication in the *Federal Register*) are severely inadequate.

Third, oftentimes policies that appear straightforward will have unintended consequences which can create problems as severe as those with which the regulations were intended to deal. For example, the Wagner Act meant to encourage the development of unions and collective bargaining, but its concept of "exclusive representation"—where the employees in a unit decide which union, if any, they want to represent them in bargaining with management—contradicted the traditional union principle of "exclusive jurisdiction"—in which all workers in a particular craft or industry are legitimately represented by one union. The Wagner Act had the effect of encouraging competition among unions for members, hence creating disputes among unions, and changing the internal governance of organized labor, an entirely unintended effect. Article 20 of the AFL–CIO constitution was later adopted to provide a method for mitigating these disputes through limited arbitration; competitive elections, rational bargaining structures, and union jurisdiction are not entirely compatible. It is very hard for affected groups to perceive the long-term and often unintended consequences of regulation.

Fourth, the rulemaking and adjudicatory procedures of regulatory agencies tend to be very slow, creating conflicts among the different groups involved, and leading to weak and ineffective remedies for the people the programs aim to help. Early experience demonstrated the need for the regulatory agencies' procedures to include the same sort of safeguards to insure fairness that were present in the judicial and legislative processes. The result eventually was the Administrative Procedure Act of 1946, which established formal procedures for the promulgation of rules and the adjudication of cases. The purpose was to ensure that each party affected by a proposed rule would have an opportunity to present its views, thereby limiting the possibility that regulations or decisions would be arbitrary, unworkable, or unfair.

Common sense recognizes the importance of these procedures, but
while they are designed to make regulation fair, they can also make it rigid. When a regulatory program is imposed immediately upon passage and the administrative agency lacks authority to adjust the law to fit the realities of business practice—as is the case with some requirements of the pension law, the Employment Retirement Income Security Act (ERISA)—the result is often rules based upon abstractions which are fair and effective in some settings and pointless and burdensome in others: In the case of one ERISA provision the Department of Labor received over 220,000 individual requests for exemption, some taking more than 12 months to process. The procedure is lengthy and complicated: If an exemption is proposed, it is then published in the *Federal Register* and comments are solicited; a public hearing can be requested and if as a result the exemption is modified, then the procedure may be repeated. The process is often prolonged by different groups taking advantage of procedure to advance their interests; thus, a legitimate exemption may take months to obtain.

Fifth, the rulemaking and adjudicatory procedures do not include a mechanism for the development of mutual accommodation among the conflicting interests. Opposing interests argue their case to the government and not to each other. Direct discussions and negotiations among opposing points of view where mutual accommodation is mutually desirable—as in collective bargaining—force the parties to set priorities among their demands, trading off one for another and creating an incentive for them to find common ground. The values, perceptions, and needs of each become apparent. And some measure of mutual understanding is a by-product. As compulsory arbitration undermines the willingness of the parties to bargain conscientiously over their differences, so regulation lessens incentives for private accommodation of conflicting viewpoints. Public hearings encourage dramatic presentations and exorbitant demands, and the government's disclosure rules and the Advisory Committee Act inhibit private meetings between the affected parties and the agency.

The regulatory agency is thus ignorant of the parties' true positions, and is forced to guess each interest's priorities and needs from the formal and often extreme public statements the parties have presented at public hearings. The regulatory process encourages conflict rather than reconciliation of opposing interests. Moreover, there is a sense that it is wrong for the regulatory agency to try to bring parties together and develop consensus. Relying on public and highly formal proceedings makes the development of consensus extremely difficult, if not impossible. And unless this consensus can be developed, neither party has any stake in the promulgated rule, thus remaining free to complain that the rule is biased, stupid, or misguided. Moreover, each side is free to continue the controversy in the form of endless petitions for review, clarification, and litigation before the agency and the courts. Nothing is ever settled because true settlement can come only through agreement, consent, or acquiescence.

A *sixth* problem is that regulatory efforts are rarely abandoned even after their purpose has been served. As James Q. Wilson has pointed out: "Both business firms and regulatory agencies operate on the basis of a common principle: Maintain the organization . . . for the agency that means creating and managing services (or a public image of services) that please key Congressmen, organized clients, and the news media." A parallel problem affects the agency's body of regulations; repealing or modifying those rules is a lengthy and complicated process and is rarely done. Thus the code becomes bloated with anachronistic and rarely enforced regulations that nonetheless have the force of law and could be applied at the convenience of a compliance officer. Trivial and important regulations are mixed: To the regulatee the program appears irrational and arbitrary. Also, as the body of rules expands, it becomes increasingly more difficult and expensive for the regulatees to figure out what is required of them. In this way, the agency and its rules remain in place long after their usefulness has been served.

A *seventh* problem involves the legal game playing between the regulatees and the regulators: The tax law is the classic example, but it is typical of regulatory programs in general. The regulatory agency promulgates a regulation. The regulatees challenge it in court. If they lose, their lawyers may seek to find another ground for administrative or judicial challenge. Congressional amendments may be developed. Between a challenge to the regulation's basic legality, pressure on the agency for an amended regulation, and administrative and judicial enforcement proceedings, there is ample opportunity for tactical strategies, allegations of ambiguity, pleas of special circumstances, and the like. It should be a first principle that no set of men/women is smart enough to write words around which others cannot find holes when the stakes are high.

An *eighth* problem with regulation concerns the difficulty encountered by small- and medium-size firms in complying with the regulations of the various agencies, and the problems the government has in trying to enforce compliance. Many regulations do not well fit the circumstances of small enterprises. It is often difficult if not impossible for small- to medium-sized firms to keep track of the large number of regulations issued by various agencies. And there is little reason to do so. The chances of a small- or medium-sized firm being inspected are minute, and if it is inspected and found to be in violation, fines for a first offence are usually small. Thus, it may make practical business sense for a firm to put off the expenses required to achieve compliance until after an inspection has specified those changes which have to be made. Compliance cannot be compelled through a police effort in every workplace given any practicable levels of funds and personnel. To a degree "public examples"—where a company found in violation is given harsh and visible treatment—encourage other companies to come into compliance. But this tactic is generally unsuccessful for several reasons. Nearly every company—particularly small ones—has a good or plausible excuse for not being in compliance (e.g., they were not aware of the regulations). Thus, a large fine tends to get whittled down to a small one through the successive stages of administrative review. Also, such tactics are perceived to be unfair and generate strong resentment in public opinion and the press, and create hostility to the program and attempts to change it in the political arena.

Ninth, over time as the rule-making and compliance activities of regulatory agencies become routine, it grows increasingly difficult for the President and the agency to attract highly qualified and effective administrators into leadership positions. As the quality of leadership declines, problems often receive increasingly less imaginative treatment or no attention at all.

Tenth, uniform national regulations are inherently unworkable in many situations because the society is not uniform. There are significant differences among industries, sectors, and regions of the country. Consequently, a regulation may be unrealistically harsh in one industry, sector, or part of the country and too lenient in another.

An *eleventh* problem is what is called "regulatory overlap," where a number of different regulatory agencies share some of the same responsibilities. Although the creation of a new, specialized agency probably heightens effectiveness in one field, the danger is that a series of uncoordinated steps, each quite sensible in themselves, can setup a feedback of unanticipated consequences that is overwhelmingly negative. No one regulatory agency is ever able to see the problems through the eyes of those subject to regulation, and the total consequences of regulatory programs on the firm or industry are never perceived. There is no mechanism in government to add to these consequences. Moreover, jurisdictional conflict among agencies, even with the best of good will, consumes vast amounts of time and energy and stimulates general disrespect for governmental agencies.

OVERCOMING REGULATORY PROBLEMS

It is not realistic to expect any significant reduction in the number of federal regulatory programs in the immediate future: In fact, it is likely that the political processes and the Congress will seek to add new ones. Regardless of the theoretical merits of regulation, it is important as a practical matter that more attention be given towards improving the quality of regulation. In a sense, accommodation with practical reality has always occurred. While some inspectors in the field enforce the letter of the law, others develop an array of informal operating rules of thumb which drafters of the regulations never thought of, or indeed rejected. Sometimes these rules of thumb call for nonenforcement in trivial cases or where application of a rigid rule would be unreasonable. Policy makers would do well to address explicitly that which lower-level implementers will do anyway—though unevenly—through the application of common sense or prejudice. The following suggestions are designed to make the regulatory process more responsive to the problems cited *supra.*

First, the parties who will be affected by a set of regulations should be involved to a greater extent in developing those regulations.

The way regulations are currently developed is inherently contentious and acts to maximize antagonism between the parties. The result is poorly framed rules, lawsuits, evasion, and dissatisfaction with the program by all parties. In our society, a rule that is developed with the involvement of the parties who are affected is more likely to be accepted and to be effective in accomplishing its intended purposes.

There is no single way by which the parties can be involved in the rulemaking process, but a method is suggested by the Department's experience with Section 13(c) of the Urban Mass Transportation Act (UMTA). UMTA gives grants to cities to take over failing private transit systems. Section 13(c) requires that funds not be granted until the Secretary of Labor has certified that employees would not be adversely affected by the federally funded activities. This requirement has caused substantial delays and confusion as unions and private managers or city officials haggled over what constituted equitable compensation. Rather than prepare regulations, the Department brought together union and transit representatives and got them to prepare a three-year agreement as to what protection employees should receive as a consequence of the federally funded activities. The Department mediated and provided technical assistance helping to create the standards to apply to individual cases presented to it. Processing time will be very noticeably reduced.

This approach is not necessarily applicable without modification to, say, OSHA or ERISA, but it represents a useful spirit of reliance on private mechanisms which sometimes can achieve a program objective most efficiently.

Second, anachronistic and unnecessary regulations should be repealed and, in the future, rules should be promulgated with greater reluctance. It is an open question as to how many regulations a business, particularly one of small or medium size, can absorb. Not only is it difficult for the regulatee to figure out what is required, but it is equally hard for compliance officers to determine violations. Often they rely on a small percentage of the rules with which they are familiar: Thus the trivial rules are enforced as often as the important ones. This causes annoyance with the program without producing substantial benefits.

Third, greater emphasis should be placed on helping regulatees achieve compliance, especially through consultation. Trying to force compliance primarily through threats of inspections and stiff fines has not proved successful. It has worked against acceptance of the programs by isolating the regulators (and their expertise) from the regulatees and creating antagonism and distrust between the two. As pointed out earlier, the chances of a small- or medium-size business ever being inspected are minute and the cost of coming into compliance is often high. If the business executive asks the agency for technical assistance, in effect the person is asking to be inspected: At least this is the common perception. The regulatory agencies have the expertise to deal with complicated, technical problems such as pollution and occupational disease. But because the programs appear punitive, there is little constructive interplay between the regulators and the regulatees.

Fourth, the activities of the various regulatory agencies need to be coordinated better. As it is now, a single firm may be under the purview of OFCC, OSHA, the Wage and Hour Administration, and a variety of other programs. Simply the number of forms required poses a substantial burden, again, encouraging antagonism for the programs. More significantly, the jurisdictions may overlap. As a long-range goal, perhaps some consolidation and more coordination and sensitivity can occur.

Fifth, regulations must be made to reflect differences between industries, sectors, and geographic regions. A rule that is fair and workable in New York may be excessively severe or unnecessary in Utah. Similar problems exist between industries and types of enterprises, and labor organizations. Uniform, national rules may assure equity but they do not reflect the reality of the workplace.

And *sixth*, the actions of the various regulatory agencies need to be brought into greater harmony with collective bargaining. Many of these programs undermine relations between organized labor and management, as when issues of safety and health, apprenticeship and training, and pensions are placed under government regulation. Without limiting its responsibility to administer the law, and recognizing that some laws are designed explicitly to change the results produced by private collective bargaining, there are ways to involve the parties better to achieve practical and acceptable solutions.

THE REFOSTERING AND DEVELOPMENT OF TRUST

The country needs to acquire a more realistic understanding of the limits of the degree to which social change can be brought about through legal compulsion. A great deal of government needs to be devoted to improving understanding, persuasion, accommodation, mutual problem solving, and informal mediation. Legislation, litigation, and regulations are useful means for some social and economic problems, but today government has more regulation on its plate than it can handle. As I said on the occasion of my swearing-in at the White House, in many areas the growth of regulations and law has far outstripped our capacity to develop consensus and mutual accommodation to our common detriment.

It has well been said that the recreation and development of trust is the central problem of government in our times. The development of new attitudes on the part of public employees, and new relationships and procedures with those who are required to live under regulations is a central challenge of democratic society. Trust cannot grow in an atmosphere dominated by bureaucratic fiat and litigious controversy. It emerges through persuasion, mutual accommodation, and problem solving.

NOTE

1. J. T. Dunlop, "The Limits of Legal Compulsion," Position Paper, Secretary of Labor (Nov. 11, 1975).

EDITOR'S NOTE

ISSUES ARISING FROM HEALTH CARE REGULATION

Despite Professor Dunlop's observations and recommendations as well as the continuing public outcry against "more" governmental intervention, federal and state government continues enlargement of its regulatory role. At the federal level, for example, Congress creates a number of major regulatory programs each year, while the number of regulations issued by federal agencies increases at an annual rate still estimated to be greater than 20 percent.

Many of the new regulatory functions are intrusive in regard to private behavior. Yet most would argue that public intervention is required to achieve such societal ends as workplace health and safety; affirmative action; job opportunities; protection of the natural environment; and food, drug, and consumer product safety. The general problem is how to create programs which yield predictable cost-effective results capable of being implemented by regulators.[1]

Health care regulatory problems are only one of the five or so clusters of interrelated issues of concern in the formulation of a national health policy. (The others are cost control or inflation restraint; character and financing of health care delivery arrangements; distribution of care and minimum standards thereof; and, the recruitment, training, and management of health personnel and institutions.) However, the regulation of health care delivery seems to be the most difficult to come to grips with insofar as study, analysis, and recommendations or prescriptions for the future are concerned. It does seem pointless to continue the ideological debate between regulatory and free-market points of view. But as suggested previously (see Noll, Chapter 2 *supra*), there are an increasing number of crucial health care issues which need to be examined on a case-by-case basis with respect to the continuing nature of government intervention. These include:

192

1. Provisions for calculation of actual cost reimbursement for certain types of patients.

2. Problems associated with various regional and local health agencies concerned with CON, licensing, and planning of facilities and equipment.

3. Provision for peer review of various medical institutional services and procedures through PSROs.

The proliferation of health care regulation raises important questions of public policy. How effective are regulatory approaches going to be over the long term? What are the costs as well as the consequences of various regulatory interventions? Are there alternative means for reasonably achieving the social purpose of the underlying legislative or administrative program without continuation of the delays, uncertainty, bureaucratic constrictions, and loss of local initiative and influence involved in the regulatory approach? What is the best way to conduct the long-term development of health care delivery so that it is of quality, accessible to all, and yet at a cost that our society finds acceptable?

Accordingly, a general task facing scholars is the development of consistent and comprehensive data on which to base proposals for health care regulatory programs. Such a data base might prove helpful in reducing litigious controversies. Yet building a data base requires some framework around which to consider the effectiveness of various approaches. There are two complications:

1. Given the number of agencies involved and the number of legislative mandates extant, health regulatory programs tend to act independently of each other, not only adding to the cost and complexity of the regulatory process, but making the process of analysis much more difficult.

2. Necessary time is required to consider the effectiveness of new technologies such as heart surgery, kidney treatment, and other applications of the explosion in scientific discovery in the life sciences.

So not only does the continuing flow of discoveries flag the problem of obsolete regulation (in common with other fields), it also highlights the debate on how to establish federal standards for adoption of new technology and medical procedures (as well as the continued evaluation of "accepted" practice) in every jurisdiction in the nation—federal, state, regional, and local. (See for example "The CAT Scanner Controversy," pages 13–15.)

Such matters obviously go beyond biomedical expertise and involve issues of cost containment, the nature of medical care delivery, and governmental intervention therein as well as fundamental matters of ethics, religion, and politics. Certainly such intertwining of specific and general issues suggests that no clear or "best" way to regulate health care delivery will be described very soon. Rather, as suggested by preceding chapters, one has to consider the alternatives available to achieve a range of possible goals.

Regulation of health care on a massive scale has been a relatively recent phenomenon just at a time when regulation is under increasing scholarly and political attack. This strengthens the view that the considerable regulatory experience from other spheres of government would be useful to apply to health care from both the positive side (what works?) and the negative point of view (what are the predictable pitfalls associated with any particular regulatory approach or device?)

The next chapter by Stephen Breyer outlines classical problems associated with major forms of economic regulation and suggests some alternatives thereto. Although his discussion centers almost entirely on regulation outside the health care sphere, his work can be applied successfully to health care regulatory problems as discussed in Chapter Six.

NOTE

1. Of course, as pointed out by Feldman and Roberts in Chapter Two, the difficulty of placing a quantitative value on health care benefits makes it questionable whether conventional cost/benefit analysis is ever possible. Some new approach for health care analysis is urgently needed.

CHAPTER FIVE

Proposals for Regulatory Reform

EDITOR'S NOTE

For a considerable period of time, Senator Edward Kennedy has given much thought to the reform of regulation in the United States. As Chairman of the Subcommittee on Administrative Practice and Procedure of the Senate Committee on the Judiciary, he chaired the investigation of the Civil Aeronautics Board (CAB) in 1975. This investigation ultimately led to the drafting and passage of the Airline Deregulation Act of 1978. Professor Stephen Breyer served as staff director of the CAB investigation. Most recently he has taken leave from the Harvard Law School to serve as Chief Counsel to the Senate Judiciary Committee.

Accordingly, it seems appropriate to ask Senator Kennedy as chairman of the Judiciary Committee to introduce this chapter, which outlines Professor Breyer's approach to the reform of economic regulation in the United States. In what follows, Senator Kennedy poses the policy and legislative issues that must be removed if the current regulatory burden is to be lightened. Basically, the Senator argues that easing the regulatory burden can only proceed on a case-by-case basis.

STRIKING A REGULATORY BALANCE

Edward M. Kennedy,[1] *United States Senator, The Commonwealth of Massachusetts*

My own concern with regulatory reform is not new, and neither is the country's. Regulation touches all of us because the cost of transportation and energy; the safety of food, drugs, jobs; and the quality of the environment are crucial for all of us. If Americans are to believe in their government, regulation must be—and seem to be—fair, reasonable, and effective.

Yet we hear that regulation may cost the economy between $25 and $50 billion in paperwork alone; that the regulatory establishment grew 115 percent between 1975 and 1978, incurring annual budget costs of nearly $5 billion; that industry's regulatory compliance costs may be over $100 billion; and that regulation may cost jobs, hit small business more heavily, be partly responsible for inflation, and at the same time may be ineffective.

However, we must remember social regulation brings benefits and not just costs: clean air, a safe working place, promotion of minority employment, control of sickle cell anemia, and safe automobiles. The difficulty of measuring these benefits is no argument that they do not exist.

Nor do these costs of regulation mean that we should plunge head-long into deregulation in every area of governmental activity. The history of unregulated markets too clearly shows that they often can prove detrimental to consumers and businesspeople alike. Recent revelations indicate that major asbestos firms were well aware of their product's harmful effects on workers and school children but covered up that knowledge for generations. The power company's behavior at Three Mile Island scarcely justifies a benign faith in the workings of the market.

The procedures of government must clearly be updated and re-vamped to achieve greater speed, openness, fairness, and efficiency. But procedural changes in regulation are unlikely to achieve change in its substantive results. Procedure alone will not give us lower prices, better health and safety, or a cleaner environment—and it is results that count.

196

How then are we to bring about meaningful change? I am convinced
the key lies in agency-by-agency examinations of specific regulatory programs. Government bodies outside the agency concerned must take the time and effort needed to force change; they need the help of outside groups committed to fundamental reform. In this endeavor they should be guided by a "regulation as last resort" philosophy. I would call this approach "least restrictive alternative" regulation.

That is the basic rule of our antitrust laws. Under these laws, when firms enter into an agreement, a court asks whether it will interfere with competition. It then asks whether the agreement is necessary to achieve an important public purpose, and it allows the agreement only if it is "the least restrictive alternative" available to achieve that purpose.

This approach applies to government regulation too. If we start out in favor of a competitive, unregulated marketplace, the government should intervene only when that market does not work properly—when it fails to fulfill an important public need. And when the government does intervene, it should choose the least restrictive means available before turning to self-perpetuating commands-and-controls. At the very least, it should examine available alternatives in a regular, structured manner before choosing that route.

Practical consequences flow from this view. First, in the area of social regulation—traffic safety, food purity, drug efficacy, environmental protection, job safety, and health—deregulation is unlikely to be an answer. There are too many powerful reasons rooted in fairness, social justice, and relief for the disadvantaged and underrepresented that will not allow such regulation to be wiped away. We can never stop trying to make social regulation more effective and incorporate new approaches. But past experience with unregulated drugs, pollution, and job conditions shows that relying on totally free markets here would invite chaos. Consumers do not have the knowledge or power to protect their best interests, and the protective efforts of more conscientious firms would be driven to the lowest common denominator. Here the choice will be how to regulate—not between regulation or none.

Second, where health and safety are not paramount, and the industry consists of several firms in a reasonably competitive market, the most likely answer is not to regulate. Instead we should rely on the discipline of that market backed by antitrust policy. This has proved true for airlines. It also applies to trucking and other regulated industries.

In other regulatory areas, however, the answer will not be to wipe the slate clean, but to make regulation less intrusive, less bumbling and bureaucratic. There are many tools the government can use to stop short of—or supplement—direct command-and-control regulation. The government can institute regulatory taxes. It can require more disclosure and it can encourage bargaining among private parties. The practical difficulties with these techniques should not be understated. But they may well make health, safety, and environmental regulation more effective and less cumbersome.

In the environment, for example, the goal is to encourage industry to use less polluting production methods. Environmental taxes *as supplements* to direct standards have long been advocated by many environmentalists and some in industry. The Environmental Protection Agency is currently experimenting with systems of "marketable rights" under which new firms can buy rights to pollute from older firms, creating a profit motive for existing and new firms to reduce emissions in the most cost-effective ways. Regulatory taxes have been used to increase the price of throw-away cans and nonreturnable bottles, encouraging buyer shifts to more socially desirable products. They might also be used to regulate the price of cigarettes with dangerous levels of tar and nicotine or to raise the prices of automobiles with low gasoline efficiency.

We might also use increased disclosure to warn consumers away from products we do not want to forbid. We use mandated disclosure as a regulating technique in drug labelling, in food packaging, at the gas pump, and in the stock market. It is less restrictive and sometimes more effective than banning a substance or product. As we discover that more and more necessary food substances also carry risks, we may want to require food labels warning consumers to eat what they want, but not too much of any one thing. Some have suggested a "dangerous food" area in each grocery store for products whose intake should be restricted though not banned entirely. And as a result of the saccharin mess, the Federal Drug Administration itself is exploring the possibility of regulating only "involuntary exposures" to food additives, not the hopeless task of regulating exposures which consumers with full knowledge still desire.

We might also make more use of informal bargaining to attain regulatory goals. In some European countries workplace safety problems are negotiated between unions, management, and a government representative. Certain firms have quietly begun to work with the Occupational Safety and Health Administration to explore such techniques here. This process can take place on an informal plant-by-plant basis, producing more effective regulation as well as freedom from unwieldy requirements. It can also make direct government enforcement a matter of last resort rather than one of first instance.

Finally, in some areas it will not be possible to avoid direct regulation. Thalidomides must be banned. Nor would it be wise to rely solely on the marketplace for the purity of our air or drinking water. Effective regulation is as important to parents filling a prescription as to the worker who breathes the air in his plant. Government safety standards are equally important to the traveler in his plane and the machinist at his workbench. There must be a Federal Aviation Administration and there must also be direct government concern with worker safety. Reform here will be complex. It may involve giving agencies more resources or changes in procedure. It may involve increased enforcement or systems that encourage more voluntary compliance. It may also involve an admission that what works for General Foods is not right for the corner grocer.

But in all these cases we can do more. We can encourage others to

follow the same case-by-case approach and to do so by procompetitive means. We can legislate a system that will encourage a scrutiny of individual agencies and require detailed reform plans. And we can promote regular examination of less restrictive alternatives to attain legitimate regulatory ends.

As we approach the 1980s, the issue of government credibility—its ability to respond sensibly and effectively, to know when to stay out as well as leap in—has grown larger.

Our citizens and businesses feel overregulated. But to most Americans, regulation is not the President. It is not the Secretary of Energy or HEW. It is not even Washington. It is the energy allocation guidelines no one can understand. It is the government contract officer who puts people through hoops before he will look at their applications. It is the inspector from the Federal Aviation Administration, the Federal Drug Administration, or the Occupational Safety and Health Administration who may hold life and death power over their businesses but does not seem to understand their operations and acts unwilling to learn.

Striking the proper balance between compulsion and choice for individual citizens must be our focus. That is where gains must be made if we are to make a real difference.

The high cost of regulation and inflation, the general public feeling that government intervenes too much in our lives, and the breakdown of classical rationales for federal regulations are the mainsprings of the current debate over regulatory reform. They are the reasons this subject has become more than the preserve of academics and commissions.

The answers to this debate will require new approaches and much hard work. Let us renew America's fearless belief in new ideas. Let us strive together to make government work better for all the people.

NOTE

1. Based on an address of Senator Edward M. Kennedy to a conference on regulatory reform sponsored by the American Enterprises Institute and the National Journal. A condensation of the article was published in the *St. Louis Dispatch* and several other newspapers in July 1979.

EDITOR'S NOTE

If one adopts the attitude that regulatory reform is like an earlier decade's "war on cancer," i.e., there is no one cure and one must deal with each case on its own merits, how does one analyze each regulatory situation? The framework for such an analysis is precisely what Professor Stephen Breyer develops. It might be helpful to the reader to summarize the intellectual problems with which Breyer wrestles in order to suggest proposals for the reform of economic regulation.

The framework consists of three basic elements: Justifications for regulation; modes of classical regulation (and the problems they entail); and "less restrictive alternatives" to regulation, including taxation and disclosure.

One problem will immediately present itself to the reader of this volume. Breyer does not directly treat problems of health care. Our major premise is that Breyer's analysis, which seeks to categorize and describe different forms of economic regulation, will be helpful to those interested in any area of regulation. It was the particular belief of the joint sponsors of the work that led to this volume that the creation of a "road map" or a general analytic approach to regulation would be applicable to some but not all areas of health care regulation. Chapter Six following Breyer's analysis provides explicit commentaries by experts concerning the applicability of his approach to health care. The reader interested in health care should know that it was a shared concern of government officials, Harvard faculty, and key foundation executives that at the very time when classical approaches to regulation are being looked at skeptically, health care agencies seem to be relying increasingly on classical regulatory approaches. Yet the fact that a perfect market does not exist, particularly in health care, is often used as a justification for regulation. While there are well-known systematic accounts of the defects of competitive markets, what Breyer attempts is a first account of regulatory failure, suggesting that "perfect regulation" also does not exist any more than a "perfect" practice of medicine or "perfect" administration of a hospital.

To understand the problem of categorization and description, consider that persons charged with creating or administering systems of health care regulation must be able to examine and learn from the experience of others in administering a large variety of other regulatory schemes. But, how can they learn? Each regulatory program is complex and unique, and often cannot be understood thoroughly without mastering vast detail. Would it not help to attempt to create useful descriptions about types of regulations?

The key word here is "useful." How does one avoid becoming either too detailed in describing particular systems or too abstract to the point where the generalizations appear obvious—or too general? The answer presented here by Breyer is to try to draw up a useful set of regulatory categories that distinguish among types of regulation but are few enough so that a description of typical examples and typical problems appears to have impact beyond the example cited.

Obviously, the way to begin is to list the major economic problems that have been thought to call for government intervention. Next, typical problems are listed that arise with classical forms of government regulation. Despite the many accounts of typical failures of free markets, up until now there has not been any systematic treatment of the recurring difficulties that are associated with regulation.

The value of the analysis will also depend upon the identification of seven categories that divide economic regulation into specific types or forms such as cost-of-service ratemaking and historically based price setting.

This chapter will illustrate each form of regulation and discuss how regulators deal with typical problems. Using contemporary regulatory programs such as Federal Communication Commission television licensing and National Highway Traffic Safety Administration automobile safety standard-setting as examples, Breyer argues that many such programs are ill-designed to meet their objectives. Further, he believes that the problems inherent in regulatory regimes can be quite severe.

If the examples chosen in fact illustrate modes of regulation in widespread use, and if the problems discussed under each heading are in fact typical, the typology or analytical structure created should prove helpful to those analyzing regulatory proposals for health.

The second focus of this chapter, based on the premise that regulation has problems as typical as those experienced by the free market, shows that the way to create better results is to optimize the problem/weapon fit. One should choose that form of regulation, or some other nonregulatory form (such as antitrust, taxes, collective bargaining), that will best suit the economic problem at hand given the typical strengths and weaknesses of the various governmental weapons, rather than perpetuate the many "mismatches" that are extant today.

Breyer describes "mismatch" guidelines or "rules of thumb" for identifying those regulatory approaches (weapons) which do not suit, in fact may exacerbate, specific economic or market problems. Finally, through the use of specific examples, Breyer suggests how to proceed to bring about some measure of regulatory reform, using as an example the recent change in airline regulation (based on Breyer's experience as staff director of the CAB investigation by the Subcommittee on Administrative Practice and Procedure of the Senate Committee on the Judiciary). The reader is challenged to think of situations in his own experience which exemplify what Breyer outlines.

PROPOSALS FOR REGULATORY REFORM: AN INTRODUCTION[*][1]

Stephen Breyer, *Professor of Law, Harvard University*

Proposals for reform of government regulation tend to fall into four categories recommending:

1. Changes in agency structure (i.e., replacing a multimember commission with a single head);[2]

2. Improvements in agency procedure (i.e., increasing the use of rulemaking or paying legal fees for public interest advocates);[3]

3. Improvements in the quality of appointments,[4]

4. Change in the substance of regulation itself (e.g., "deregulating" airlines[5] or taxing natural gas producers instead of regulating them).[6]

The first three types of reform are often inadequate or incapable of producing significant change. Proposals of the last type—calling for major shifts in the substance of regulation—can result in significant effects on regulated enterprises. But such proposals are difficult to formulate because of the detailed knowledge they require about the regulated industries and the actual effect of a particular regulatory system upon them.

Proposals of the fourth sort are considered here. A framework is suggested for analyzing economic regulation thus enabling one to progress from analysis of current systems to proposals for substantive change.

This framework applies to economic regulation broadly conceived as governmental efforts to control or to affect decisions about price, output, product quality, or production processes. Such regulation includes both traditional rate and entry regulation and more recent efforts to regulate health, safety, and the environment.

The framework is designed to isolate existing regulatory areas that are particularly likely to need reform. It also seeks to help in determin-

---

ing when, how, and whether new regulatory programs should be designed or whether reliance should be placed upon alternatives to traditional systems of regulation.

The framework is built upon a simple approach to creating and implementing any program: Determine one's objectives, examine the alternative methods of obtaining those objectives, and choose the best method for doing so. Use of the framework will help to identify candidates for serious substantive reform and will help to weed out methods which, given a particular primary problem, are likely to prove unsatisfactory.

Too many arguments made in favor of government regulation assume that regulation, at least in principle, is a perfect solution to any perceived problem with the unregulated marketplace.[7] But regulation embodies its own typical defects. One of this chapter's objectives is to present these defects systematically. However, not every factor—historical, political, administrative, economic—that affects the success or failure of individual regulatory programs need be considered from the outset. Rather, one should analyze the comparative merits of alternative methods in terms of the justifications underlying the choice of a regulatory program and *then* introduce historical, political, procedural, or administrative consideration to see if, and how, they change one's judgment about the best method. Very often they will not.

In the pages that follow is a skeletal framework for analysis of economic regulation. The framework is discussed in three separate articles. The first article describes those market defects that typically give rise to a call for regulation. The second discusses the several different modes of classical regulation, along with the major problems that typically accompany each of them. Finally, the third lists certain alternative regimes that may sometimes be employed with greater success than classical regulation.

The third article will also illustrate the framework and explore some of its details and implications by applying it to several regulatory programs. But the framework and the general rules which flow from it serve only to identify certain "candidates" for regulatory reform. Before a final decision can be reached on any specific regulatory program, it is necessary to explore in detail all the benefits and harms of and justifications for regulation and deregulation. The process by which reform can occur is a political process, and the third article will briefly describe how one might proceed with a regulatory "candidate" to determine what sort of reform is desirable and how to achieve it.

NOTES

1. This section and the three that follow essentially summarize the main points of Professor Stephen Breyer's forthcoming book, *The Reform of Economic Regulation*. Professor Breyer's work was supported by the Commission on Law and the Economy of the American Bar Association (for which he acted as a consultant) and was used as a source for many of the ideas expressed in Chapters Three and Four of the exposure draft of that Commission's report,

his article in 92 *Harvard Law Review* 549 (1979). Excerpts from the book manuscript were used as part of the program and conference proceedings, *Regulation as an Instrument of Public Administration* conducted by the John F. Kennedy School of Government (under contract from the Health Resources Administration) which also supported the preparation of summaries of Breyer's work useful to health care personnel (contained in the final report to that agency).

These sections represent an amalgamation of all versions. The Editor is grateful to the editors of the *Harvard Law Review* and to the Commission on Law and the Economy, American Bar Association, for permission to utilize without continuing attribution their versions where such seemed most appropriate for this volume.

This Editor can only add that the wide circulation that Breyer's thoughts have already achieved only attest to their importance and general usefulness.

2. E.g., J. M. Landis, *Report on Regulatory Agencies to the President-Elect* (1960); also printed as *Report on Regulatory Agencies to the President-Elect, Chairman of the Subcomm. on Administrative Practice & Procedure of the Senate Comm. on the Judiciary*, 86th Cong., 2nd Sess. (1960).

3. E.g., *Study on Federal Regulation, II–V Senate Comm. on Governmental Affairs*, 95th Cong., 1st Sess. (1977).

4. E.g., *Study on Federal Regulations, Senate Comm. on Government Operations*, S. No. 95-25, 95th Cong., 1st Sess. (1977).

5. *Report on Civil Aeronautics Board Practices and Procedures, Staff of the Senate Subcomm. on Administrative Practice & Procedure of the Comm. on the Judiciary*, 94th Cong., 1st Sess. (1975), hereinafter cited as *CAB Report*. The report is also known as the *Kennedy Report* (Senator Kennedy served as chairman of the Subcommittee).

6. S. Breyer and P. W. MacAvoy, "The Natural Gas Shortage and the Regulation of Natural Gas Producers," 86 *Harvard Law Review*, 941 (1973).

7. See Douglas, "The Case for the Consumer of National Gas," 44 *Georgia Law Journal* 566 (1956); A. Kahn, "Economic Issues in Regulating the Field Price of Natural Gas," 50 *American Economic Review* 506 (1960).

MARKET DEFECTS*

Stephen Breyer, *Professor of Law, Harvard University*

THE FRAMEWORK FOR ANALYSIS
OF ECONOMIC REGULATION

In order to appraise our system of governmental intervention analytically, four fundamental questions are posed:

1. What are the fundamental economic benefits of the competitive marketplace?[1]

2. What are the traditional reasons which have been urged in support of, or appear to underlie, a demand for regulation?

3. What are the classical types of regulation, and what are their inherent characteristics?

4. Which alternatives to these classical regulatory processes could possibly answer the need with less adverse impact on the economy?

The framework for analysis employed assumes that an unregulated marketplace is the norm and that those who advocate government intervention must justify it by showing that it is needed to achieve an important public objective that an unregulated marketplace cannot provide. This assumption, and the traditional "market failure" analysis that it suggests, are sometimes justified by appealing to basic societal values such as freedom of individual action and minimization of governmental coercion. The justification for the assumption here, however, does not rest on the adoption of a particular set of values; it lies in its ability to generate demonstrably desirable results by identifying regulatory problems, predicting regulatory failures, and suggesting alternatives.

This traditional market failure analysis turns out to be a powerful tool for determining not only whether but also how much and what sort of regulation is called for. Moreover, one finds its justification not simply by reference to basic societal values such as freedom of individual

---

action or dislike of governmental coercion, but more importantly by the concrete results that a total system of government regulation based on this assumption is likely to achieve.

THE FUNDAMENTAL ECONOMIC BENEFITS OF COMPETITIVE MARKETS

The intrinsic advantages offered by a well-functioning, competitive free market system have traditionally been identified as:

1. Minimization of economic waste by continuous "individual balancing of costs and benefits by consumers and producers;"

2. The "carrot and stick" incentive for greater production efficiency; and

3. The incentives for and socially desired channeling of innovations.[2]

In achieving these ends, competitive markets reduce the need for the central collection of information.[3] Their price signals allow producers and consumers to adapt quickly to change, and the impersonality of the decision-making process in competitive markets prevents those injured in the process (when, for example, their goods are no longer in demand) from obstructing change.[4]

To these advantages may be added a competitive market's tendency to decentralize power and to make decisions that are "fair" in the sense of being impersonal.[5] Finally, as Charles Schultze has noted, "Relationships in the market are a form of unanimous consent arrangement . . . minimizing the need for coercion as a means of organizing society."[6]

The normative approach to regulation[7] that is taken obviously differs markedly from the analyses of those who argue that as a matter of historical fact or present political reality, regulation is or was designed to further private interests of special groups.[8] The framework used here assumes, for the reasons mentioned above, that regulation is *justified* only if it achieves policy objectives that a consensus of reasonable observors would consider to be in the public interest. Even if the creation (or administration) of existing programs is best explained by the political power of special groups seeking selfish ends—which is doubtful—those who seek to justify those programs must appeal to the "public interests." Legislators, administrators, judges, critics, reformers, and the public at large wish to know whether regulatory programs are justified.

TYPICAL JUSTIFICATIONS FOR REGULATION[9]

The most important justifications for government regulation of the economy are well described as instances of classical market failure.[10] Most of the market defects that give rise to a demand for regulation can be classified as follows.

A traditional, persistent rationale for price and profit regulation is based on the need to control the exercise of power by a "natural monopolist."[11] Where economies of scale are so great as to make it inefficient for more than one firm to operate, that firm can increase its profits by restricting output and charging higher than competitive prices. Regulators have traditionally sought to keep the prices charged by the telephone company or electric utilities at a "competitive" level.

In part, such regulation is aimed at allocative efficiency.[12] To the extent that the prices are set at a competitive level,[13] they accurately reflect comparative costs in terms of real resources used. If monopolistically high prices are set, however, consumers will tend to substitute for the monopolist's product X a second product Y, which, in terms of real resources may cost the economy more to produce.[14]

The rationale for the regulation of monopoly power rests not only upon a desire for allocative efficiency, however, but also upon such other political justifications as fairer income distribution, avoiding discrimination in price or service among customers, and distrust of the social and political (as well as the economic) power of an unregulated natural monopolist.

Control of Windfall Profits

Windfall profits (rents) may occur as the result of sudden increases in the price of a commodity without a simultaneous change in the producer's cost. The profits may benefit any firm that holds a stock of that commodity or controls any nonduplicable low-cost source of supply.

Thus, those who own large stocks of oil are in a position to obtain windfall profits when the OPEC countries raise the price of their new oil; owners of old natural gas, if free to raise their prices, can obtain a windfall when the costs of finding new natural gas rise;[15] and those who own existing housing can reap windfall profits as long as construction costs rise faster than other costs. Such profits are common in competitive and noncompetitive industries alike. Ordinarily they are not regulated, but they may give rise to a demand for regulation.[16] The object of the regulation is to transfer allegedly undeserved profits from producers (or owners) of the scarce resource to consumers (or taxpayers).

Correcting for Spillovers (External Costs)

Regulation is frequently justified by the need to compensate for the fact that the price of a product does not reflect the major costs that its production and use impose upon the economy.[17] The price of steel does not reflect the spillover or external costs that it imposes in the form of air pollution that harms or irritates those who live near the plant. As a result, more steel may be demanded than is warranted in light of its adverse side effects.

Regulation must therefore rest on a judgment that some extra production cost, e.g., the cost of clean air scrubbers, is warranted by the resulting reduction of pollution harm. This judgment reflects the belief that steel users and pollution sufferers would agree to pay for pollution reduction if they could readily bargain among themselves. Regulation in the presence of spillover costs can be seen as a way of correcting for the fact that bargaining among affected parties is difficult.[18]

Correcting for Inadequate Information

For competitive markets to function well, consumers need information sufficient to evaluate competing products. This information is itself a commodity, the supply of which will reflect costs and demand. However, the market for information is imperfect. Consumers as a class have an interest in obtaining information, but there is no satisfactory way for them to share the costs. Each is unwilling to pay enough for information from which all will benefit but for which only some will pay. In addition, some products are so complex that individual consumers need the assistance of experts to evaluate them.[19]

Government regulation is sometimes designed to compensate for inadequate information or to lower the costs to the consumer of obtaining adequate information.[20] In particular, government action may be called for when:

1. Suppliers seek to mislead consumers.

2. Consumers cannot readily evaluate the information available, such as the comparative abilities of doctors or lawyers or the potential effectiveness of a drug.[21]

3. The market on the supply side is insufficiently competitive to furnish all the information needed or demanded, as when automobile companies or airline firms "tacitly agree" not to advertise comparative safety records.

In the latter instances, government may seek to provide more or better information or through substantive regulation make up for its lack.

Excessive Competition: The Empty Box

A commonly advanced justification for the regulation of airlines, trucking companies, and shipping firms is the asserted need to control "excessive," "destructive," or "unfair" competition.[22] In fact, this notion of need refers to several different sorts of justification, all of which assume that if prices fall too low, firms will go out of business and products will end up being too costly.

This particular set of justifications is labelled the "empty box" because no existing regulatory program can be justified by reference to it. Analysis of the different problems to which this rationale for regulation refers makes it clear how empty the box really is.

This rationale may refer to an historical problem. For example, when airlines originally received large government subsidies (from the 1920s to the 1950s), they had an incentive to cut prices well below costs to increase their size, while making up the additional losses through additional subsidy.[23] Though the problem was caused by government intervention (through subsidization), it required additional intervention to counteract it. Protection was provided in the form of minimum price regulation by the Civil Aeronautics Board (CAB).[24] Similarly, minimum price regulation of trucking was historically responsive to claims by the railroads that it was "unfair" to regulate them while leaving unregulated truckers free to compete for the railroads' most lucrative business.[25]

Other rationales refer to the problems faced by industries with large fixed costs and cyclical demand or to the possibility of "predatory pricing."[26]

Moral Hazard: Avoiding the Distortions Caused When Buyers Do Not Pay the Entire Bill

The term "moral hazard" applies to a situation in which someone other than the buyer makes purchasing decisions for him or helps to pay for his purchase, or both. When this happens, market forces may be distorted, generally causing greater consumption than if the buyer had to make the purchase and pay for it entirely by himself.

The most salient example is escalating medical costs.[27] If the government or private insurers pay for all or most of the expenses, the prescribing physician may lack the incentive to minimize the cost of treatment and the patient's own "pocketbook constraint" is reduced, making the patient oblivious to the resource cost he or she imposes upon the economy.[28] As medical care is purchased to an ever greater extent by the government or by large private insurers, medical costs have accounted for an ever greater proportion of the GNP.[29] When ethical or other institutional constraints or direct supervision by the payer fail to control purchases, government regulation may be demanded.

The fact that purchases are paid for by others frees the individual from the need to consider that using more medical care means less production of other goods; thus he or she may unnecessarily or excessively use medical resources. If one believed that too much of the GNP is accounted for by medical treatment and also believed that the problem of "moral hazard" prevents higher prices from acting as a check on individual demand for those resources, which in turn reduces the incentive to hold down prices, one might advocate regulation to keep prices down, improve efficiency, or limit the supply of medical treatment.[30]

Rationalization: Restructuring Particular Industries to Promote Economies of Scale or Other Benefits

Government intervention is occasionally justified on the ground that without it the firms in an industry would not produce their products in an economically efficient manner.[31] It would seem natural to expect an industry composed of numerous small and inefficient firms to be gradually transformed into an industry of fewer, more efficient large firms.[32] However, social or political factors may inhibit such change.[33] Hence, European governments have sometimes intervened to overcome conservative business practices by "rationalizing" an industry, such as steel.

Regulatory agencies in the United States have sometimes sought to engage in industrywide planning. In the 1960s, for example, the Federal Power Commission sought to reduce the unit costs of electricity by urging private electric utilities to coordinate the planning and operation of generating and transmission facilities.[34] The result was relatively unsuccessful.[35]

Minor Justifications for Regulation

Several additional justifications have on occasion been advanced for government regulation. While not in themselves persuasive, they often provide partial justifications for regulatory action.

Unequal bargaining power   The assumption that the "best" or most efficient allocation is achieved by free market forces rests in part upon an assumption that there is a "proper" allocation of bargaining power among the parties affected. Where the existing division of such bargaining power is "unequal" in this sense, it may be thought that regulation is justified in order to achieve a better balance. The usual congressional response is to grant an exemption from the antitrust laws, thus allowing the weaker parties to organize in order to deal more effectively with the "stronger." This rationale underlies the exemption granted not only to labor, but also to agricultural and fishing cooperatives.[36]

Scarcity   Regulation is sometimes justified in terms of scarcity.[37] Such regulation reflects a deliberate decision to abandon the market and to use regulatory allocation to achieve a set of (often unspecified) public interest objectives,[38] such as in the case of licensing television stations. Sometimes regulatory allocation is undertaken because of sudden supply failures which create consumer financial hardships due to skyrocketing prices (e.g. the Arab oil boycott of 1973). A shortage may also be the result of the workings of an ongoing regulatory program, as when natural gas must be allocated because of windfall control.

Paternalism   Some kinds of regulation have an element of paternalism, and are partially justified on the grounds that government has certain responsibilities to protect individuals from their own irresponsibility. An example is the mandating of secondary school education.

Although full and adequate information needed to reach a rational decision may be available to the decision maker in the marketplace, some may argue that government regulation is needed to avoid the wrong decision. This justification is one of pure paternalism. Distrust of purchaser capability may be based on the layperson's inability to evaluate information, as in the case of purchasing professional services, or on the belief that irrational human tendencies prevent him from evaluating information accurately. The latter may be the case where small probabilities are involved, such as small risks of injury, or where matters of life and death are implicated, such as when those suffering from cancer will purchase a drug even though all reasonably reliable information indicates that it is worthless or even harmful.

Paternalism based on mistrust of consumer rationality may be inconsistent with notions of freedom of choice, but it seems to play an important role in some government decisions.

Multiple-Asserted Justifications

It is important to bear in mind that many regulatory programs, in fact, have multiple-asserted justifications. Thus, for example, one might favor regulation of workplace safety for several reasons. One might recognize that employers and employees can bargain for improved workplace safety (greater safety expenditures), but argue that accidents impose costs on others who are not represented at the bargaining table. Thus bargaining alone will produce inadequate expenditure upon safety devices and regulation through standard-setting is needed. This is a *spillover* rationale. On the other hand, one might believe that workers do not know enough about the risks or consequences of accidents to insist upon added safety expenditures. This is to argue that there is an *informational defect* in the market. One might also feel workers are too poor or too weak to bargain for the safety they need— that they have *unequal bargaining power*. Finally, workers may overlook the likely seriousness of accidents and health hazards. They inevitably underestimate the risk. If regulation is an effort to give them what they ought to want, a *paternalistic rationale* is at work. Each rationale may, of course, suggest a different remedy. Identification of the real rationale will assist in choosing the regulatory tool best suited to the problem at hand. One who believes the primary problem is informational will favor government efforts to provide more information, not classical regulation, while another who accepts a paternalistic rationale may disagree with that solution. A clear statement of the parties' points of difference could lead to some constructive empirical work. The resulting data should suggest basic rationale and the choice of the best regulatory weapon.

1. The economist's ideal of a free market rarely exists. Thus "competitive marketplace" means a market policed only by antitrust policy.

2. Seen generally C. Schultze, *The Public Use of Private Interest* 16–27 (Brookings Inst., 1977).

3. *Ibid.* at 19–21.

4. *Ibid.* at 21–25.

5. See C. Kaysen and D. Turner, *Antitrust Policy: An Economic and Legal Analysis* (1959).

6. C. Schultze, n. 2 *supra* at 16–17.

7. The framework assumes, for the reasons mentioned above, that regulation is *justified* only if it achieves policy objectives that a consensus of reasonable observers would consider to be in the public interest. Even if the creation (or administration) of existing programs is best explained by the political power of special groups seeking selfish ends—which is doubtful—those who seek to justify those programs must appeal to the public interest. Legislators, administrators, judges, critics, reformers, and the public at large wish to know whether regulatory programs are justified.

8. See, e.g., G. Kolko, *Railroads and Regulation, 1877–1916* (Princeton Univ. Press, 1965); S. Peltzman, "Toward a More General Theory of Regulation," 19 *Journal of Law and Economics* 211 (1976); G. Stigler, "The Theory of Economic Regulation," 2 *Bell Journal of Economics and Management Science* 3 (1971).

9. This analysis assumes that those who advocate governmental intervention must justify it by showing it is needed to achieve an important public objective that an unregulated marketplace cannot provide. That there are those who argue that as a matter of historical fact regulation in some instances was designed to serve the private interests of special groups in discouraging competition and maintaining profits. However, each of these groups must attempt to justify regulation through an appeal to the public interest. The initiative for regulation is not crucial to the analysis.

10. See, e.g., E. Mishan, *Economics for Social Decisions* 85–111 (1975) (externalities as one type of classical market failure); Bator, "The Anatomy of Market Failure," 72 *Quarterly Journal of Economics* 351 (1958).

11. See R. Posner, *Economic Analysis of Law* 139–149, 163–165, 268–269 (1973).

12. See A. Kahn, *The Economics of Regulation,* Vol. 1, pp. 65–70 (1970–1971).

13. The "competitive price" may be defined loosely as the price that would be set were the industry in fact capable of sustaining competition. The ambiguity of this definition in part accounts for some of the difficulties facing classical regulation.

14. Whether this allocative goal can be achieved through regulation of the prices charged is debatable. The fact that the regulated price is set high enough to cover the natural monopolist's fixed costs automatically makes it higher than the incremental cost price that would produce allocative efficiency. Moreover, some would argue that in the absence of regulation, natural monopolists would set prices that, by discriminating in price

among customers, are allocatively more efficient. Nonetheless, as long as one believes that without regulation the firm will raise prices *substantially,* one can reasonably argue that regulated prices will *help* achieve allocative efficiency. (See Posner, "Natural Monopoly and its Regulation," 21 *Stanford Law Review* 548, 569–573 (1969)).

15. See Breyer and MacAvoy in "Proposals for Regulatory Reform: An Introduction," n. 6 *supra* at 950.

16. See, e.g., Douglas in "Proposals for Regulatory Reform: An Introduction," n. 7 *supra*; Note, "A Proposed Response to the Energy Crisis: Windfall Profits Taxation," 49 *Notre Dame Law* 867 (1974).

17. See E. Mishan, n. 10 *supra* at 93–95.

18. See generally G. Calabresi, *The Costs of Accidents: A Legal and Economic Analysis* (Yale Univ. Press, 1970); G. Calabresi, "Optimal Deterrence and Accidents," 84 *Yale Law Journal* 656 (1975); Calabresi and Melamed, "Property Rules, Liability Rules, and Inalienability: One View of the Cathedral" 85 *Harvard Law Review* 1089 (1972); Coase, "The Problem of Social Cost" 3 *Journal of Law and Economics* 1, 11–12 (1960).

19. A fuller treatment of defects in the market for information may be found in N. Cornell, R. Noll, and B. Weingast, "Safety Regulation," in *Setting National Priorities: The Next Ten Years* 465–470 (H. Owen and C. Schultze, Eds., Brookings Inst., 1976).

20. See, e.g., 15 U.S.C. §§ 1681–1681t (1976) (fair credit reporting requirement for consumer credit protection).

21. See Bates v. State Bar, 433 U.S. 350, 373–375 (1977); Virginia State Bd. of Pharmacy v. Virginia Citizens Consumer Council, Inc., 425 U.S. 748, 769–770 (1976).

22. See A. Kahn, Vol. 2, n. 12 *supra* at 172–250 (1971).

23. *CAB Report* in "Proposals for Regulatory Reform: An Introduction," n. 5 *supra* at 60–62.

24. *Ibid.* at 31–34.

25. See A. Kahn, Vol. 2, n. 12 *supra* at 14; S. Rep. No. 482, 74th Cong., 1st Sess. 2–3 (1935).

26. See S. Breyer, 92 *Harvard Law Review* 557 (1979).

27. See Gibson and Mueller, "National Health Expenditures, Fiscal Year 1976," *Social Security Bulletin* 3 (Apr. 1977).

28. For a descriptive example of the "moral hazard" situation, see K. Arrow, *Essays in the Theory of Risk Bearing* 142–143 (1971).

29. See M. Feldstein and A. Taylor, *The Rapid Rise of Hospital Costs,* Staff Report of the Council on Wage & Price Stability, Executive Office of the President (Jan. 1977).

30. See Conference on Health Planning, Certificates-of-Need, and Market Entry, *Regulating Health Facilities Construction* (1974).

31. See, e.g., S. Breyer and MacAvoy, "The Federal Power Commission and the Coordination Problem in the Electrical Power Industry," 46 *Southern California Law Review* 661, 680–682, 685–687, 688–694 (1973). See generally A. Kahn, Vol. 2, n. 12 *supra* at 64–77.

32. See Breyer and MacAvoy, n. 31 *supra* at 665–669.

33. See generally F. Scherer, *Industrial Market Structure and Economic Perfor-mance* 163–64, 437–439, 490–494 (1970).

34. *U.S. Fed. Power Comm'n, National Power Survey* (1964).

35. See Breyer and MacAvoy, n. 31 *supra*.

36. 15 U.S.C. § 17 (1976) (labor organizations); Capper-Volstead Act of 1922, 7 U.S.C. §§ 291–292 (1976) (farming); Fisherman's Cooperative Marketing Act, 15 U.S.C. §§ 521–522 (1976) (fishing).

37. Brannan, "Prices and Incomes: The Dilemma of Energy Policy," 13 *Harvard Journal of Legislature* 445, 447 (1976).

38. See Federal Communications Act, 47 U.S.C. §§ 151–609 (1970).

DIFFERENT MODES OF CLASSICAL REGULATION AND THEIR PROBLEMS*

Stephen Breyer, *Professor of Law, Harvard University*

THE REGULATORY WEAPON: THE CLASSICAL TYPES OF REGULATIONS AND THEIR INHERENT CHARACTERISTICS

The great variety of regulatory problems makes it tempting to conclude that each program or system of regulation is unique. This is not the case, however. Almost all classical examples of regulatory programs can be grouped into seven types or "forms:"

1. Cost-of-service ratemaking

2. Historically based price setting

3. Allocation under a public interest standard

4. Historically based allocation

5. Standard setting

6. Individualized screening

7. Disclosure regulation

Any one regulatory program may involve several of these activities. Regulators soon discover that each of these forms is usually accompanied by certain typical problems which often cannot be resolved successfully and should be recognized in advance as defects characteristic of that particular regulatory regime.

Each individual regulatory form is applied in widely divergent substantive contexts. Public interest allocation, for example, describes the allocation of broadcasting licenses, airline routes, liquor licenses, and certain scarce natural resources.

In addition, all regulatory programs are subject to the following institutional constraints:

216

First, the relationship between the regulator and the affected industries is often adversary.

Second, the regulator is itself an institutional bureaucracy operated by people who prefer to design rules which they can administer with relative ease.

Third, despite the talk of sudden growth,[1] regulation has emerged gradually over many years, and new programs usually copy old ones. Thus, the framers of the Civil Aeronautics Act (1938),[2] precursor of today's Federal Aviation Act,[3] copied the language of the Interstate Commerce Act (1887)[4] which in turn was modeled after the British Railroad Act (1845).[5] Those devising new programs have always been the prisoners of history.

Fourth, regulatory agency decisions are subject to the requirements of administrative law, chiefly codified in the Administrative Procedure Act (APA).[6] At a minimum, agencies may make decisions only after (1) giving advance notice; (2) allowing affected parties "some kind of hearing;" and (3) providing a public record of the reasons for their actions. Agencies must always act so that they may justify their decisions before a court of law, which may decide whether an agency's decision in a particular case was rational and fair.

Cost-of-Service Ratemaking

Whenever regulators are asked to set industry prices, they are more likely than not going to use cost-of-service ratemaking, whether the justification be control of monopoly power, rent control, or excessive competition. This system has been most often used to set rates for public utilities such as electricity producers.[7] But agencies have also used it to set rates for airlines, natural gas producers, and others.[8]

The system involves determining a firm's costs and then allowing the firm to set prices sufficient only to cover those costs. The regulator determines the firm's revenue requirement by. (1) Selecting a test year; (2) adding together that year's operating costs, depreciation, and taxes; and also (3) adding a reasonable profit determined by multiplying a reasonable rate of return times the rate base, i.e., investment, which is determined by taking historical investments and subtracting prior depreciation. Prices are then set so that revenue yield equals revenue requirement. The regulator must also determine a rate structure—the price to be charged for each different service or to each class of customer.

Cost-of-service ratemaking is often used where the object of regulation is to replicate those prices that would exist in well-functioning competitive markets. But certain inherent defects in the cost-of-service ratemaking system make this objective impossible to achieve.

Use of historical costs Regulators determine the investment upon which the firm is allowed to earn a return on the basis of historical cost or actual dollars invested instead of replacement costs. This distinguishes regulated firms from firms competing in an open market, since the latter are materially affected by rising (or falling) reproduction costs. Regulators use historical costs, however, because reproduction costs would usually produce higher rates and also because such costs are difficult to measure.[9]

Calculation of a rate of return There is no scientifically correct method of determining the cost of capital or a "just and reasonable" rate of return. The two methods typically used—the "comparable earnings" method and the "discounted cash flow" method[10]—provide only a very rough approximation of the rate of return required to attract capital in a competitive rather than regulatory environment.[11]

Creation of efficiency incentives Insofar as cost-of-service ratemaking manages to hold prices close to costs, it provides little incentive for efficiency.[12] A variety of ad hoc measures are substituted for the carrot and stick ("increased profit" versus "loss of business to others") that a competitive marketplace provides. These measures include "bonus points" in allowable rate of return,[13] deliberate delays in ratemaking proceedings during noninflationary periods (with firms keeping any extra profits made during the interval), and efforts to supervise major expenditures—efforts that may call for more expertise than most commissions possess. Yet it is often extremely difficult to determine whether increased profits result from greater efficiency, changing market conditions, or market defects producing monopoly profits. Indeed, the more the agency attempts to supervise the firm's production processes directly, the more it simply replicates within itself the staff of the regulated firm.

Recognition of changes in cost of demand Commissions find it unusually difficult to adjust rates to reflect likely changes in cost or demand. Probable inflation in future costs is often regarded as too "speculative" to warrant price increases.[14] Similarly, commissions are aware that changes in price will affect demand and thereby affect revenues. Yet they often ignore probable demand changes. It is hard to estimate the effect of price changes on demand (demand elasticity) since consumers adapt gradually and differently to price changes over time; therefore, it is particularly difficult for commissions to choose among models of demand elasticity presented by adversary parties.[15]

The problems of ratemaking are especially acute during periods of falling or rising costs. Under most regulatory statutes, it is procedurally difficult for commissions to force firms to lower existing rates, although they have considerable power to delay or modify requested rate increases, and are usually under political pressure to resist them. Hence, whereas when costs are falling regulation often appears to be ineffective, when costs are rising it appears to be unreasonable.

Allocation of costs Finally, it is difficult for regulators to determine a
proper rate structure, for there is virtually no way to determine what proportion of fixed costs or joint costs each class of customer should bear. This problem does not arise in a competitive market where allocation of joint costs is determined primarily by comparative demands for final products. The butcher charges less per pound for chicken necks than breasts not because less grain is needed to grow a neck but because people do not want chicken necks as much as they want chicken breasts.

It can be argued that, for reasons of efficiency, the regulator should distribute fixed costs among classes of customers in inverse proportion to their elasticity of demand (i.e., let those whom a higher price is most likely to discourage pay the least). But this formula runs into practical problems surrounding the making of estimates of demand elasticity.[16] Furthermore, the correct distribution of fixed costs and corresponding markups changes over time as markets, consumer preferences, and technologies change.

Even worse, those charged the higher markups under the inverse proportionality rule will have strong incentives to find alternative sources of supply. As technologies proliferate, their chances of successfully finding such alternatives will increase sharply. The stability of price discrimination imposed by regulatory fiat is thus likely to be under constant attack and to be particularly susceptible to erosion in areas of rapid technological change. This susceptibility will increase as the gap widens between costs and the prices established by regulation.

In general, any joint cost allocation scheme and associated price discrimination in regulated markets will be plagued by the uncertainties surrounding market technological developments. Such practices will also be affected by the fact that different regulatory bodies (say, state and federal, in the case of the telephone company) may have jurisdiction over different end services, some of whose costs are joint. Divisions of cost then tend to reflect political or other arbitrary factors rather than an effort to achieve an "economically efficient" outcome. Furthermore, some commissions find it particularly difficult to experiment with different price systems which contain economic incentives that allow for more efficient use of existing plants (although some commissions have adopted off-peak pricing plans, with lower prices when full capacity is not being used).[17]

In a nutshell, the need for rules that are administratively practical and the difficulty of making economic predictions about changes in demand and costs (particularly about the effect of price changes on demand) make it impossible for the regulator to replicate the price and output results of a hypothetically competitive world. For various reasons, the competitive world is one in which prices can adjust fairly rapidly. Prices are based on present costs and not those of a "test year," changes in demand resulting from changes in price are taken into account as they occur, and firms can experiment with different price structures. The regulated world, on the other hand, is one in which prices remain stable for fixed periods of time. Although prices may not yield the amount of revenue that the regulator expects, and although costs will increase or decrease due to changes in efficiency, prices will not change quickly nor will those changes reflect increases or decreases in the cost of supplying similar service. In short, regulated firms find price experimentation difficult. This is due in large part to the rigidity required for administrative, legal, and political reasons.

Two conclusions can be drawn from this discussion. First, attempts to obtain economic precision in the regulatory process are unlikely to be worth the effort expended. Second, insofar as one advocates price regulation (or cost-of-service ratemaking) as a "cure" for market failure, one must believe the market is working very badly before advocating regulation as a cure. Given the inability of regulation to reproduce the competitive market's price signals, only severe market failure would make this regulatory game worth the candle.

Historically Based Price Regulation

When the government seeks to control the prices of large numbers of firms with disparate costs, as is true of economywide price controls, the only practical method is an historically based system.[18] Each firm is allowed to charge the price it charged on a particular historical date plus, for example, "additional costs," or "8 percent extra per year." The system works in the short run because historical price is readily ascertainable, the same rule applies to all firms, and the basics of the system are easily understood by the industry and the public. It thus tends to be self-enforcing.

Over time, however, the system is plagued with problems that become ever more serious. First, the regulator must decide how to price new products, how to deal with existing firms that are earning low profits or are losing money, and how to treat new plant investment (what "additional cost" does it impose?).[19] These problems begin to require consideration of individual firms or industries, and the problems associated with cost-of-service ratemaking begin to reappear.[20] Second, different items of the same type costing different dollar amounts to produce will come to have different prices, and the existence of different price "vintages" will lead to an allocation problem: Who gets the lower-priced product? Third, enforcement becomes ever more difficult as varieties of evasion become widespread. Credit, payment, terms of delivery, and discounts can be tightened. Product quality may deteriorate: Supermarkets may sell their "free" parking lots to developers, or lawyers may accomplish less work-per-hour billed. Customer services can be reduced. Evasion schemes may arise as they did, for example, during World War II when some butchers insisted that chicken buyers take (and pay extra for) the skin. As with other sorts of price regulation, those subject to it will search for unregulated markets in which to sell their products: Natural gas producers will try to sell

their gas in intrastate markets; cattle raisers will ship their beef to
Canada; medical equipment producers will make models just cheap
enough to fall outside the category of medical expenditures subject to
government control. Fourth, it becomes difficult to direct new investment to where it is most needed, for prices are not allowed to rise in
response to increased consumer demand or producer need.

In sum, the system becomes more and more complex as the regulator
seeks to meet each problem with additional price, quality, or allocation
regulation. It tends inevitably to evolve towards cost-of-service
ratemaking in which firms or industries are regulated individually in
accordance with classical principles.

Allocation Under a Public Interest Standard

Regulators frequently must allocate scarce resources such as television
licenses, liquor licenses, airline routes, certificates-of-need for hospitals, or natural gas among competing applicants. When the regulator
cannot legally use a market-based system (e.g., an auction) or a lottery
to do so, and when supply is too limited to satisfy all the applicants who
meet minimum standards of qualification, the regulator often develops
a procedure, such as hearings, for comparing applicants to determine
which is the "best."

This method of awarding scarce items is characterized by the need to
decide (in chronological order): (1) What precisely will be given away;
(2) what threshold criteria will eliminate those who are not minimally
qualified; (3) which of the remaining applicants is "best;" and (4) how
long the successful applicant is to retain the license or right to a commodity. The most difficult decision typically is the third—who is the
"best" among those minimally qualified? To make this decision, regulators usually promulgate a lengthy list of conflicting criteria, but
ultimately rely upon subjective judgment to apply and to balance those
criteria in individual cases.[21]

At the heart of the regulator's problem is the tension between a
desire to find standards that will "objectively" select the winner and a
belief that the exercise of subjective judgment is inevitable. The Federal
Communication Commission's (FCC) efforts to develop standards for
awarding television licenses, for example, have led it to emphasize
"diversity of media ownership" and "integration of management and
ownership" as the key factors determining selection.[22] Yet if rigorously
applied, the first of these would favor General Motor's acquisition of a
Detroit station over that of an Albuquerque newspaper owner. The
second would tend to favor managers rich enough to put up their own
capital. The FCC will modify the application of these standards by
considering and subjectively balancing other factors, such as past experience, trustworthiness, plans, and financial backing, in order to
meet the original goal of the regulatory statute; but then it is subjective
judgment that tends to decide close cases.

The task is managerial, rather like selecting an executive; objective criteria simply cannot be applied determinatively if one wishes to find the best person for the job. This tension between the need for objective standards and the importance of subjective judgment spawns several problems that typically plague public interest allocation, which can be illustrated by airline route allocation.

First, it is difficult to separate "what" is being allocated from the question of "who" will get it. As in the writing of job descriptions, one can shape the "what" so that the "who" is also decided. To avoid this, the CAB will hold massive hearings covering route selections for the entire South in which "what" and "who" questions are simultaneously at issue. Delta Airlines might argue, for example, that the Board should award a "Tucson/Los Angeles route" (for which Delta believes itself to be the most logical candidate), while National Airlines could argue for an "El Paso/Los Angeles route with a Tucson stopover" (for which National considers itself to be the most logical candidate). The number of proposed combinations and permutations in a single set of such area hearings can be very large.

Second, the selection process, once past the minimum qualification stage, runs into the major standard-setting problem discussed *supra*; there are simply too many relevant standards and no clear rules as to how they apply to individual cases or how they are to be weighed against each other. When awarding routes, the CAB takes into account such diverse factors as: (1) Whether the carrier will render effective service desired by the public; (2) whether it can provide benefits to "beyond segment" traffic; (3) whether there will be "route integration"; (4) the needs of local communities; and (5) the carriers' need for financial strengthening.[23] Yet the Board has not, and really cannot, make clear precisely how these criteria apply or how they are to be weighed against each other.[24]

The result of having standards which simply list "factors" without clear priorities is unmanageable agency hearings.[25] The number of issues remains open; each applicant argues for the preeminence of criteria that favor its cause; evidence on each point is voluminous (for who knows what final argument will spell the difference in a close case). Inconsistent decision making may also result, for there is no way the public or the courts can determine whether the agency is balancing consistently from case to case. Indeed, the CAB's staff described the results of the Board's carrier selection processes as "random."[26] Finally, the public may even suspect that routes, permits, or commodities are being awarded without clear standards by political appointees to repay political debts.[27]

Third, the renewal process favors incumbents. The FCC has refused to renew television licenses only twice in its history.[28] This is not surprising since it pits actual performance against unsubstantiated promises. It forces the regulators to notice that an identifiable party has relied upon continuing possession of a license regardless of possible warnings by regulators not to do so.[29] The deep-seated regulatory tendency to protect such identifiable reliance interests—whether or not

incumbents have received advance warnings—may reflect political, **223**
legal, or moral factors. When the other factors governing selection of an *Different Modes*
applicant conflict, incumbency tends to carry the day, for it points to a *Regulation*
of Classical
single applicant.

Historically Based Allocation Regulation

Just as history can provide a simple standard for temporarily circumventing cost-of-service ratemaking, so it can help to circumvent the
complexity of public interest allocation—but at a price. Goods temporarily in short supply (such as oil in 1973, California water in 1976, or
natural gas in 1977) can be allocated provisionally according to historical
usage in a specific preceding year, less a designated percentage of that
usage. This system has many of the same virtues and vices of historically based price regulation. It, too, is unstable and tends to evolve
towards public interest allocation.

A first major problem arises out of the progressively greater need to
make exceptions. Strictly historical allocation will appear increasingly
unfair over time. While one family, growing in size, needs an increasing supply of water, another, stable in size, needs it for watering its
lawn. Firm A could easily use nearby coal instead of oil; Firm B could
not. Some account must be taken of new entry. To ignore the new
family is unjust; to ignore the new firm threatens anticompetitive stag-
nation. Finally, unless quotas are shiftable, existing industrial patterns
are frozen, and an industry is unable to react to shifting consumer
needs or to new technologies. As exceptions are made, factors justifying
more exceptions proliferate and, again, one is faced with an ever more
complex system that evolves towards public interest allocation.

Second, historical allocation of goods in scarce supply typically requires price controls. Once price controls are instituted, one encounters
the problems previously discussed.[30] If price controls are not instituted,
allocation simply allows those with historical rights the power to earn
windfall profits as they sell, for example, taxi medallions or liquor
licenses to those who will pay the most for them. Only where controls
are temporary and resale is impractical (as in the case of water rationing
in California) can this problem be avoided.

Third, widespread allocation controls (like widespread price controls) are usually temporary. Out of this arises the perverse incentive to
raise prices or to increase consumption before controls are imposed, so
that the user's base is higher when they take effect.

Standard-Setting

At the outset it needs to be recognized that in certain areas standard-
setting is essential. Certain dangerous chemicals or pharmaceuticals
must be altogether prohibited or their use or availability regulated.
Even when such substances involve unknown risks, standards greatly
limiting or prescribing their use may be necessary. But in other areas,

one might ideally expect standards to be set through application of cost-benefit principles. The regulatory agency would first define the adverse effects caused by an industrial product or process and then try to identify the particular causal element that it seeks to control. It would obtain relevant information and write a standard with maximum benefits (in terms of stopping adverse effects), minimum costs (the standard's undesirable side effects), and acceptable distributional consequences. The agency would then enforce that standard, revising it in the light of careful monitoring of results.

The actual process—whether it involves such difficult problems as the setting of safety standards for automobiles or the development of environmental standards for smelters—differs radically from this "policy planner's ideal." It usually relies heavily on political debate to specify the problem (e.g., auto safety) and the elements to be controlled (e.g., brakes and seatbelts, but not outside signal lights to call the attention of the police to excessive speed). Furthermore, political considerations or statutory requirements frequently force regulatory agencies to act hastily, thus resulting in undue reliance on existing precedents for the creation of initial standards. The Occupational Safety and Health Administration (OSHA), placed under a statutory deadline, simply republished hundreds of existing safety standards culled from the rulebooks of other organizations, including such outdated rules as the one forbidding ice in drinking water because the ice might be cut from polluted ponds.[31] The process relies for the formulation of standards to a considerable degree on a form of negotiation among the affected parties in which political factors play an important role.

The procedure is also subject to a lengthy delay. The development of safety standards for automobiles, for example, has dragged on for years; more than ten years for passive restraints, seven for brakes, and nearly eight for tires.[32] The resulting standards have proven surprisingly inflexible and resistant to change. The National Highway Traffic Safety Administration (NHTSA), for example, found in 1976 that its 1969 "head restraint" standard for automobiles was ineffective, but has not yet been able to change it.[33]

The most typical and most serious of the standard-setter's problems is the need for and the difficulty in obtaining accurate and complete information.[34] The regulator's sources of information are normally limited and have characteristic flaws.[35] The industry may provide relevant data, particularly about technology, probable costs, and likely economic impact. But the adversary posture of the industry often leads the regulator to distrust industry-provided information, for the industry has an incentive to supply that information most favorable to its cause.[36] Since the industry need respond only with information relevant to a specific proposed standard, the adversary relation also hinders the production of complete information useful in developing alternative standards. Only occasionally can regulators overcome these problems by exploiting potential adversary relationships among different elements of the industry or industries before them.[37]

The agency can instead turn to its staff for expertise and information.

Yet much of the needed information is so detailed that only by replicating the industry's expertise could the agency obtain it.[38] How else is the agency to determine, for example, precise characteristics of an all-weather track that can be used to test the comparative wear and tear, blowout, and stopping distance characteristic of tires? Will a 5,000-mile test, instead of a 10,000-mile test, discriminate against tires that wear out quickly for the first 5,000 miles but then more slowly? NHTSA was able to answer such detailed but important questions in its 8-year tire standard-setting effort only after hiring a retired vice president of Uniroyal.[39] Aside from the conflict-of-interest problems inherent in such an approach, it is both impractical and wasteful to try to replicate vast amounts of industry expertise.

The agency can also seek help from outside experts such as academic authorities or consultants.[40] But often these experts themselves must rely for their information upon industry. Finally, consumer groups often in an adversary posture toward industry tend to share the government's difficulty in acquiring adequate information.

Moreover, the information available *anywhere* may be less than complete. To avoid reliance upon past standards, agencies may be tempted to guess the extent to which industry will be able to develop new technology to meet the standard.

The need to develop information in an adversary mode makes the exploration of alternative standards time-consuming and the coordination among overlapping standards difficult.[41] The adversary method of information gathering produces back-and-forth question and answer, related to a specific proposed standard, which can undergo modification only over time. And insofar as the same firms are affected by several standards at issue, answers to requests for information may depend on other agency action, particularly if different agencies are involved.[42]

A second problem raised by standard-setting is enforcement. Regulators must have standards that are practicably and readily enforceable. Tests to determine compliance must be capable of simple application by the industry and agency staff. This need tends to bias the standard towards enforceability rather than relevance. For example, NHTSA's passive restraint standard must be designed to apply to a readily buildable test "dummy" even if doing so means requiring features not relevant to the protection of a human being.[43] Regulators often will have to choose between "design" standards which are readily enforceable and "performance" standards which encourage the development of new technology.[44]

The need for enforcement will bias their choice in the former direction. And the smaller the agency's resources, the more the agency must rely upon voluntary compliance for enforcement—which biases choice further in the direction of simple standards which the industry finds reasonable.

Third, standard-setting adversely affects competition within the regulated market. It makes the cost of doing business more expensive, raising entry barriers in the process.[45] At the same time, the specific standards chosen will favor some companies over others, often in unpredictable ways. For example, the selection of a bumper standard requiring no dent in 5-miles-per-hour crashes would favor rubber bumper manufacturers, while a standard allowing slight dents would keep steel bumper manufacturers in business.[46] Existing firms usually can influence regulators to write standards sufficiently flexible to keep them in business through specific exemptions or "grandfather" rights.[47] Potential entrants are unlikely to be persuasive. Accordingly, standards may create entry barriers inhibiting new competition.

Fourth, these standards must survive judicial review. Review ordinarily consists of a check by the courts to see whether the statute has been complied with to assure that the regulator has not acted arbitrarily or capriciously, and to make certain he or she has used fair procedures.[48] Since in practice courts usually uphold the agency's action,[49] at first blush it may seem surprising that these minimal requirements create problems.

Initially, the adversary process together with notice and opportunity for argument and counterargument (comment), which strikes a lawyer as basic to any fair procedure, aggravates the problems of standard-setting by making it more difficult to consider alternatives not included in the rulemaking notices to modify initially proposed standards,[50] and to coordinate one set of standards with another. To coordinate auto fuel economy standards with pollution exhaust standards, for example, or to determine which among the vast number of potential brake standards is best, involves regulators in what Lon Fuller described as a "polycentric," or "management" problem.[51] This problem is best solved through informal give-and-take among many knowledgeable and affected parties, with exploration of alternatives and patterns of overlapping standards, and with continual modification and revision. The back-and-forth nature of the notice-and-comment rulemaking process, with its requirement of new notice and a new round of comments with each significant change, does not lend itself easily to such an approach.[52] Recent court decisions restricting informal access to regulators by forbidding ex parte communications may further aggravate this back-and-forth problem.[53] (See Wright, Chapter Two, pages 145–146.)

Moreover, the requirement of judicial review necessitates compilation of a defensible record which draws the agency toward standards that can be documented[54] and supported by existing studies rather than toward new standard development which will lack apparently objective support. Finally, judicial review is time-consuming. Hearings, records compilation, and review, particularly for decisions involving highly complex technology, often take far longer than Congress expects in setting statutory deadlines.

These four types of problems—information, enforcement, competition, and judicial review—explain to a considerable degree why the standard-setting process so often deviates from the planner's ideal and

why in setting standards an agency is so often attracted to "negotiated"
or "mutually satisfactory" solutions.[55] Given the complicated and
time-consuming nature of these problems, an agency's accommodation
with adversary parties has obvious advantages. The agency's temptation to base its work on preexisting standards is understandable in light
of the difficulty of developing information needed to allow radical
departures. Preexisting rules also provide the regulator with security.
They are probably workable and enforceable and have been accepted as
nonarbitrary. Finally, one can easily see why rules tend to be rigid,
resisting modification or abolition, once one understands the time and
effort needed to work through the complex process of making a new
rule.

Individualized Screening

Vague standards (e.g., "qualified doctors") or scientific uncertainty
(e.g., products that cause cancer) require regulators to screen out on a
case-by-case basis those individual products or persons that do not
meet the vague or complex regulatory standards. Such individualized
scrutiny has been applied to airline pilots, lawyers, doctors, food additives, prescription drugs, toxic substances, pesticides, and nuclear
power plants. Appendix 5-A *infra* illustrates the special types of problems that arise with individual screening.

NOTES

1. A recent Brookings Institution report documents the growth of federal
   administrative organizations and concludes that there is little in the way of
   affirmative steps available to check the increase. H. Kaufman, *Are Government Organizations Immortal?* 47–52, 70–77 (1976).

2. Ch. 706, 52 Stat. 973 (*repealed* 1958).

3. Pub. L. No. 85-726, 72 Stat. 731 (1958) (current version at 49 U.S.C. §§
   1301–1551 (1970 & Supp. V 1975)); see, e.g., 49 U.S.C. § 1373b (Supp. V
   1975); 49 U.S.C. § 1374b (1970).

4. Ch. 104, 24 Stat. 379 (codified at 49 U.S.C. §§ 2, 3 (1) (1970).

5. 8 Vict. c. 20 (1845); 17 & 18 Vict. c. 31 (1854).

6. 5 U.S.C. §§ 551–559, 701–706 (1976).

7. See A. Kahn, Vol. 1, in "Market Defects," n. 12 *supra* at 25–35.

8. See generally *ibid.* at 150–153 and ns. 67, 69.

9. See Smyth v. Ames, 169 U.S. 466, 546–547 (1898); Missouri *ex rel.* South-
   western Bell Tel. Co. v. Public Serv. Comm'n, 262 U.S. 276, 289–312 (1923)
   (Brandeis, J., dissenting).

10. See generally A. Kahn, Vol. 1, in "Market Defects," n. 12 *supra* at 25–58.

11. The "comparable earnings" method suffers because earnings as a percent-
    age of book value in comparable industries vary over time and therefore
    provide only an approximate value; because industries being compared

may themselves earn higher than competitive returns; and because the returns needed to induce investment depend upon risk—and risks vary widely between industries and over time. The "discounted cash flow" method, on the other hand, lacks precision because it is based on measurable variables which cannot correlate precisely with "investor expectations;" because those objective factors which led investors to predict a certain growth rate in the past may not produce such a growth rate; because expected returns may change radically with changing economic conditions, governmental policies, or stock market expectations; and because regulatory policies themselves will affect investors' expected return.

12. To the extent that ratemaking is based on actual costs and is performed accurately and promptly, firms will not benefit by adopting cost-saving devices; the total saving produced by increased efficiency will flow to the consumer.

13. Firms judged to be more efficient are given a "bonus" by being allowed some extra profit above the cost of capital.

14. For a description of methods used by commissions to adjust to inflation, see *Public Utility Fortnightly,* July 20, 1978, p. 48; Jan. 19, 1978, p. 38; and Jan. 17, 1974, p. 49.

15. See e.g., Taylor, "The Demand for Electricity: A Survey," 6 *Bell Journal of Economics and Management Science* 74 (1975). See also Nordin, "A Proposed Modification of Taylor's Demand Analysis: Comment," 7 *Bell Journal of Economics and Management Science* 719 (1976); *CAB Report* in "Proposals for Regulatory Reform: An Introduction," n. 5 *supra* at 111. One expert who has spent much of his professional career estimating demand elasticity for air travel stated, "There has never been a study which satisfactorily removed the nonprice determinants of demand while successfully freezing the price determinants for a sufficiently long period of time to produce results which could be deemed extrapolable." *Oversight of Civil Aeronautics Board Practices and Procedures: Hearings before the Subcomm. on Administrative Practice and Procedure of the Senate Comm. on the Judiciary,* 94th Cong., 1st Sess., 2234 (1975) (statement of Harry A. Kimbriel) (hereinafter cited as *CAB Hearings*).

16. See, e.g., *CAB Report* in "Proposals for Regulatory Reform: An Introduction," n. 5 *supra* at 123–124 (1975).

17. See generally Joskow, "Electric Utility Rate Structures in the United States: Some Recent Developments (1977)," in *A Current Evaluation of the Performance of Public Utility Regulation* (W. Sichel, Ed., forthcoming).

18. See T. Manning, *The Office of Price Administration* (1960).

19. See generally Slawson, "Price Controls for a Peacetime Economy," 84 *Harvard Law Review* 1090 (1971).

20. See pp. 517–519 *supra.*

21. See Anthony, "Towards Simplicity and Rationality in Comparative Broadcast Licensing Proceedings," 24 *Stanford Law Review* 1, 26–38 (1971).

22. See *ibid.* at 28–29.

23. L. Keyes, "A Survey of Route Entry Awards by the CAB, 1969–1974 (1975)," in *Oversight of Civil Aeronautics Board Practices and Procedure: Appendix to Hearings Before the Subcomm. on Administrative Practices and Procedures of the*

Senate Comm. on the Judiciary, 94th Cong., 1st Sess., 2545 (1976) (hereinafter cited as *Appendix to Hearings*).

24. *Bureau of Operating Rights, Civil Aeronautics Board, The Domestic Route System: Analysis and Policy Recommendations* 50–52 (1974), reprinted in *Appendix to Hearings*, n. 23 *supra* at 2235, 2290–2292.

25. See Anthony, n. 21 *supra* at 46–48.

26. *Bureau of Operating Rights, Civil Aeronautics Board, The Domestic Route System: Analysis and Policy Recommendations* 63 (1974), reprinted in *Appendix to Hearings*, n. 23 *supra* at 2293.

27. See Schwartz, "Comparative Television and the Chancellor's Foot," 47 *Georgia Law Journal* 655 (1959).

28. WHDH, Inc., 16 F.C.C.2d 1 (1969), *aff'd sub nom.*, Greater Boston Television Corp. v. FCC, 444 F.2d 841 (D.C. Cir. 1970), *cert. denied*, 403 U.S. 923 (1971); In re Alabama Educ. Television Comm'n, 50 F.C.C.2d 461, 32 Rad. Reg. 2d (P & F) 539 (1975). See generally Citizens Communications Center v. FCC, 447 F.2d 1201 (D.C. Cir. 1971).

29. See, e.g., Hearst Radio, Inc., 15 F.C.C. 1149 (1951).

30. See pp. 220–221 *supra*.

31. R. Zeckhauser and A. Nichols, "The Occupational Safety and Health Administration—An Overview (1977)," reprinted in *Study on Federal Regulation, VI Senate Comm. on Governmental Operations*, 95th Cong., 2nd Sess., 169, 201 (1978).

32. J. Gotbaum, L. Seale, R. Barusch, M. Delikat and L. Masouredis, *The Standard-Setting Process in the National Highway Traffic Safety Administration* (Dec. 1977) (unpublished paper on file with author) (hereinafter cited as J. Gotbaum).

33. *Ibid.*, head restraints section at 9–19.

34. See H. & H. Tire Co. v. United States Dep't of Transp., 471 F.2d 350 (7th Cir. 1972) (government standards overturned where they were based on inadequate information); National Tire Dealers & Retreaders Ass'n v. Brinegar, 491 F.2d 31 (D.C. Cir. 1974); J. Gotbaum, n. 32 *supra*, Introduction at 26–27.

35. See Green and Nader, "Economic Regulations vs. Competition; Uncle Sam the Monopoly Man," 82 *Yale Law Journal* 871, 875 & n. 28 (1973). See also United States v. Automobile Mfrs. Ass'n, CCH Trade Cas. 87, 456 (C.D. Calif. 1969) (consent decree); R. Noll. *Reforming Regulation* 99–100 (1971).

36. See National Tire Dealers & Retreaders Ass'n v. Brinegar, 491 F.2d 31, 39–40 (D.C. Cir. 1974). See also United States v. Automobile Mfrs. Ass'n, CCH Trade Cas. 87, 456 (C.D. Calif. 1969) (consent decree enjoining, inter alia, conspiratorial "restrict(ion of) publicity of research and development relating to devices"); 117 *Congressional Record* 15, 626–27 (1971) (remarks of Rep. Burton).

37. See Chrysler Corp. v. Department of Transp., 515 F.2d 1053, 1060–1061 (6th Cir. 1975) (General Motors' initiative in gaining approval of its specifications for rectangular headlamps gives it permissible competitive advantage over Chrysler); J. Gotbaum, n. 32 *supra*, Introduction at 13, 14.

38. See sources cited n. 35 *supra*; J. Gotbaum, n. 32 *supra*, Introduction at 18.

39. Preliminary draft of J. Gotbaum, n. 32 *supra* (on file with the author).

40. See Automotive Parts & Accessories Ass'n v. Boyd, 407 F.2d 330, 342 (D.C. Cir. 1968); Morris, "Motor Vehicle Safety Regulation: Genesis," 33 *Law and Contemporary Problems* 536, 557, 560 (1968); J. Gotbaum, n. 32 *supra,* head restraints section at 11–12, fuel economy standards section at 4.

41. See J. Gotbaum, n. 32 *supra,* fuel economy standards section at 11, 13–14 (tension between fuel economy and auto emission control standards); Comment, "Regulatory Reform: Will an Injection of Competition Cure the Patient?" 52 *Tulane Law Review* 362, 375 & n. 72 (1978).

42. See Cutler and Johnson, "Regulation and the Political Process," 84 *Yale Law Journal* 1395, 1406–1407 (1975); Loevinger, "Regulation and Competition as Alternatives," 11 *Antitrust Bulletin* 101, 122 (1966). For a discussion of the arguments for and against forcing more cooperation between regulatory agencies, see R. Noll. n. 35 *supra* at 30.

43. Chrysler Corp. v. Department of Transp., 472 F.2d 659, 675–678 (6th Cir. 1972).

44. The Highway Safety Act of 1966, 23 U.S.C. § 402 (1976), mandates the use of performance standards, but such standards can be written so that in practice they compel the use of a particular design. See Chrysler Corp. v. Department of Transp., 515 F.2d 1053, 1058 (6th Cir. 1975). See generally J. Gotbaum, n. 32 *supra,* Introduction at 25–26.

45. See Green and Nader, n. 35 *supra* at 879–880; R. Noll, n. 35 *supra* at 23; J. Gotbaum, n. 32 *supra,* Introduction at 22; cf. Radiant Burners v. People's Gas, 364 U.S. 656 (1951) (private association's establishment of a seal of approval creates impermissible barriers to entry).

46. J. Gotbaum, n. 32 *supra,* bumper standards section at 35–38.

47. See Chrysler Corp. v. Department of Transp., 472 F.2d 659, 679 (6th Cir. 1972) (flexibility to keep different kinds of cars—specifically sports cars—on the road); R. Noll. n. 35 *supra* at 25–27; Stewart, "The Reformation of American Administrative Law," 88 *Harvard Law Review* 1669 (1975). If the agencies do not make standards flexible enough to keep going concerns in business, courts may interpret the statutes so as to provide the required flexibility. See H. & H. Tire Co. v. United States Dep't of Transp., 471 F.2d 350 (6th Cir. 1972); S. Rep. No. 1301, 89th Cong., 2d Sess., 6 (1966).

48. See Administrative Procedure Act § 10, 5 U.S.C. § 706 (1976); Chrysler Corp. v. Department of Transp., 472 F.2d 659 (6th Cir. 1972).

49. See, e.g., Chrysler Corp. v. Department of Transp., 515 F.2d 1053 (6th Cir. 1975); Automotive Parts & Accessories Ass'n v. Boyd, 407 F.2d 330 (D.C. Cir. 1968). But cf. Wagner Elec. Corp. v. Volpe, 466 F.2d 1013 (3d Cir. 1972) (agency order invalidated because it changed a rule without adequate notice and opportunity to comment).

50. See Stewart, n. 47 *supra* at 1772–1773. See also Wagner Elec. Corp. v. Volpe, 466 F.2d 1013 (3d Cir. 1972).

51. Fuller, "The Forms and Limits of Adjudication," 92 *Harvard Law Review* 353, 394 (1978).

52. See Wagner Elec. Co. v. Volpe, 466 F.2d 1013, 1019–1021 (3d Cir. 1972) (notice is inadequate where it fails to alert interested parties to all issues to be considered in rulemaking); cf. International Harvester Co. v. Ruckelshaus, 478 F.2d 615, 632, n. 51 (D.C. Cir. 1973) (rejecting endless rounds of notice and comment as absurd).

53. See Home Box Office, Inc. v. FCC, 567 F.2d 9, 51–60 (D.C. Cir. 1977) (ex parte communications must be made part of public record).

54. See National Tire Dealers & Retreaders Ass'n v. Brinegra, 491 F.2d 31, 50 & n. 44 (D.C. Cir. 1974). See also J. Gotbaum, n. 32 *supra*, head restraints section at 4, 5.

55. See Jaffe, "The Federal Regulatory Agencies in Perspective: Administrative Limitations in a Political Setting," 11 *Boston College Industrial and Commercial Law Review* 565, 565–566 (1970); Stewart, n. 47 *supra* at 1714.

APPENDIX 5-A: INDIVIDUALIZED SCREENING

The special types of problems that can arise with individual screening are well-illustrated by efforts to screen food additives in order to weed out low-risk carcinogens. As in standard-setting, the initial problem is to develop more precise standards or practical tests for identifying cancer-causing substances. Testing procedures are expensive, costing up to half a million dollars per chemical tested.[1] Because of the expense and time involved, only a few substances can be thoroughly tested for toxicity. Moreover, the tests adopted are, for practical reasons, unlikely to be convincingly tailored to the general regulatory goal. For example, suspected carcinogens are tested by using extremely high doses on laboratory animals over a short period of time when the real concern is over the effect of small doses on humans over a long period of time.[2] Such tests therefore rarely give results sufficiently accurate to warrant basing regulatory decisions upon them. Thus regulators find that test results will not relieve them of the need to make highly subjective, highly judgmental decisions in the face of inadequate information. This seems to be the inevitable result of the scientific uncertainty that calls for the use of individualized screening in the first place.

Second, there is an informational problem as in cases of ordinary standard-setting. The problem is aggravated in the case of individualized screening because regulators will often try to delegate the decision to a group of outside experts.[3] Often those who are most qualified to serve on such a panel are those who have the greatest potential conflict of interests—representatives of the producing industry or regulated profession.

Third, it is often more difficult to determine the benefits of a particular substance than to determine its risks. Determining health benefits in the case of a chemical additive, for instance, raises difficulties equal to determining its risks, with the added problem of assessing the health risks of potential substitutes to which consumers may turn.[4] Similarly, if one is not to license a nuclear plant because of potential dangers, one must also consider the benefits of providing additional power, the dangers posed by power shortages, and the dangers posed by alternative sources of power such as coal.[5] Each of these decisions, as well as the initial decision regarding potential dangers of the power plant, requires considerable expertise and the application of vague

232

standards. Furthermore, it is clear that both food additives and nuclear plants
provide nonhealth benefits, and these benefits must be assessed and weighed
against the danger to health.

Fourth, agencies evaluate existing products with criteria different from those used for new entrants. In the case of food additives, regulators often cope with other regulatory problems by imposing a strict burden of proof upon manufacturers who seek to introduce new substances.[6] The effect of imposing rigid test requirements is to make such products more expensive, and to reduce the likelihood they will be approved. Thus a new product may be screened out even though in fact it poses less danger and may provide greater benefits than a product already on the market. In the case of an existing product, significant groups of consumers or workers have expressed some preference for it, and presumably some benefit has been shown, so the regulator will be wary of banning it.

Finally, the problems posed by judicial review and limitations on administrative procedures are more pronounced in the case of individualized screening, since the process by its very nature is more like adjudication than rulemaking.

NOTES

1. For a discussion of the high cost of such testing see U.S. Council on Environmental Quality, *Sixth Annual Report* 26–28 (1975).

2. See Freedman, "Reasonable Certainty of No Harm: Reviving the Safety Standard for Food Additives, Color Additives, and Animal Drugs," 7 *Ecology Law Quarterly* 245, 277–78 (1978) (citing J. Verret and J. Cooper, *Eating May Be Hazardous To Your Health* 51–65 (1974)); Doniger, "Federal Regulation of Vinyl Chloride: A Short Course in the Law and Policy of Toxic Substances Control," 7 *Ecology Law Quarterly* 497, 512 (1978).

3. Doniger, *ibid.* at 514.

4. *Ibid.* at 516 (noting that the banning of a certain chemical in aerosols in 1974 led to the increased use of fluorocarbons, which have been found to be a threat to the environment themselves).

5. See Plumlee, "Perspectives in U.S. Energy Resource Development," 3 *Environmental Affairs* 1 (1974) (benefits of nuclear power source); Cockrell, "Coal Conversion by Electric Utilities: Reconciling Energy Independence and Environmental Protection," 28 *Hastings Law Journal* 1245 (1977) (problems involved in the use of coal as a power source). See generally S. Breyer, "Vermont Yankee and the Courts' Role in the Nuclear Energy Controversy," 91 *Harvard Law Review* 1833 (1978).

6. See Freedman, n. 2 *supra* at 256–259.

ALTERNATIVE REGIMES AND THE FRAMEWORK APPLIED*

Stephen Breyer, *Professor of Law, Harvard University*

ALTERNATIVE REGIMES

The merits of classical regulation, like old age, can be judged only after asking "compared to what?" A simple comparison with unregulated markets is inadequate; deregulation is not the only choice. There are a number of tools that may be used as alternatives or supplements to classical regulation. In any analysis carried out to identify cases of regulatory failure, the following alternatives should be considered.

Unregulated (Competitive) Markets Policed by Antitrust Laws

In deciding whether to regulate one should compare the likely defects of the unregulated market with the potential effectiveness, and the likely defects, of classical regulation.[1] But one should recognize that unregulated markets are subject to the antitrust laws—a form of government intervention designed to maintain a workably competitive marketplace.[2] Antitrust enforcement is a form of government regulation, but unlike classical economic regulation, it seeks to achieve the *conditions* of a competitive marketplace, rather than replicate the *results* of competition or correct for its defects.

The antitrust laws are most effective in prohibitions on mergers.[3] Effectiveness of the law is more debatable when enforcement requires discovery of surreptitious conduct such as price fixing among competitors. Nonetheless, these laws are generally thought to stop much price fixing, boycotts, market divisions, and other similar conduct, including instances in which individual firms charge below-cost predatory prices. The greatest strength of the antitrust laws lies in their ability to preserve competition in markets that are *already* structurally competitive.

Many would argue that antitrust effectiveness is minimal when enforcement requires lengthy litigation, as in monopolization cases.[4]

234

Moreover, the law itself, as traditionally interpreted, allows antitrust
enforcers to restructure markets only when a single firm monopolizes a market. It does not allow restructuring of highly concentrated industries in which a handful of major firms may together exercise significant market power.[5]

Antitrust enforcement is not a useful tool for controlling the market power of a natural monopolist, for the ordinary antitrust remedies of dissolution or divestiture are inappropriate. Moreover, antitrust enforcement is not directly relevant to the problem of spillover costs, or to the failure of the market to supply adequate information to consumers (unless the failure is conspiratorial). Antitrust is more useful in dealing with the problems of excessive competition insofar as those problems amount to concern with predatory pricing.

Disclosure Regulation

When used for economic regulatory purposes, disclosure[6] typically helps buyers make more informed choices. Regulators must set standards governing what is to be disclosed, where, and how. They must decide how these standards will be enforced. In setting those standards, they will have to deal with those very problems of information, enforcement, anticompetitive effects, and judicial review that affect other forms of standard-setting.[7] Additional discussion and examples of disclosure regulation for tires are presented in Appendix 5-B *infra.*[8]

Taxes As A Substitute for Classical Regulation

Taxation ordinarily seeks to raise revenue or to encourage conduct through special deductions or credits. The tax system has also been used as a means of stimulating socially or economically desirable action that otherwise might have been sought through more direct governmental regulation.[9]

Tax-free municipal securities are an example of an attempt by government to stimulate voluntary allocation of private capital to public projects at the state and local level and to reduce the cost of capital to those lower levels of government.

Only rarely have taxes been designed as a specific substitute for regulation. But taxation could certainly be used where regulation is aimed simply at transferring income, as when cost-of-service ratemaking is used to control windfall profits received by those who control scarce, low-cost sources of a commodity, such as oil or gas. Taxes might provide a more efficient way to transfer this income. Second, taxes might be used to deter socially undesirable conduct, such as pollution. Thus, a tax system could supplement or substitute for classical standard-setting by providing incentive for ever more technological changes and innovation in a socially desired direction.[10]

In applying taxation to the problem of spillovers, it will often be difficult to determine the correct rate of taxation in order to achieve the desired result. This and other problems involved in using taxes to control spillovers may be overcome to some extent through the use of a closely related system of market-based incentives: A limited number of rights to engage in the conduct (such as pollution) are established, and these are then bought and sold on the free market. Eventually those willing to pay the most for the privilege of engaging in the conduct, usually those for whom the costs of avoiding or limiting the conduct would be the greatest, will buy up the rights. Although such a system raises the problem of the initial allocation of rights (which could be accomplished by a market system such as an auction), the subsequent operation incorporates the flexibility and freedom of choice inherent in the competitive market.

Systems based on this principle have been employed in Germany's Ruhr Valley. Though the system originated to deal with pollution, it might be used whenever it is desired to limit artificially the amount of a certain activity, and it is not necessary that the allocation of the right to engage in the activity be on a public interest basis.[11]

For the allocation of a privilege such as an FCC license, it might well be preferable to give qualified applicants an equal chance to be selected by lottery rather than to apply arbitrary standards. Another alternative would be to conduct an auction among qualified applicants, inasmuch as the government now assigns licenses which may be sold for large sums after only a brief period of operation. An auction permits the government to be paid for the value of the privilege it is granting. This is precisely how the federal government now licenses offshore exploration for oil. To avoid dominance of the market by the richest firms, joint bidding ventures among large firms could be prohibited and the number of broadcast stations or oil exploration licenses awarded to any one firm could be limited.

Bargaining

The major advantage of bargaining as a method of dealing with regulatory problems is that it achieves consensus. Agreement among those affected by regulation tends to avoid the distortions and difficulties arising out of classical regulation's adversary mode and its formal back-and-fourth procedures.[12] Bargaining also helps the various parties to maximize the benefits they can obtain at the expense of others: Each side must set its own priorities and then trade-off those desired less for those desired more. With bargaining it is easier to tailor different rules to special needs, and voluntary compliance is thus more likely.

The major weaknesses of bargaining are three. First, there must be some way to force the parties to reach agreement, and that way may affect their comparative bargaining strengths.[13] Second, the intended beneficiaries of regulation too frequently are not organized or lack the requisite bargaining power to make the process meaningful. Third, and perhaps most importantly, the final decision may affect others who are not at the bargaining table and who cannot protect themselves.[14] Despite these problems, collective bargaining is thought to work well in labor relations, where the need to achieve consensus is primary. As applied to regulatory matters, however, consensus may be thought less important. In principle, the government can impose a solution. Moreover, affected parties may agree most readily only about "worst" cases—the most obvious examples of the evil at which the regulatory program is aimed. Obtaining agreement about how to proceed against lesser evils may be more difficult. But as one abandons the goal of perfect regulation and begins to understand the serious problems embedded in each mode of classical regulation, the use of bargaining becomes an attractive alternative.

Other Possible Alternatives

Changes in liability rules   In certain instances of spillovers, such as accident safety and environment pollution, scholars have suggested changes in tort law that would encourage the production of safer products or the greater use of pollution-free processes.[15] The notion behind these proposals is to increase the risk of liability (and thus the cost) for those who can most readily reduce the risk of accidents or the level of, for example, air pollution. To rely upon changes in liability rules, however, has often not been thought sufficient.[16] The costs of using the courts are high, and those harmed may have inadequate incentive to bring suit. Results are likely to vary from court to court, at least when damages are measured.[17] Finally, court decisions inevitably reflect moral[18] and legal considerations that may conflict with the regulatory goals.

Nationalization   Nationalization as an alternative is less utilized in the United States than elsewhere, although publicly owned utilities are an example of its application. In principle, it offers a preferable solution to many market defects because it eliminates the adversary relation between regulator and firm. In practice, however, it has been felt to suffer from two serious political defects. Its critics have feared that staffing would reflect political considerations. The writer Ambrose Bierce, for example, defined a lighthouse as a "tall building on the seashore in which the government maintains a lamp and the friend of a politician."[19] Second, there is the risk that government may view the nationalized industry as an instrument for carrying out a variety of desirable social objectives. British and French nationalized airlines were forced to buy the Condorde for reasons of "national prestige" despite the fact that doing so was economically unsound.[20] PanAm and TWA were not under comparable pressures and did not buy the Concorde.

This section discusses the implications for substantive reform of the analytical framework outline in "Market Defects" *supra*. It will outline several rules of thumb which the framework suggests for selecting candidates for a change in regulatory regime. Finally, it will describe the preliminary work which is essential if analysis is to be followed by action.

The Framework in Relation to Existing Programs

The proposed framework, then, consists of three sets of considerations:

1. Typical market defects thought to call for regulation.

2. Modes of classical regulations with typical accompanying problems.

3. Alternative regimes.

The application of this basic framework may alert an administrator, or one who is proposing new regulatory programs, to problems he or she is likely to encounter and may guide him toward alternative solutions.

The contemporary problem of controlling rising medical costs provides one example. One possible problem with relying on a free market, as explained *supra*, is "moral hazard," which results in a lack of incentive on the part of hospitals to hold down costs. The Carter administration has proposed a regulatory program that would hold hospital prices to "historical costs plus a percentage fixed by statutory formula (9 percent per year)."[21] Those considering such a program should be aware that the historical system of price-setting evolves toward cost-of-service ratemaking as the need for exceptions forces consideration of individual cases.[22] In the case of hospitals, considerations giving rise to exceptions might include new units, special historical need, unusually costly items required by the nature of the service or by the needs of the users, and the inability to stop wage increases. Given the ability of hospitals to appeal directly to legislatures, the regulator is unlikely to be able to ignore justifiable claims for exception.

The resulting cost-of-service ratemaking in turn brings with it the classical set of problems accompanying that regime, including those problems associated with the test year, inefficiency, and rate structure. Since those creating such a program are doing so in an effort to improve efficiency, knowledge of the inability of cost-of-service ratemaking to promote efficiency—perhaps its greatest single weakness—calls into question the regulatory scheme.

An alternative way of controlling medical costs directly is to impose a limit on capital expenditures, but requiring hospitals to obtain a Certificate-of-Need (CON) before making such expenditures also raises problems.[23] The framework suggests that the regulator will then face a serious set of allocation problems—at least if the number of CONs is limited and must be allocated to hospitals with exclusive demand for them. The regulator may try to find a set of standards that automatically

and objectively selects the "winning" applicants for CONs—standards, for example, that allow hospitals to maintain what they presently (historically) operate, that categorize and allocate through some form of numerical quota ("all in category X get Y percent increase"), or that share the CONs among competitors equally (Hospital A gets an additional allocation in category X, but Hospital B gets an additional allocation in category Y). Experience would indicate that the agency will not find any set of standards that can obviate the need for a multitude of special exceptions ("special historical programs with special needs," "special program quality," "unusual need of population served," "unique opportunity to obtain necessary land," "special importance of new equipment X," etc.), particularly if a meaningful limit is to be placed on an area's total expenditure.

Accordingly, the regulator must inevitably move toward public interest allocation. It will then be faced with the usual problem of many factors relevant to a decision and no clear way to balance or weigh them. This tends to result in lengthy proceedings and to cause inconsistent decision making amid suspicions of favoritism. To avoid these problems, which are typically associated with public interest allocation, the program might (as in some cities where the CON program is now being administered)[24] allow hospitals to negotiate among themselves on how CON entitlements will be allocated. Such negotiation may work to the disadvantage of community interests who do not participate in the bargaining: It may not be totally rational, and it will reflect political considerations. But it is also true that negotiation leads to consensus among those directly affected, that knowledgeable parties make the allocation decision, and that the worst cases of waste are likely to be stopped. These advantages may make this form of bargaining solution preferable to the alternatives when there is a demonstrable need for entitlements at all existing hospitals.

The above example suggests several general principles that follow from the framework. First, regulation should seek simple rules directed at "worst cases." Efforts to cure every minor defect or to close every conceivable loophole are ultimately counterproductive. In fact, United States experience suggests that attempts to do this are impossible and constitute one of the major weaknesses of classical regulation.

Second, regulators should rely upon incentives and bargaining when possible to induce more acceptable behavior. Incentives provide a practical method for reconciling the need for simple regulatory rules with the diversity and complexity of the industrial world.[25] Bargaining provides a practical method for identifying "worst cases" and obtaining effective cooperation in dealing with them.

Finally, the focus on problems accompanying classical regulation supports the notion of looking at economic regulation through a procompetitive lens and adopting a "least restrictive alternative approach. The unregulated market should be relied upon in the absence of a significant market defect. Where the harm produced by the unregulated market is serious, one should turn first to incentive-based (tax) or disclosure regulation. Only where that will not work should classical regulatory modes be adopted.

The Selection of Candidates for Reform: The Mismatch of Objective and Regime

Efforts at reform are likely to prove most fruitful in those cases where the harms caused by the regulation are serious and either the rationale for regulation is not compelling or there exists regimes less restrictive than classical regulation that will obtain its purported objectives.

AVOIDING THE MISMATCH OF OBJECTIVE AND REGIME

The framework suggests several maxims or rules of thumb that may help a legislator or administrator avoid a "mismatch" between a regulatory objective and the means chosen to achieve it.

The advisability of reliance on market forces in structurally competitive industries   Where classical price and entry regulation is applied to a structurally competitive industry, one should consider abolishing regulation and rely instead upon an unregulated market policed by antitrust laws. Three arguments support this conclusion. First, application of classical price and entry regulation is likely to produce unnecessary anticompetitive harms. In particular, cost-of-service ratemaking inhibits price cutting and price competition. Firms in a competitive industry subject to cost-of-service ratemaking will compete by providing excessive service or a higher quality product, giving the consumer more service or quality than he or she wants, and charging a higher price for doing so.[26] Second, regulators find it particularly difficult to apply cost-of-service ratemaking to an industry with many firms.[27] Third, the rationale for price regulation in such industries is ordinarily weak. The commonly given justification—excessive competition—is simply an empty box.[28] Insofar as one legitimately fears predatory pricing, alternatives to regulation such as the antitrust laws are available.

Appendix 5-C considers the case of the airline industry prior to the recent dramatic reform in airline regulation. This analysis of the difficulties in using classical regulation for the airline industry serves to illustrate why it is inappropriate, in general, to attempt to regulate price and entry in a structurally competitive industry.

Problems inherent in classical price and entry regulation   Classical price and entry regulation does not deal effectively with the need to control windfall profits over a long period. Although it is recognized that in emergencies regulation may be politically necessary, a tax system should be considered as a substitute, for the objective of windfall control is to capture profits earned by producers and to transfer them to consumers. The problems of using a classical regulatory sys-

tem to deal with windfall profits are severe. They are great enough
to warrant detailed exploration of tax or comparable income transfer alternatives, for the problems inherent in these other methods seem less severe. If it is impossible to secure adoption of the alternative, the magnitude of the problems associated with classical regulation makes deregulation preferable to continued cost-of-service ratemaking.

Alternative approaches to classical standard-setting Controlling dangerous conditions and substances usually requires classical standard-setting. However, in dealing with problems of spillovers such as environmental pollution or safety, less restrictive tools such as taxes, disclosure, or bargaining should be considered as supplements to or as partial substitutes for classical standard-setting. Appendix 5-D *infra* discusses the feasibility of a tax regime or "marketable rights" system as a promising alternative to regulation in the pollution control area. Appendix 5-D shows that the needs for balancing the extent to which resources are put to conflicting use for providing incentives, for producing a broad variety of different end-results, and for dealing with a large number of enterprises all point toward the use of a tax[29] or similar incentive-based system. These advantages, weighed against the problems of standard-setting, make the effort to devise a practical complementary or alternative regulatory taxation mechanism important to substantive regulatory reform.

A stronger case for standard setting can be made with regard to workplace health and safety than pollution control. Workers exposed to toxic or carcinogenic agents will never, it is argued, have the information or background necessary to evaluate risks rationally, nor do they have the mobility to change jobs if knowledge of risks in alternative places or employment were fully available. Thus, some toxic substances must be banned altogether, but the total elimination of all risks is not feasible. OSHA's early experience suggests that the wholesale adoption of standards leads inevitably to inflexibility. A proper balance would include creation of incentives to avoid the more dangerous activities, products, and production processes, and to invent safer technology.

Inadequate information is often part of the problem, and disclosure requirements would provide a useful supplement to standard-setting. Where union contracts are in place, the bargaining system may help to resolve some safety problems in particular plants. An improved system of workers compensation would be a useful adjunct to safety standards by providing employers with enhanced incentives to improve safety conditions. These and other mechanisms used as supplements to safety standards would allow those standards to be used only for the most severe problems, where standards are both essential and practical.

Problems of cost-of-service ratemaking when applied to complex industries Cost-of-Service ratemaking seems reasonably well-suited to the natural monopoly problem, but its use in one portion of a complex industry radically alters the terms of the debate over regulation elsewhere in that industry. Classical cost-of-service ratemaking is reasonably capable of dealing with a single large firm with costs and demands that stay fairly constant. Its problems there, while serious, are less imposing than when the system is applied to markets with many firms and fluctuating costs and demand. In the former case, the system can hold prices somewhere near cost, offer some incentive for efficiency, and provide some guarantee of fair dealing for the customer.[30] More important, there is no obvious alternative regime that offers promise of significant improvement.[31]

One must be pessimistic about the likelihood that an alternative regime can effectively supplant classical regulation in this area. Whether the added costs of regulation are outweighed by the possibility that unregulated prices might significantly exceed regulated prices is a political question.

One of the economic difficulties encountered with the regulation of so-called natural monopolies is the tendency of the government to reach out and regulate enterprises which are not natural monopolies at all, but which in some way affect the regulated natural monopoly. The concern of the regulator is to protect the regulated entity from the risks of free competition; thus, for example, regulation of railroads led to regulation of the trucking industry, and regulation of broadcast television channels led to the regulation of the cable television business.

To decide that a firm is a natural monopolist with respect to one of its products and that it should be regulated does not decide the extent to which classical regulation should apply to other related products of the firm. Since most regulated firms are complex entities selling many different services, it is possible that regulation may be appropriate for some but not for others. Yet the very fact that the firm is regulated in part significantly affects the question of whether, or what, regulation is appropriate elsewhere. It distorts the competitive framework in related areas and makes the question of whether competition or regulation is appropriate in those other areas difficult to answer.

How should the natural monopoly be regulated when it is operating outside its noncompetitive area? How can cross-subsidies between monopoly and competitive businesses be prevented? How can full and fair competition be achieved in the nonmonopoly fields while protecting the interests of the monopoly consumers? Appendix 5-E *infra* uses the recent controversy surrounding the FCC's efforts to introduce competition into longline communications in an attempt to illustrate some of these problems posed. While the discussion in the appendix is not sufficient to determine whether competition should be allowed in private longline telecommunication, it does suggest that if one regulates a firm on grounds of natural monopoly, that fact will complicate the question of how far regulation should extend into related areas.

Skeleton for Regulatory Reform

In sum, the framework of primary problems, coupled with the mode of and problems with classical regulation and suggested alternative re-

gimes, helps to establish certain tentative linkages which may in turn
guide a program of meaningful regulatory reform. In particular, the
framework suggests the following matches between problems and solutions:

Problem	Tentative Solution
Natural monopoly	Cost-of-service ratemaking
Windfall control	Taxes or deregulation
Spillover	Taxes, market-based incentives, bargaining
Excessive competition	Deregulation (with antitrust enforcement)
Inadequate information	Disclosure regulation

The virtue of these tentative linkages is that they suggest where the
most serious mismatches may lie, and in some instances they suggest
the advisability of replacing classical regulatory programs with less
restrictive regimes.

FROM CANDIDATE TO REFORM: GENERAL SUGGESTIONS FOR INSTITUTING REGULATORY REFORM

The framework for analysis presented in this article does not conclu-
sively demonstrate in any individual case that reform should be made.
Rather, the framework helps to identify "candidates" (existing programs that should be considered as potential subjects) for individualized reform efforts. Appendix 5-F *infra* outlines the suggested steps
involved in the process of instituting regulatory reform which, in summary, calls for: (1) Identification of a candidate for reform; (2) a detailed
empirical study of the regulatory industry; (3) the gathering of the
necessary political support to pass reform programs; and (4) the development of a practical plan for implementation.

The most instructive case of how a procompetitive framework such
as that advocated here can guide reform to the point of achieving
practical results is that of airline regulatory reform. It is important to see
that the very process of making the issue of regulatory reform "visible"
can itself help to develop political coalition and bring it to the public's
attention. Thus airline deregulation, for example, was brought to the
public's attention in part through Senator Edward Kennedy's hearings
on CAB regulation in 1975.

It is also important to recognize the bipartisan nature of the regulatory reform issue. Airline deregulation has been strongly supported by
both the Ford and Carter administrations. Both Presidents have supported legislative proposals and have made procompetition appointments to the Board. Senator Thurmond, a conservative, and Senator
Kennedy, a liberal, both urged such reform.

Moreover, the political coalition was reinforced by consumer groups
supporting reform as a means to lower prices, business groups as a

return of free enterprise and good government groups as bringing about administrative improvement.

The hearings helped to depict the reform as an effort to help the consumer ("low prices" and "consumer protection") and to lessen the burdens imposed by a regulatory bureaucracy. Once the issue became one of "regulatory reform," it received support from many who would not have concerned themselves if the interest were depicted as "economic rationality," "higher airline profits," or "changing outmoded airline regulation."

The development of a supporting political coalition in this area was not overwhelmingly difficult, for the issue could be readily depicted in a manner appealing to a set of diverse political instincts. Indeed, political support is in part a function of how one sees the issue—how it has been characterized—and that is a matter partly but not wholly within the control of those who are seeking to bring about reform.

The detailed discussion of this CAB model for successful reform, illustrating the steps outlined in Appendix 5-F, is contained in Appendix 5-G *infra*. The experience outlined in Appendix 5-G suggests that Congress and more particularly a congressional committee, is an effective institution for bringing about major individual programs of substantive regulatory reform. A committee can combine its power to gather information with the power to develop significant political support. The executive branch possesses superior ability to do sustained detailed work, but it may be less capable of carrying out certain of the necessary political tasks. Moreover, the experience of the Subcommittee on Administrative Practice and Procedure suggests there may be an advantage in placing initial responsibility for reforming a particular program in the hands of a committee that does not ordinarily supervise the agency concerned. Although one thereby loses expertise, one is also freed from some of the political or institutional constraints that may make it difficult for the regular congressional committee to carry out the investigation.

The experience also suggests that reform of a particular substantive area requires an intellectual framework that will both identify a candidate for reform and guide a later detailed investigation. Candidates for reform are best treated individually once identified by the framework suggested in this article. The subsequent investigation may take months or years, but it is a necessary part of any effort to bring about significant change.

Finally, the airline reform example in Appendix 5-G suggests that a "transition plan" need not always be drawn up formally and presented in advance, nor is such a plan impossible to create. In part, the legislative process automatically tends to produce such a plan, for groups adversely affected by proposals for change seek amendment of it and will settle after negotiating for some form of protection. Moreover, time itself tends to ease transition. Several years elapsed between the initial Kennedy investigation, the publication of the Subcommittee's conclusions, and its implementation in the form of regulatory order and legislation. This fact itself helped the industry and others to adjust and plan for what they began to see as the growing risk of a significant change in the status quo.

SUMMARY AND CONCLUSION

The value of this study depends in part upon the usefulness of the categorization as outlined that divides economic regulation into specific modes. These are, in review:

1. Cost-of-service Ratemaking

2. Historically Based Price Setting

3. Allocation under a Public Interest Standard

4. Historically Based Allocation

5. Standard-Setting

6. Individualized Screening

7. Disclosure Regulation

This article illustrates how each form of regulation works and how regulators deal with typical problems. The article examines certain maxims or rules of thumb which emerged from the analysis, and which should help to determine when old regulatory programs should be abandoned and new programs designed.

This work suggests that in lieu of governmental intervention in the economy, more reliance should be placed, when feasible, upon the competitive market as regulator supported by the antitrust laws. If governmental intervention is required, consideration should be given to disclosure or to incentive-based modes of regulation before turning to the classical command-and-control modes.

Careful analysis is essential to avoid a mismatch between a particular need for governmental intervention and the regulatory method used to meet that need. In such analysis, four rules of thumb are useful.

1. In structurally competitive industries, consideration should be given to greater reliance on market forces in lieu of classical price and entry regulation.

2. Classical price and entry regulation does not deal effectively with the need to control windfall profits over a substantial period. Although it is recognized that in emergencies this type of regulation may be politically necessary, consideration should be given to substituting a tax system.

3. Cost-of-service ratemaking appears to be reasonably suited to the "natural monopoly" problem, but when applied to complex industries, it may create substantial difficulties.

4. Classical standard-setting is needed to protect the public by controlling dangerous conditions and substances. Where possible, however, in

dealing with problems of spillovers (such as environmental pollution or safety), less restrictive tools (such as taxes, disclosure, or bargaining) should be considered as supplements to or as partial substitutes for classical standard-setting.

Substantive reform of government regulation might begin with those programs which exhibit most clearly the problems inherent in classical regulation. Some of the examples used here suggest the areas of transportation, energy, health, safety, and environmental regulation as candidates for efforts to develop "less restrictive alternatives" to classical regulation. Appendix 5-H *infra* discusses why these areas are logical candidates for reform.

The framework for analysis developed and applied here may aid those charged with the responsibility of developing, administering, operating, and monitoring those regulatory activities. At the least, this analysis suggests abandoning the simplistic view that "imperfect" free markets call for the introduction of "perfect" governmental regulation.

Apart from the analysis, experience shows that effective action in the arena of regulatory reform requires strong political sponsorship, detailed empirical study, a mechanism to bring about public awareness, and careful attention to problems of transition.

Overall, regulatory reform is both a vital issue and a practicable goal. There is an immense amount of experience on which lawmakers and administrators in the executive branch can draw to avoid mismatches between demands for regulation and the means chosen to regulate a particular situation. Nevertheless, the question remains, even with such experience can the framework for analysis developed here help to avoid needless repetition of past mistakes? Can it assist in the reexamination of existing regulatory structures?

NOTES

1. See P. Areeda and D. Turner, 2 *Antitrust Law,* ¶ 401, p. 37 (1978). But see Kaysen and Turner in "Market Defects," n. 5 *supra* at 82 (rejecting notion of workable competition as an "undesirable policy standard").

2. See, e.g., Clayton Act §§ 2, 3, 15 U.S.C. 13, 14 (1976); Federal Trade Commission Act 5, 15 U.S.C. § 45 (1976).

3. Areeda and Turner, Vol. 2, no. 1 *supra* at ¶ 406b (realistic antitrust policy contents itself with inhibiting creation or extension of market power by merger).

4. Posner, "A Statistical Study of Antitrust Enforcement," 13 *Journal of Law and Economics* 365, 374–381 (1970).

5. Kaysen and Turner in "Market Defects," n. 10 *supra* at 110–111.

6. Regulation that requires disclosure of certain information is so common today that it may be regarded as another form of classical regulation. It is presented here as an alternative regime, however, because it does not regulate the production processes; the output, price, or allocation of products; or otherwise restrict the influence of individual choice in the marketplace as directly as do the classical regulatory forms discussed *supra.*

Moreover, like antitrust regulation, it can be viewed as helping to achieve a more competitive market.

7. See Breyer, "Different Modes of Classical Regulation and Their Problems," at 223–227 *supra*.

8. Of course the issue widely debated is whether consumers of health care can ever receive enough information to make intelligent choices. It is probably helpful to distinguish between information relative to individual medical treatment (the patient-doctor relationship) and information relative to institutional arrangements. In the former case, consumers will probably continue to rely on peer review and physician licensing. The thrust of much recent legislation which focuses on provider costs and services suggests that citizens should be able to exercise the same degree of control over health care institutions as they now do over local school systems—Ed.

9. For example, under the Tax Reform Act of 1969 taxpayers were permitted to amortize over a five-year period a portion of the cost of business machinery and equipment of longer useful life qualifying as pollution control facilities. Similar incentive provisions have been included in the tax laws to stimulate such divergent investments as child-care facilities, railroad cars, rehabilitation of low-income housing, and the employment of welfare recipients. See Pub. L. 91-172, § 704(a), and Internal Revenue Code 40 (employment of welfare recipients), 167 (low-income housing rehabilitation), 184 (railroad rolling stocks), 188 (child-care facilities) (1954). See also S. Surrey, "Federal Income Tax Reforms: The Varied Approaches Necessary to Replace Tax Expenditure with Direct Governmental Assistance," 80 *Harvard Law Review* 352 (1970).

10. The design of a tax to replace cost-of-service ratemaking in health care seems, on the surface, to be a difficult proposition given the not-for-profit nature of many of the institutions open hither to unexplored options. See S. Breyer's extended discussion of this idea in 92 *Harvard Law Review* 581–582 (1979) and "Taxes as a Substitute for Classical Regulation, in *Federal Regulation: Roads to Reform* 61, Exposure Draft, Comm'n on Law & Economy, ABA (1978)—Ed.

11. The idea of marketable rights might well be transferred from its present experimentation with effluent limits to purchase of rights to offer a specific service in a particular health service area—Ed.

12. For two seminal pieces on the virtues of collective bargaining, see Cox and Dunlop, "The Duty to Bargain Collectively During the Term of an Existing Agreement," 63 *Harvard Law Review* 1097 (1950); and Cox and Dunlop, "Regulation of Collective Bargaining by the National Labor Relations Board," 63 *Harvard Law Review* 389 (1950). Also see Dunlop's remarks in Chap. 4 *supra*.

13. See generally A. Cox, D. Bok and R. Gorman, *Cases and Materials on Labor Law* 531–563 (8th ed., 1977).

14. *Ibid.* at 567–572.

15. See, e.g., G. Calabresi in "Market Defects," n. 18 *supra*.

16. See Calabresi and Melamed in "Market Defects," n. 18 *supra* at 1089–1124 (urging a unified approach to property and torts by which "entitlements" would be protected).

17. *Ibid.* at 1115–1124.

18. See, e.g., Fletcher, "Fairness and Utility in Tort Theory," 85 *Harvard Law Review* 537 (1972).

19. A. Bierce, *The Devil's Dictionary* 107 (1957).

20. M. Stewart, *The Jekyll And Hyde Years: Politics and Economic Policy Since 1964* 32 & n. 1 (1977).

21. S. Rep. No. 1391, 95th Cong., 1st Sess., § 111, *Hospital Cost Containment Act of 1977: Hearings Before the Subcomm. on Health and Scientific Research of the Senate Comm. on Human Resources,* 95th Cong., 1st Sess., 3, 7–9 (1977) (died in committee).

22. See Breyer, "Different Modes of Classical Regulation and Their Problems," 220–221.

23. Cf. Public Health Service Act § 1532, 42 U.S.C. § 300n-1 (1976) (establishing procedures and criteria to be used by state health planning agencies in considering proposed health delivery system changes).

24. See, e.g., J. Howell, Chap. 1 *supra* at pages 13–15 and n. 4. See also J. Howell's case study, "CAT Scanner Policy in Boston," which is Appendix B to "Certificate of Need in Massachusetts" in *Regulation as an Instrument of Public Administration,* vol. 2, 48–68 (February 27–28, 1978), on file at the J. F. Kennedy School of Government, Harvard University.

25. J. Dunlop, "The Limits of Legal Compulsion" Position Paper, Secretary of Labor, 8–9 (Nov. 11, 1975). See also Chap. 4 *supra.*

26. *CAB Hearings* in "Different Modes of Classical Regulation and their Problems," n. 15 *supra* at 97 (statement of Alfred C. Kahn).

27. See *ibid* at 84–87 (prepared statement of Roger G. Noll).

28. See Breyer, "Market Defects," 209–210.

29. A number of economists have strongly urged the use of taxes to control pollution. See, e.g., A. Kneese, *Economics and the Environment* (1977); A. Kneese and C. Schultze, *Pollution, Prices and Public Policy* 85–111 (1975); Buchanan and Tullock," "Polluter's Profits and Political Response: Direct Controls Versus Taxes," 65 *American Economic Review* 139 (1975); Baumol, "On Taxation and Control of Externalities," 62 *American Economic Review* 307 (1972); Freeman and Haveman, "Residual Charges for Pollution Control: A Policy Evaluation," 177 *Science* 322 (1972). See generally S. Surrey, "Appendix: A Note on Regulatory Taxes" in *Pathways to Tax Reform: The Concept of Tax Expenditures* 155–174 (1973). An expanded version of this subsection appeared as "Taxes as a Substitute for Regulation," *Growth and Change,* 10, 39 (1979).

30. See A. Kahn, Vol. 1, in "Market Defects," n. 12 *supra* at 24, n. 11.

31. Nationalization has severe drawbacks and, while accepted in Europe, is politically unpopular here. Unregulated markets would allow the single "natural monopolist" to raise prices well above cost. The pressing need for telephone service and electricity allows for a reasonable fear that without regulation or the threat of it, unregulated prices would significantly exceed regulated prices. A tax on excess profits of less than 100 percent would lead the firm to increase its price rather than attempting to produce more efficiently, and would raise the difficult question of the profit level at which

the "excess" tax rate should apply. But see T. G. Moore, "The Effectiveness of Regulation of Electric Utility Prices," 36 *Southern Economic Journal* 365 (1970); G. J. Stigler, "The Theory of Economic Regulation," 2 *Bell Journal of Economics and Management Science* 3 (1971). Their studies, however, failed to take into account both the fact that a currently unregulated company may choose not to raise prices too high for fear that it too may become subject to regulation, and the fact that their data was drawn from the 1960s when technological advances lowered costs so significantly that prices remained constant.

APPENDIX 5-B: EXAMPLE OF REGULATION BY DISCLOSURE STANDARD

Consider the problems faced by NHSTA in deciding what combination of stopping distance, treadwear, and blowout resistance characteristics for auto tires would be disclosed, and how.[1] The Agency had great difficulty gathering the information needed to develop a meaningful rating system, and developing a fair testing system for enforcement purposes was difficult. The rating system, some feared, would unfairly favor certain firms over others, and preparing the necessary support to survive judicial review was time-consuming. The whole process took eight years.[2]

Nonetheless, there remains one important difference between disclosure standards and ordinary standards governing primary conduct. When ordinary standards forbid or dictate the type of product that must be sold or the process that must be used, they interfere with consumer choice and impede producer flexibility. And to the extent that those standards deviate from the "policy planner's ideal" (as they inevitably do), these restrictions on choice and conduct are clearly undesirable. Standards governing disclosure, however, do not restrict conduct beyond requiring that information be provided. The freedom of action that disclosure regulation allows vastly reduces the cost of deviations from the "policy planner's ideal." At worst, too much or the wrong information has been called for. It does not stop buyers from obtaining products or producers from making them. Thus when regulators seek disclosure, they need not fine-tune standards quite so precisely. They themselves need less information from industry, there are fewer enforcement problems, there is less risk of anticompetitive harm, and there is greater probability of surviving judicial review. Although NHSTA faced many problems in trying to set tire disclosure standards, its problems would have been still worse had it been seeking to set ordinary standards directing what sorts of tires could or could not be manufactured. Similarly, those who work in the securities industry seem to feel that the Security Exchange Commission's efforts to stop fraud by administering standards that require only disclosure are more successful and more efficient than state efforts to do so through blue sky laws, which often set substantive standards.[3]

Of course, disclosure is effective only where the public can understand the information disclosed and is free to choose on the basis of that information.

Where these conditions exist, disclosure standards often offer a less restrictive means than standards governing primary conduct to obtain a regulatory end.

NOTES

1. J. Gotbaum in "Different Modes of Classical Regulation and their Problems," n. 32 *supra*, Appendix D at 7 and n. 9.
2. *Ibid.*, uniform tire quality grading section at 11–20.
3. L. Loss, 1 *Securities Regulation* 121–128 (2d ed., 1961 and Supp. 1969).

APPENDIX 5-C: THE CASE FOR REFORM OF AIRLINE REGULATION

Recent government studies show that the airline industry is *competitively structured*, consisting of ten major firms which provide more than 90 percent of domestic scheduled airline service.[1] But it also contains local service carriers, supplemental carriers, and commuter carriers.[2] The industry can support several, perhaps many, firms of efficient size.[3] Moreover, entry barriers are not very high.[4] Although airplanes are expensive, new entrants can lease them. And entry into new routes by firms already in the industry is inexpensive. Economic conditions in the industry are *volatile*. Demand for air travel is strongly affected by change in personal income, and profits are very sensitive to the number of passengers.[5] As the number of passengers increases, the cost per passenger decreases. The industry cost structure is highly complex, for more than 20,000 city-pair combinations receive scheduled air service, and the cost of serving them varies with such factors as distance, congestion, equipment, time, amount of traffic, and relation to the rest of the service network.[6]

Application of classical price and entry regulation to this industry caused the airlines to compete in services offered rather than price.[7] Airlines not only provided gourmet meals but also scheduled more flights than necessary on popular routes—to the point where transcontinental flights, for example, were only 39 percent full on average.[8] Fares rose to cover the cost of extra capacity caused by limited price competition.[9] Thus, for example, California intrastate carriers (unregulated by the CAB), which flew fuller planes, charged about $26 for the 456-mile, 65-minute San Diego–San Francisco trip. On the comparable interstate, the CAB-regulated Boston–Washington 399-mile, 67-minute flight, the carriers (flying fewer passengers in the same planes) charged $42.[10]

Classical price regulation also tended to protect the existing firms and their market shares. The CAB allowed no new firms into the industry after 1950.[11] The market shares of the major airlines in 1975, compared with those in 1938 when the industry was 1/435 its later size, showed remarkable stability.[12] Finally, there appeared to be little incentive to perform more efficiently. Airlines that had lower costs were not allowed to seek more business by charging lower prices or, for that matter, by offering wider (and fewer) seats.[13] Those with higher costs and lower profits were frequently rewarded (in order to "balance" the industry) through the granting of more lucrative new routes.[14]

252

The industry was also plagued by a host of typical regulatory problems: Delay,
lack of standards, favoritism in awarding routes, interminable proceedings, and
secret determination of major policies without hearings.

To those familiar with the classical regulatory process and problems set out in "Different Modes of Classical Regulation and their Problems" *supra*, these complaints and adverse effects are not surprising. How is the CAB supposed to apply cost-of-service ratemaking in so complex, volatile, and competitive an industry? There are far too many firms, too many routes, and too many changes to do so firm by firm, route by route. For a time the Board attempted to negotiate changes in rates privately with the industry's trade association: This method—secret, informal and lacking consumer participation—was held unlawful.[15] The Board then developed, after elaborate and open hearings, a set of rules that automatically determined prices, pegging them to changes in cost on an industrywide basis.[16] Although those rules were "fair" and administratively workable (for they dispensed with the need for individualized hearings), they froze fares and prohibited price competition, further channeling the airlines' energies into service competition.

Similarly, the familiar problems associated with public interest allocation surfaced in the Board's difficulties in allocating route certificates. The Board found it difficult to separate the "who" and "what" questions, it found no single set of consistently usable standards, its proceedings were lengthy and unmanageable, and its decisions were attacked as unfair and possibly corrupt.[17]

Nor is it hard to understand the inability of the Board to stimulate greater industry efficiency. The efficiency problem plagues all cost-of-service ratemaking. In addition, need for an administrable price system led the CAB to adopt such rules as "equal fares for equal miles."[18] Since "equal miles" might have unequal costs, the Board then found it difficult to determine whether lower profits meant inefficiency or an undesirable route structure.[19]

The problems of classical regulation often lead to still greater regulation. In the 1970s, the CAB sought to solve the "excess service, empty plane" problem by imposing "capacity standards." If it could persuade airlines to restrict their schedules to an appropriate degree, the airlines would fill their planes and increase their profits, and the CAB could reduce fares. This approach was at least arguably sound from an economic point of view,[20] but it reckoned without the administrative and bureaucratic problems inherent in the standard-setting process. The CAB was unable to determine an appropriate level of service. It found it could not obtain the agreement of all the airlines, nor could it adequately enforce the agreements that were made. These and other problems led to less service at the same price.

The weakness of the "excessive competition" rationale was confirmed by the CAB studies.[21] Between the 1920s and the mid–1950s, when most airlines were subsidized, the rationale might have referred to a tendency to cut prices below cost in order to expand routes, making up the loss with the aid of the subsidy. However, the subsidy program was effectively ended for the major carriers by the mid–1950s. Although the airlines argued that more competition on popular routes would destroy the extra profit used to finance service to smaller communities, the studies showed that any such extra profit was not significant and that there was little "cross-subsidization."[22] The airlines, in fact, had long since discontinued most of their unprofitable routes. Insofar as "excessive competition" referred to a fear of predatory pricing, the antitrust laws were available to deal with the problem.[23]

Thus, airline regulation presented a case in which the justification for classical regulation was unusually weak; the problems inherent in applying the relevant regulatory modes (cost-of-service ratemaking and public interest allocation) were unusually severe; and, in any event, an unregulated market policed by antitrust presented an acceptable alternative.

The CAB studies discussed above have led to a significant reform in airline regulation. The CAB is in the process of reducing regulatory barriers to entry into the industry and has proposed greater price competition, all without change in the existing statutory framework. There is strong support in the Congress for legislation confirming these reforms.

NOTES

1. *CAB Report* in "Proposals for Regulatory Reform: An Introduction," n. 5 *supra* at 29.

2. *Ibid.*

3. *CAB Hearings* in "Different Modes of Classical Regulation and their Problems," n. 15 *supra* at 50 (prepared statement of Thomas E. Kauper), 65 (prepared statement of Gary L. Seevers and James C. Miller, III), and 453–454 (testimony of William A. Jordan). See also G. Douglas and J. Miller, *Economic Regulation of Domestic Air Transport: Theory and Policy* 178 (1974).

4. See *CAB Report* in "Proposals for Regulatory Reform: An Introduction," n. 5 *supra* at 49. See also *CAB Hearings* in "Different Modes of Classical Regulation and their Problems," n. 15 *supra* at 10 (testimony of Acting Secretary of Transportation Barnum).

5. *CAB Hearings, ibid.* at 2240–2263 (statement by Herbert H. Moser).

6. *Ibid.* at 42–46 (but concluding that these factors do not explain differences between intra-California and East Coast fares). See also 49 U.S.C. § 1482(e) (1970) (factors which CAB must consider in determining rates).

7. *CAB Hearings* in "Different Modes of Classical Regulation and their Problems," n. 15 *supra* at 104–105.

8. *CAB Report* in "Proposals for Regulatory Reform: An Introduction," n. 5 *supra* at 64.

9. *Ibid.* at 38–40.

10. *Ibid.* at 43 (1975 fare schedule).

11. *Ibid.* at 78–79.

12. United Airlines had approximately 20 percent of the market in 1938, and still had 20 percent of the market in 1975. Despite mergers and other changes, the industry is still comprised of the original 16 firms (now reduced to 10). See *CAB Report, ibid.* at 87–88; Moss v. Civil Aeronautics Bd., 521 F.2d 298 (D.C. Cir. 1975).

13. See *CAB Report, ibid.* at 87–88.

14. *Ibid.* at 119.

15. Moss v. Civil Aeronautics Bd., 521 F.2d 298 (D.C. Cir. 1975).

16. See *CAB Report* in "Proposals for Regulatory Reform: An Introduction," n. 5 *supra* at 109–112.

17. *Ibid.* at 95–96.

18. *Ibid.* at 111–112.

19. *Ibid.* at 118–120.

20. W. E. Fuhan Jr., *The Fight for Competitive Advantage: A Study of the United States Domestic Trunk Air Carriers* 177–183 (Harvard Univ. Press, 1972).

21. See *CAB Report* in "Proposals for Regulatory Reform: An Introduction," n. 5 *supra* at 60–62.

22. A detailed examination of United's route system revealed that at most 0.1 percent of

United's revenue passenger miles received cross-subsidy. See *CAB Report, ibid.* at

65–68. Moreover, the Boston-Washington route, charging the high fare of $42, did not generate revenues for a cross-subsidy. American Airlines estimated its fully allocated cost for a Boston-Washington flight at $5752 per trip while averaging revenues of $5544 for an average net loss of $208. *Ibid.* at 45–46.

23. 15 U.S.C. 2 (1976). See generally P. Areeda and D. Turner, 3 *Antitrust Law* 711 (1978); Areeda and Turner, "Predatory Pricing and Related Practice Under Section 2 of the Sherman Act," 88 *Harvard Law Review* 697 (1975).

APPENDIX 5-D: TAXATION: AN ALTERNATIVE TO STANDARD–SETTING?

The four problems to which standard-setting is prone are well-illustrated by the case of pollution control. The need to balance harms and benefits, to tailor solution to each polluter's production processes and locale, and to avoid undue advantages for existing competitors suggests particularized standards dependent on obtaining detailed and accurate information.[1] But the variation in standards and the many points to be policed would then make enforcement difficult. The different costs of alternative technologies in various locations and industries, combined with information-gathering problems, would make it difficult to avoid anticompetitive consequences. And the many different standards needed, combined with the large number of potential plaintiffs, exacerbate the problems of judicial review.

A tax system immediately occurs to many economists as a promising alternative to spillover problems such as pollution.[2] Since the problem is that the price of a product does not reflect the important social cost it imposes (i.e., pollution), why not simply raise the price through a tax to reflect the harm? The response of the classical regulator is that no one knows *how much* to raise the price, and it is no easier to decide the *amount* of the tax than to decide how much smoke the maker of the product should be allowed to emit. Why not, therefore, just tackle the latter question directly through standards?[3]

The true virtue of a tax regime, however, lies not in its ability to measure pollution's "cost" but in its ability to provide incentives to direct behavior in a socially desirable direction—without freezing current technology or eliminating a degree of individual choice. Several factors suggest its suitability to an environmental spillover problem.

First, the problem in its very statement suggests that the answer is not an outright ban of polluting products and processes, but rather, a better balance between the two competing goals—a clean environment and industrial production—which are in part mutually exclusive, but both of which are desired. The solution requires both a balancing among goods and strong incentives (1) to consumers to shift away from pollution-causing products and (2) to producers to shift to or to develop pollution-free processes. Relative prices perform just such functions throughout the economy.[4] Except where especially serious health hazards exist thus justifying an outright prohibition on polluting substances, a price tag on pollution allows buyers to balance the competing "environmental" and "industrial" goods and provides incentives in the right direction. A tax allows those with a special need or desire for the polluting item to obtain it (thus permitting continuous individual balancing) while providing a continuing incentive to manufacturers to find less polluting production methods.[5]

Second, "proper" solutions are likely to vary substantially depending upon thousands of products and processes and thousands of locations. Hence one needs a method that allows for that variation. Imposing a tax and hence allowing use of the process or production method, if consumers are willing to pay the price, can to some extent deal with this need for flexibility.[6]

Third, the large number of industrial pollutant sources suggests the desirability, from an enforcement point of view, of a fairly simple rule. And a tax system offers the prospect of a system that is fairly simple in application yet can produce variation and flexibility in result.[7]

It is important to remember that a pollution tax is only one possible market-based approach to the problem. Under this approach, an agency would set a tax per unit of pollutant emitted. A firm would be free to pollute provided it paid the tax. Another market-based approach is for an agency to set an absolute limit on the amount of pollutant that can be emitted in a given region and to issue marketable rights to pollute up to this level. Those rights could be sold by the government to firms which would either use them or sell them to others. To pollute without a permit would be unlawful.

Each of these market-based systems has its own typical uncertainty. A regulatory agency that instituted a tax system would not know in advance how much pollution would be eliminated, since an unknown number of firms would choose to pay the tax rather than eliminate pollution. A marketable rights system offers more certainty on this score, for the agency would set an absolute limit on pollution. But the agency would be less certain of the extent to which it was imposing a cost burden on firms within the region, a matter about which the tax gives greater certainty.[8]

When compared with classical standard-setting, however, either market-based system seems more efficient. A tax, for example, would encourage firms to buy nonpolluting equipment up to the point where the equipment's cost exceeded the amount of the tax. Thus, units of pollution would be eliminated in rank order of least cost. Under such a system the only pollution remaining would be that which was the most expensive to eliminate. Similarly, marketable rights could be sold and exchanged until they fell into the hands of those to whom they were most valuable—namely, the creators of those units of pollution that were the most expensive to prevent. Moreover, as previously pointed out, both market-based solutions provide a continuous incentive to adopt production methods that pollute less.

NOTES

1. R. Stewart and J. Krier, *Environmental Law and Policy* 556–557 (2d ed., 1978).

2. See, e.g., A. Kneese and C. Schultze, *Pollution, Prices and Public Policy* 5–9 (1975); C. Schultze in "Market Defects," n. 2 *supra* at 50–51; J. Senaca and M. Taussig, *Environmental Economics* 218–245 (1974); Ruff, "The Economic Common Sense of Pollution," 19 *Public Interest* 69, 78–81 (1970); Solow, "The Economist's Approach to Pollution and Its Control," 173 *Science* 498, 501 (1971).

3. See Roberts and Stewart, "Book Review," 88 *Harvard Law Review* 1645, 1653 (1975). On the difficulty of measuring the costs of pollution, see Lave, "Air Pollution Damage:

Some Difficulties in Estimating the Value of Abatement," in *Environmental Quality Analysis* 213 (A. Kneese & B. Bower, Eds., 1972).

4. Stewart and Krier, n. 1 *supra* at 103–107, 351; Ruff, "Price Pollution Out of Existence, *Los Angeles Times*," Dec. 7, 1969, p. G7, col. 3.

5. W. Baxter, *People or Penguins: The Case for Optimal Pollution*, 73–78 (1974); C. Schultze in "Market Defects," n. 2 *supra* at 53–54; Ruff, n. 2 *supra* at 79–80.

6. See W. Baxter, n. 5 *supra* at 65–68, 75.

7. C. Schultze, E. Fried, A. Rivlin and N. Teeters, *Setting National Priorities: The 1973 Budget* 368–373 (1972); W. Baxter, n. 5 *supra* at 76–77.

8. Roberts and Stewart, n. 3 *supra* at 1653–1654; see R. Stewart and J. Krier, n. 1 *supra* at 587–602.

APPENDIX 5-E: THE ATTEMPT TO INTRODUCE COMPETITION INTO LONGLINE TELECOMMUNICATION MARKETS

Initially, the FCC's intention (as expressed by the chief of its Common Carrier Bureau) was "to use competitive market forces as an alternative to regulation, which was largely ineffective."[1] Such "ineffectiveness" may be traced, in large measure, to the serious problem of allocating AT&T's costs among its various services.[2] AT&T has significant costs which are joint and common to more than one service and often subject to regulation by both federal and state regulatory commissioners. For example, telephone handsets in homes and offices and local exchange facilities connecting those telephones into the local exchange network are used for both local and interstate service. Moreover, long-distance communications facilities (cable, microwave, or satellite) provide numerous offerings: Ordinary message toll telephone service (MTS), wide-area telephone service (WATS)—for which a flat rate per month is charged—and a variety of private line services (typically provided over facilities connecting two points in distant cities with a continuously open line between them).

The problem of how to allocate the costs of fungible plant among the services—local, intrastate, and interstate—that use them pervades cost-of-service ratemaking. Regulators, for practical reasons, tend to use methods that are economically arbitrary.[3] Moreover, the joint and common cost problem is exacerbated by the fact that the FCC regulates interstate communications while state regulatory commissions have jurisdictional authority over intrastate and local exchange telephone service.[4] The allocation of costs of plant used jointly to provide interstate and intrastate services—such as buildings, land, handsets, and local exchange facilities—between state and federal regulators is determined initially by jurisdictional separation procedures prescribed by a joint board of federal and state regulators subject to a final decision by the FCC. The Communication Act of 1934, as amended, mandates this jurisdictional allocation process but, in practice, the process reflects not simply economic costs but also an added noncost factor based upon political considerations which have determined that revenues from interstate MTS and WATS should be set at levels to help defray the costs of providing local exchange service. The result is that AT&T must include significant amounts of local exchange plant costs in its interstate rate base and set interstate rates to recover these costs.

Whether such rates have been properly set has proved to be a matter of continuing controversy within the regulatory process, especially with the entry into the telecommunications field of new so-called "specialized carriers" initially desired to compete with AT&T in providing long-distance private line services.

The FCC staff argued that the enormous problem of how costs should be allocated among long-distance services might be avoided to some extent and the benefits of competition could be realized if private microwave companies were allowed to set up their own "longline" service (based upon microwave stations), interconnect with AT&T's local exchanges, and compete with AT&T to provide long-distance private line service[5] (for example, direct open lines between, say, General Motors' San Francisco office and its Detroit plant). For one thing, the new competitors might provide long-distance private line service at a lower cost. For another, they might provide more innovative service. In any event, they would put pressure on AT&T to cut its prices for similar, competing private line services and hence its cost of providing them. Finally, new entry would provide a practical test of AT&T's price competition, which might itself show that longline telecommunications service was not a natural monopoly.

Since the FCC is uncertain about whether existing, new low-cost technology makes longline communications service a natural monopoly, it might allow new firms to enter, allow all firms to charge prices that reflect "incremental" costs (the additional cost to the firm of providing the additional service at issue), and let the most efficient firm survive. New competition would drive prices towards incremental costs and allow customers to choose among the competing firms on the basis of lowest cost or best service.

The Bell System's response is important, for it shows how the existence of regulation in one conceded area of natural monopoly (in this case local telephone service) complicates decision making in other, related areas. Bell points out that, given the existence of this regulation, new entry into private long line markets will not necessarily lead to free and open competition.[6] Rather, the fact that *some* of AT&T's services (e.g., local telephone service, local exchange service) will continue to be regulated by both federal and state governments will prevent AT&T from competing effectively with the new competition. More specifically, the regulatory rules developed in these other areas will inhibit AT&T's competing in price with new competitors, because they prevent AT&T from cutting its price to reflect only the additional cost of providing longline service (i.e., the incremental cost). The rules effectively hold a price umbrella over the new firms. AT&T argues that were it free to charge prices for these services that reflected incremental cost, it could easily drive the new competitors from the market. Given the rest of its system, longline telecommunications (or private longline services) is a natural monopoly, for the additional cost of providing such service is very low.[7]

The small competitors argued, however, that AT&T should not be allowed to cut its price to incremental cost, for, given the complexity of AT&T's accounting system, no regulator could determine whether a low AT&T longline telecommunications price in fact reflected a low natural monopoly cost or whether it constituted a predatory price—a price *below* the incremental cost of providing the service.[8]

Once new competition appeared, AT&T responded by cutting its prices, and the FCC had to determine whether those new prices were below AT&T's costs. Thus, the FCC did not escape the "cost determination" problem. It has had to allocate joint costs, and in so doing it has effectively required AT&T to charge prices on competitive longline services that are closer to average than to incremental costs. Moreover, since AT&T is required by the interstate/intrastate "separations" rules to include some of the costs of its local handsets and wires in its interstate rate base, while its longline competitors need not include such costs in their interstate charges, AT&T starts at a pricing disadvantage.[9] For these reasons, in AT&T's view, the notion that it will be able to compete vigorously and fairly with its competitors is illusory. Rather, regulatory rules will force it to charge prices higher than its incremental costs. In allowing new entry, the FCC runs the risk that higher cost carriers will attract a portion of AT&T's business, and if it loses many customers, AT&T's unit costs may rise, for it will not have sufficient volume to provide service at lowest cost.

Those favoring the introduction of competition make several arguments in reply to AT&T. First, whether or not longline communications does or will continue to enjoy the cost characteristics of a natural monopoly is uncertain. New technology may always change those cost characteristics. And the competitive pressures brought by new firms makes the introduction of new technology more likely. Second, some add that the regulatory rules which prevent AT&T from responding to new competition by cutting its prices to its incremental cost should be abandoned. Regardless of the economic merits of this goal, however, it is unlikely to be attained as a practical matter as long as jurisdiction is divided between state and federal agencies, for the local regulatory commission will seek to keep its own rates low by allocating as much of AT&T's costs as possible to its interstate rate base. Finally, it might be claimed that some small inefficiency (some small amount of higher cost facilities) in private longline telecommunications is simply a price worth paying in order to obtain new competitors and the pressure they put upon AT&T to innovate, to operate more efficiently, and to try to cut its prices.

In fact, there was initially little risk that new competition would raise AT&T's unit cost of service, for the FCC authorized entry only into a very small market—the market for long-distance private line telecommunications.[10] Thus even if AT&T's prices were maintained at high levels to protect new competitors in that area, its loss of business would be small, and the corresponding risk of eroding economies of scale would be small as well.[11] But as a practical matter, it has proved difficult to confine the new entrants to the relatively small private line market. Initially, these carriers received FCC permission to interconnect with AT&T's local exchanges,[12] allowing any subscriber to take advantage of their private line services. Thereafter, they received regulatory approval to sell and resell "portions" of the private lines (for example, three minutes' worth), effectively allowing them to offer ordinary long-distance service. Then recently, one of these companies (MCI) filed a tariff offering ("Execunet") that would allow any subscriber to call any other—an offering which AT&T alleges duplicates its ordinary long-distance service. The FCC rejected the tariff in an effort to restrict to private lines the area in which the new entrants offered competition but was reversed in the Court of Appeals (and the Supreme Court declined to consider the case further).[13] Thus, the threat to AT&T's entire longline system is potentially severe. Accordingly, AT&T again would appear to have a competitive disadvantage if it alone must include in its charges for long distance calls a "separation determined" portion of local equipment costs.

On the other hand, the FCC strongly believes that its policies will prove to be in the public interest. The agency has argued that competition will lead to lower prices and new and innovative services. The FCC also has contended, at least prior to Execunet, that new entry is authorized only in a small market (private line) which has no natural monopoly characteristics. Finally, the FCC has indicated that the problem of competitive disadvantage, if it indeed exists, can be dealt with effectively by appropriate changes in the separations procedures.

NOTES

1. B. Strassburg, *Organization Analysis of Regulatory Process: A Comparative Study of the Decision Making Process in the Federal Communications Commission and the Environmental Protection Agency* (Nov. 30, 1977) (report prepared for the National Science Foundation). As FCC Chairman Richard Wiley stated:

> the issue is whether the American consumer is better served by unfettered access to suppliers of diverse and specialized communications services than by artificial regulatory barriers limiting his or her access to a single, sole-source monopolist. In this comparative evaluation, the Commission has concluded that the public interest is better served by the open marketplace.

   Competition in the Telecommunications Industry: Hearings Before the Subcomm. on Communications of the House Comm. on Interstate & Foreign Commerce, 94th Cong., 2d Sess., 738 (1976) (hereinafter cited as *Telephone Hearings*).

2. See J. Sechter, *Separations Procedures In The Telephone Industry: The Historical Origins Of a Public Policy* 3–7 (1977).

3. *Telephone Hearings*, n. 1 *supra* at 77 (testimony of Paul H. Henson). The separation of intrastate and interstate telecommunications property, revenues, and expenses was mandated by the Supreme Court. Smith v. Illinois Bell Tel. Co., 282 U.S. 133 (1930). The principle of separation has been incorporated into legislation regulating the telecommunications industry. See 47 U.S.C. §§ 221 (1970) and 410(c) (Supp. V. 1975).

4. The state commissions, hoping to hold down intrastate service prices, seek to allocate as much of the rate base as possible to interstate service. The allocation involves bargaining among state and federal regulators. The result is that AT&T must set rates (or interstate service higher than the incremental costs of providing that service). *Telephone Hearings*, n. 1 *supra* at 77 (testimony of Paul H. Henson).

5. See Specialized Common Carrier Servs., 29 F.C.C.2d 870 (1971); *aff'd sub nom.* Washington Utils. & Transp. Comm'n v. FCC, 513 F.2d 1142 (9th Cir.), *cert. denied* 423 U.S. 836 (1975). The development of this policy is outlined by the Commission in *Telephone Hearings*, n. 4 *supra* at 856–867.

6. *Telephone Hearings*, n. 1 *supra* at 39–40 (testimony of John D. DeBotts), and at 143–144 (testimony of Theodore F. Brophy). AT&T has pushed the incremental cost concept in American Tel. & Tel. Co. Long Lines Dep't, 61 F.C.C.2d 587 (1976). The FCC rejected the motion of long-run incremental cost and instead adopted a version of the ratemaking theory of fully distributed costs.

7. *Telephone Hearings*, n. 1 *supra* at 143–144 (statement of Theodore F. Brophy).

8. See *Ibid.* at 307, 328, 489.

9. The inclusion of these costs is partly a result of the political negotiation between federal and state regulators described in n. 4 *supra*.

10. See Specialized Common Carrier Servs., 29 F.C.C.2d 870 (1971); *aff'd sub. nom.* Washington Utils. & Transp. Comm'n v. FCC, 513 F.2d 1142 (9th Cir.), *cert. denied* 423, U.S. 836 (1975).

11. The FCC noted that private-lines business generated only 3.5 percent (or 4 percent if revenues from video tape line services were included) of AT&T's enormous interstate revenues. Specialized Common Carrier Servs., 29 F.C.C. 870, 892, 911 (1971); *aff'd sub*

nom. Washington Utils. & Transp. Comm'n v. FCC, 513 F.2d 1142 (9th Cir.), *cert. denied* 423 U.S. 836 (1975).

12. Bell Sys. Tariff Offerings of Local Distrib. Facilities for Use by Other Common Carriers, 466 F.C.C.2d 413 (1974); *aff'd sub nom.* Bell Tel. Co. v. FCC, 503 F.2d 1250 (3d Cir. 1974).

13. Regulatory Policies Concerning Resale & Shared Use of Common Carrier Services and Facilities, 60 F.C.C.2d 261 (1976); MCI Telecommunication Corp. v. FCC, 561 F.2d 365 (D.C. Cir. 1977), *cert. denied* 434 U.S. 1040 (1978).

APPENDIX 5-F: ACCOMPLISHING REGULATORY REFORM

THE ANALYTIC FRAMEWORK IS APPLICABLE UNDER VARIOUS CIRCUMSTANCES AND AT SEVERAL GOVERNMENTAL LEVELS

The application of the analytic framework can be expected to be used primarily at the legislative level. That is, it supplies a mode of systematic analysis by which Congress can consider questions of governmental intervention in the economy. Where the administration or an independent agency is called upon to recommend legislation, or does so on its own initiative, Congress could and should expect such recommendations to reflect the kind of analysis described in this article.

The framework can also be used at the administrative agency level for certain purposes, particularly by an agency that is vested with broad discretion in the regulation of a particular industry or function of the economy. The framework is usable in rulemaking proceedings where an agency is considering a new application of its regulatory powers, or in reexamining (as an agency should from time to time) the efficacy of existing regulations.

Moreover, the framework may be applicable in two quite different circumstances. First, it can be brought to bear in considering whether or not, and how, to intervene in a heretofore unregulated sector of the economy. In that circumstance, of course, the burden of the analytic framework is to put such a decision to a significant test. The "anatomy of regulatory failure" is a warning that any supposed cure can be worse than the perceived disease and, indeed, that the disease may be misperceived. If the perception survives examination and it is concluded that the competitive market cannot adjust to a real deficiency, alternatives to classic forms of regulation should be considered seriously by legislators before they enact regulatory statutes of the more traditional sort. Indeed, utilization of an analytic framework in the development of any new regulatory system might reduce the need for extensive regulatory reform in future years.

Second, the framework can be applied to existing regulatory structures. Where the analytic framework is being used for regulatory reform purposes—that is, where a candidate for reform has been identified by ascertaining the existence of a mismatch—it should be recognized that identification of the candidate is only the beginning of the process of substantive reform. Whether reform can or should take place thereafter depends upon further steps being taken, as follows.

264

A regulatory reform effort can be conducted under any of several auspices. The most likely and the most advantageous one for carrying out a substantive reform is the congressional committee that would be called upon to conduct hearings on any proposed reform legislation. That committee can be expected to combine information-gathering power with an ability to develop significant political support. Depending somewhat upon the current relationship between the Congress and the executive branch, it is also possible for the latter—which may have superior ability to do sustained and detailed work—to conduct a study and assemble the necessary political support. At different eras in the political life of the country, the initiative for such a study might be in one branch or the other. It is also conceivable that such a study could be carried out by a well-regarded regulatory agency. In recent times, there are examples of major regulatory reform efforts originating in each of these.

The most drastic recent reform effort originated in Congress and, perhaps significantly, in a committee of Congress that does not ordinarily supervise the industry and the agency involved in the reform. It was the Administrative Practices Subcommittee of the Senate Judiciary Committee that sponsored the studies of the airline industry that led to the Cannon-Kennedy Deregulation bill. The work of the Committee was strongly supported by the executive branch in two successive administrations, and the CAB's policies have undergone a change in the direction of deregulation (see Appendix 5-G *infra* for a detailed discussion of this case).

Another example of successful reform shows the interaction of the executive and legislative branches with a particularly independent administrative agency. This was the deregulation of securities brokerage commissions. The process began with extensive studies and hearings by the SEC. The Antitrust Division of the Justice Department participated in the hearings. After the initial SEC decision to deregulate, Congress turned to the subject with a broad-ranging study of various securities industry practices, including those involving brokerage commissions. The resulting legislation confirmed the deregulation of brokerage commissions and imposed a number of additional reforms on the industry. In this case the reforms were carried out by the committees of Congress which have responsibility to oversee the SEC.

A third example of reform is the national energy program which originated in the executive branch. Perhaps significantly, this reform program cuts across a number of different executive departments and regulatory agencies, deals with an especially massive and complex problem involving more than one industry, and is a matter of the highest national priority.

The last example on energy highlights the need for innovative procedures which will assist Congress in confronting some of the complex problems outlined in this article. The involvement of all the congressional committees that have jurisdiction over the industries or federal regulatory agencies involved in a novel regulatory proposal (or proposal for reform) makes multiple referrals necessary, enhances the likelihood of protective attitudes toward particular regulatory agencies, accentuates committee rivalries, and increases the possibility of delay. Recognizing this problem, the House of Representatives recently formed a special committee of senior members of each concerned standing committee to consider the President's proposed energy legislation.

A special committee like this one, cutting across traditional jurisdictional lines, can more easily develop a combination of methods for dealing with a regulatory problem, including tax incentives where appropriate.

It might also be desirable for Congress to develop improved methods for analyzing regulatory reform proposals similar to those suggested in this article. Agencies such as the Congressional Budget Office, with its outstanding reputation, might be utilized for this purpose during the course of committee consideration of such proposals.

A DETAILED, EMPIRICALLY BASED INQUIRY MUST BE MADE INTO THE EFFECTS OF REGULATION WITHIN THE INDUSTRY

Regardless of the regulatory program's basic objective (and the possible inability of regulation to achieve that objective), any existing program will in fact serve a host of subsidiary objectives. Moreover, the industry, its suppliers, and its customers will have adjusted to the existing system and the patterns of service that regulation has produced. Technology will reflect those patterns. Countless investment decisions will have been made in reliance upon them. Whether such particular factors make it unwise to introduce systematic change that might otherwise seem warranted can be known only after a detailed examination of the industry in question. A thorough factual inquiry is essential before judgments can be reached that reform is in fact desirable and about the direction that reform should take. A substantial portion of the factual inquiry should be conducted before legislative hearings are held, but legislative conclusions about the desirability of substantive reform and a particular plan for it should await the completion of hearings.

A PUBLIC LEGISLATIVE HEARING SHOULD NORMALLY BE HELD

A detailed hearing brings to the surface the major objections to change and forces proponents to deal with them. It also makes the regulatory reform issue, and its applicability to a particular industry, politically "visible" by calling it to the public's attention. An "invisible" issue will lack the support necessary for major change. If the proposed reform has validity, it will pick up support from diverse sources. Conversely, a public hearing open to testimony from all interested parties will expose whatever failings may exist in the proposed reform.

The hearing should allot sufficient time to all parties to explain their views. It should focus on a draft bill or a preliminary staff report containing a proposed plan of reform that commands intial support. Witnesses should be asked to address themselves to the plan but be allowed to offer alternatives to it.

To analogize a legislative hearing on a matter of regulatory reform to a judicial or an administrative fact-finding hearing is to miss an essential difference between them. The legislative hearing has an educational objective. One of its major functions is to allow proponents to gather political support and opponents to gather political opposition. The clash of views serves primarily to dramatize the issues. The hearings themselves are unlikely to produce detailed factual information for time is too limited. The congressional proceeding thus moves on two levels at once: (1) The gathering of masses of published and unpublished information, dry and detailed but essential to the writing of the legislative committee reports in support of reform legislation; and (2) the oral level, which should dramatize the significant issues clearly, succinctly, and in a manner comprehensible to the layperson.

The proponents of change must have a plan that appears practical and provides for adequate transition arrangements. In particular, the plan must allow workers, managers, and customers the time they need to learn how to work within the new regulatory environment. Particularly during the transition period, the plan must adequately protect those who have invested time, effort, and capital in reliance upon the existing system. Whether the transition is from an absence of regulation to the imposition of regulation or from existing regulation to an unregulated market, the timing and method of transition in either direction are as difficult problems as the basic analysis and reaching of a decision. This is not to say that the difficulty of transition is in any way a conclusive argument against change. Nonetheless, a reasonable plan that might take five years to implement and thus permit an orderly transition could be one with a practical chance of enactment, while an immediate discarding of existing structures, however inadequate they may be, is less likely to be successful.

THE JUSTICE DEPARTMENT SHOULD BE CALLED UPON TO TEST EXISTING REGULATION AGAINST COMPETITIVE STANDARDS OR TO TEST ANY PLAN FOR NEW REGULATION AGAINST SUCH STANDARDS

Since any existing or proposed regulatory structure should be tested against the competitive market alternative, the views of the Antitrust Division of the Justice Department should be solicited. The division's role was significant both in the deregulation of brokerage commissions and the proposed deregulation of air travel fares. It is important, of course, that the rather fixed lens of the Antitrust Division, whose only mission is to enforce the antitrust statutes, be recognized. The Division can not be expected to place great weight on what may be reasonable public policy considerations that lead in a different direction (and, therefore, the views of consumers should be solicited as well). Nonetheless, the thrust of a single-minded procompetitive advocate is a valuable way to evaluate other alternatives.

A DETAILED FACTUAL REPORT BASED ON THE INQUIRY SHOULD BE PUBLISHED CONTAINING THE BASIC ELEMENTS OF THE PROPOSED REFORM PLAN

The publication of such a report will show the results of the inquiry and permit reasoned study by all affected parties and by the Congress. It is important that the report be balanced and objective. It is also important that the report reach separately stated conclusions and set forth the main components of any plan for reform, including how any transition is proposed to be dealt with.

APPENDIX 5-G: REGULATORY REFORM: THE CAB EXAMPLE

By 1974, when Senator Edward Kennedy began to prepare hearings on airline regulation, considerable academic work by economists and others—including, for example, Caves, Miller, Jordan, and Levine—had been done criticizing the anticompetitive effects of airline regulation.[1] Thus the airlines were already a natural choice for deregulation. The resulting investigation was conducted in accordance with the principles set out in "Alternative Regimes and the Framework Applied" *supra*.

During 1974 and part of 1975 the staff of the Subcommittee on Administrative Practice and Procedure conducted detailed fact gathering on the airline industry. The Subcommittee then held eight days of hearings on regulation by the CAB. The hearings were followed by publication of a lengthy, detailed factual report urging abandonment of classical regulation and increased reliance on competition.[2]

The congressional hearings themselves served three separate but interrelated functions. First, they acted as a catalyst in forcing other agencies of government to focus upon the problem and develop a policy position. Thus, when the staff of the Subcommittee on Administrative Practice and Procedure began to talk to administration officials about airline deregulation in August 1974, those officials had begun to develop but had not yet decided whether to present an airline regulation reform plan. The hearings, to be held in January 1975, offered them an opportunity to announce a major policy initiative. Moreover, the hearings required that the Secretary of Transportation have an answer ready when asked to state the administration's position on reform on the first day of the hearings. The need to write testimony in response to detailed questions of the Subcommittee required the administration to work out its answers in detail. And, by calling as witnesses representatives from agencies such as the Antitrust Division of the Justice Department, the FTC, the Council of Economic Advisors, and the Council on Wage and Price Stability, all who would tend to favor competition, the Subcommittee could to a limited extent influence the making of those policy decisions within the administration.

Acting Secretary of Transportation John W. Barnum, speaking for the administration, announced a major policy change in favor of more competition.

Subsequently, President Ford appointed a new CAB chairman who began to institute such reforms. The hearings provided the opportunity for those urging reform to contact a wide range of executive and administrative officials; in short, the hearings helped develop a network of persons throughout the government who would influence policy and help each other in the movement for reform. The hearings also acted as a catalyst with respect to the regulated industry.

Individual airlines in preparing testimony would have to ask themselves how the CAB's overall regulatory policy affected the firm. They had to consider seriously the effect of major procompetitive change. In some instances airlines considered for the first time whether or not open price competition would hurt or harm them. Some simply reaffirmed their previous opposition to change; but others did not. Moreover, the hearings led still other firms to resurrect proposals for new service at low prices, such as World Airways' plan to fly coast to coast for $99, or Freddy Laker's plan to bring low-fare/full-plane service to the North Atlantic.

Thus, the threat of hearings forced each airline to reassess its position, to develop new information, and to put its own bureaucracy to work to develop and assess alternatives.

Second, the hearings served to gather the detailed factual information used to write a comprehensive report. The report did not need to produce empirical information that would definitively resolve every issue, but it had to be comprehensive. Existing studies could not answer every relevant question, so new information had to be gathered. The empirical effort had to determine who is actually being hurt or helped by the program in order to evaluate the arguments made in its favor. Doing so avoids wasting scarce political resources "reforming" programs that in practice cause minimal harm.

The airlines argued, for example, that competition would not result in lower fares.[3] As evidence that reform would result in lower prices, proponents cited the experience with intrastate carriers in California where fares on intrastate routes were only 50 to 60 percent as high as those on comparable interstate routes.[4] The controversy over the relevance and significance of the "California experience" provides a concrete example of the extent to which detailed facts are needed. Before concluding that increased competition was responsible for the lower fares in California—where entry had been freely allowed for twenty years (until 1967)—the Subcommittee had to examine airline claims that the differences reflected: (1) different weather conditions, (2) traffic density, (3) direction of traffic flow, (4) less congestion, (5) fewer costs from interlining connections with other services, (6) different aircraft types, (7) less need to provide through service, and (8) less need to support other routes in the system. The Subcommittee examined each of these factors and the industry trade association was persuaded to commission an independent study of the causes of the fare differences.

All this information was compiled and sent to the airlines requesting confirmation, refutation, or additional information. The result showed that the main cause of the cost difference was that intrastate airlines flew more passengers on each flight, thus lowering their costs. This fact supported the argument that price competition had induced the airlines to offer the lower fare (and fuller plane) service that most travelers wanted. The net result of the empirical work was that the argument against using the California experience as a comparison simply dropped out of the public debate.

Each of the major objections had to be treated in a similar manner. Airline deregulation raised a host of issues. Would new competition lead to reduced services to smaller communities? Would less regulation increase the risk of bankruptcy for individual firms? Would any such increase in risk mean less investment in new aircraft? Could airport financing arrangements be adapted to a new system? Would it be possible to change labor contracts to work within a new system? Would less regulation lead to increased industry concentration? Would more competition destroy the complex national airline network? Would it make air travel less safe?

While the hearings could not definitively answer all the questions raised, they could investigate them in detail, marshal the relevant information, and base policy recommendations on that work.

The result was a 250-page report that was circulated in draft form to all witnesses, firms, unions, and other interested parties for comment. The report was then revised to take all such comments into account. The final document, which recommended major change, was difficult to attack; it obtained a reputation for being thorough and comprehensive,[5] and that reputation in turn helped to produce a political attitude that the time had come for change. This attitude was reinforced by further hearings before Senator Cannon's Aviation Subcommittee.

Whether or not the report was read, those dealing with the issue of regulatory reform could argue that all relevant issues had been considered and dealt with and that the report showed the change would likely mean lower prices and was unlikely to produce disaster. Those opposed to change could not point to major flaws or omitted points or inaccuracies. Thus the airline issue became naturally attractive to politicians who wished to act effectively to bring about some type of "regulatory reform" in the public interest.

With the support of President Carter and CAB Chairman Alfred Kahn who began to deregulate the airlines administratively, a major deregulation bill was enacted.[6]

Third, the hearings dramatized the issue. This helped mobilize public and political support for regulatory reform. The CAB hearings had an educational objective and a political purpose, and moved on two levels at once: the gathering in written form of masses of detailed fact needed to write a report or develop a proposal and the more dramatic or educational level. This latter level illustrated the issues in a way that is both comprehensible and interesting to the general public. The hearings can communicate their message to the public only by capturing the attention of the media.

The Subcommittee hearings, for example, were structured so that they in effect told a story: Each aspect of the overall regulatory reform problem was covered on a different day, and each day of the hearings was organized to maximize the chance that an "event" of interest would occur. During the first day of the hearing, for example, the Acting Secretary of Transportation announced that the administration would propose major reform of the CAB, an event which was front page news in many newspapers. The strength of the oral hearings lay in their gradual revelation to the journalists, and through them to the public, of the way in which the CAB regulated the airline industry and the potential advantages to be wrought from deregulation.

It is crucial to understand that both the oral, dramatic level and the written, detailed factual level of the hearings are needed. A hearing can capture headlines without detailed factual work. It can look for scandal or distort issues and in doing so capture media attention. But had that been done, the hearings would have proved less effective. The distortion would have produced distrust among the airline executives, union officials, administrators, and others who must be convinced or neutralized before proposals can be enacted. Opponents

would have found grounds to discredit the Subcommittee's work. Additionally,
without the underlying detailed work in which to ground the proposals, the media attention would have proved ephemeral. Inadequate preparation on the part of the Subcommittee would also have prevented it from making its strongest points in public hearings against those who opposed reform. But to do no more than study regulatory reform issues—to do the detailed factual work without the drama that a hearing can provide—would likely have produced only one more report to be placed unread upon a shelf.

It is difficult for several reasons to draw lessons from the experience with airline deregulation. Much of the evidence is anecdotal. More important, one cannot be sure whether airline regulation is a "special case," whether the issues involved were unusually easy, the timing unusually propitious, or the political forces aligned in an unusually felicitous combination. Moreover, as with any political issue, much depends upon personalities. But one thing is clear: In October of 1978 Congress enacted the Cannon-Kennedy bill which effectively deregulated the airline industry.[7]

NOTES

1. See, e.g., R. Caves, *Air Transport and Its Regulators* (1962); G. Douglas and J. Miller, *Economic Regulation of Domestic Air Transport: Theory and Policy* 178 (1974); W. Jordan, *Airline Regulation in America* (1970); Note, "Is Regulation Necessary? California Air Transportation and National Regulatory Policy," 74 *Yale Law Journal* 1416 (1965).

2. *CAB Report* in "Proposals for Regulatory Reform: An Introduction," n. 5 *supra*. See also "Report of the CAB Staff on Regulatory Reform: General Conclusion and Principal Recommendations," 41 *Journal of Air Law and Commerce* 60 (1975).

3. See, e.g., *CAB Hearings* in "Different Modes of Classical Regulation and their Problems," n. 15 *supra* at 104 (testimony of G. W. Vans, Senior Vice President, Air Transp. Ass'n).

4. *Ibid.* at 437 (prepared statement of G. W. Douglas, Professor of Economics, Univ. of Tex.).

5. See, e.g., "The Opening Shot to Reform the CAB," *Business Week*, July 7, 1975.

6. Airline Deregulation Act of 1978, Pub. L. 95-504, 92 Stat. 1705 (1978) (primarily amending scattered sections of Federal Aviation Act of 1958, 49 U.S.C. §§ 1301–1551 (1970 and Supp. V 1975)),

7. *Ibid.*

APPENDIX 5-H: CANDIDATES FOR REFORM: PRIORITIES

One should not leave the discussion of substantive reform without a brief judgmental effort to pinpoint existing programs that appear to be logical "candidates" for such reform. The major areas that have been mentioned explicitly or implicitly in this article include the following:

Transportation Airline regulatory reform is well under way. It has proceeded along the lines drawn in this article and it should continue. A similar effort to examine Interstate Commerce Commission (ICC) trucking regulation has begun.

Trucking regulation presents many of the same features found in airlines. The industry is structurally competitive. It is unconcentrated, technical entry barriers are low, variable costs (operating costs) account for a very high proportion of total costs, and necessary investment is small. Economic studies suggest that economies of scale for less than truckload transport are exhausted by the time a firm generates $1 million per year in revenues[1] and diseconomies set in at the level of $10 million. (Total revenues of intercity truckers amounted to more than $50 billion in 1974.)[2]

To apply classical price and entry regulation to such an industry threatens the same harms as in the case of airlines. Prices may be too high. Rate bureaus (associations of private carriers which jointly determine the level of prices in tariffs to be filed with the ICC) may be able to secure approval of prices higher than competitive levels. Firms may provide "excess service" for they face inadequate price competition. It may be difficult for new firms to secure entry into the industry. Indeed, the critics of trucking regulation charge just this: Rates are too high; firms are wastefully led or forced to drive trucks empty on back hauls; the pattern of service is inefficient; and regulation wrongly favors those already in the industry.

At the same time, the rationale of "excessive competition" seems weak, as applied to today's industry. And, insofar as it is meant to refer to predatory pricing, the antitrust laws would seem capable of dealing with the problem.

Given the claims of the critics, an effort to examine the problem seriously would seem warranted. The industry and its regulation is highly complex, with different classifications of carriers, different carriage rules applying to each, different groups of shippers who may have relied upon existing rate patterns in locating their plants, and a system of labor agreements that may also depend upon existing regulation. While one cannot be certain of precise details of an eventual reform proposal, the effort should be made to see whether a shift from classical regulation to an unregulated regime (in which the market is policed by antitrust) would seem warranted.

Finally, it should be noted that regulation of the maritime shipping industry possesses some of these same characteristics: Structurally competitive markets; the use of classical regulatory systems; the rationale of "excessive competition;" and the apparent availability of unregulated markets (with antitrust) as an alternative. Hence, it suggests itself as a natural area for further work.

Energy   Natural gas regulation has been studied in detail within the executive branch and Congress. The extent to which a substitution of regimes is desirable is presently a matter of political debate.

Oil price regulation is also a candidate for reform, for in terms of the analysis presented here, it presents much the same problem as natural gas. The regulatory objectives is one of windfall profit control. The means chosen—classical regulation (in this case historically based price regulation)—seems ill-suited to the problem. A shortage has not appeared, but that is because the regulators have chosen to allocate cheap, low-cost oil through a complex "entitlement system" which, in effect, takes the windfall profit from the old, low cost oil and uses it to "subsidize additional high cost imports."[3] The system is highly undesirable: The object of windfall control is not to transfer windfalls to foreign producers. Thus, it is not surprising that both the executive branch and Congress are actively exploring alternatives— including the use of taxes as a substitute for regulation and deregulation.

Both natural gas regulation and oil regulation are topical political issues—a fact that may make those interested in regulatory reform hesitant to enter the arena. Nonetheless, one cannot avoid pointing out the unsuitability of classical regulation of both gas and oil industries as a means to secure a reasonable regulatory objective.

Health, safety, and environment   Regulatory programs in this area have been discussed throughout this article. The major problem with such programs consists of their near total reliance upon standard-setting to achieve the program's objectives. Reform consists for the most part of efforts to use other, less restrictive regimes as partial substitutes for the classical standard-setting process.

OSHA, for example, has been severely criticized both for ineffectiveness and for imposing unreasonable burdens upon industry in the form of physical safety standards that are expensive to meet and tend to freeze existing technology.[4] OSHA has, however, created an internal task force to look into major reform. And, it is to be hoped that the task force will examine alternative, incentive-based regimes. To some extent, for example, the provision of information about safety might prove more effective than detailed physical standards. Collective bargaining might be used to identify "worst cases" and to allow appropriate variations in standards between firms or industries. Taxes might be used to provide incentives. Performance-oriented standards, such as those requiring a certain "accident-free record," might be substituted for rules governing the precise height of a guardrail. Throughout, to discard the notion of "perfect regulation" to see the virtue in limiting its application to "worst cases," to see the importance of achieving consensus, to recognize the serious drawbacks of setting standards, and to look for incentive-based or other less restrictive alternatives should help to guide the process of achieving major reform.

Similarly, the Environmental Protection Agency is beginning to consider more incentive based alternatives. A variation of the "tax regime"—"marketable rights"—has been proposed that would possess many of the beneficial characteristics of the tax system discussed *supra* in "Alternative Regimes and the Framework Applied." After setting the level of pollution allowed in a region, rights to pollute—limited in total amount—could be sold by the government and freely resold or exchanged by firms doing business there. Similarly, taxes might be considered, not as total substitutes for standards but as supplements that would more readily allow the regulator to set more lenient absolute standards that would totally ban only "worst case" pollution.

The point here, however, is not to argue which particular incentive-based system is best nor to work out its details. It is rather to point out that to move away from total reliance on classical standard-setting in these areas (which potentially affect the entire economy in major ways) is of crucial importance. And it is to encourage effort in these areas to develop and to increase reliance upon the use of less-restrictive rights.

NOTES

1. *Regulation of Entry and Pricing in Truck Transportation* 137 (P. W. MacAvoy and J. S. Snow, Eds., American Enterprise Inst. for Pub. Policy Research, 1977).

2. *Ibid.* at 3.

3. R. Zeckhauser and A. Nichols, *The Occupational Safety and Health Administration: An Overview Prepared for the Senate Committee on Government Operations,* 50 (J. F. Kennedy School of Gov't, Harvard Univ., 1977).

4. See R. E. Hall and R. S. Pindyck, "The Conflicting Goals of National Economic Policy," *The Public Interest* (Spring 1977).

Reaction to Breyer's Proposal for Regulatory Reform

MATCH, MISMATCH, COMPETITION, AND REGULATION

Alain C. Enthoven, *Marriner S. Eccles Professor of Public and Private Management,*
Graduate School of Business, Stanford University

OVERALL REACTIONS: THE POSITIVE SIDE

Stephen Breyer's approach is basically sensible and useful. I believe that an "anatomy of regulatory failure" comparable to the well-developed "anatomy of market failure"[1] is badly needed. For years, an acceptable form of social criticism has been to describe a "failure" in a private market, defined as a departure from the theoretical ideal, and to recommend a regulatory solution on the implicit assumption that the regulator will have the information and the political will to act in the public interest. That is not good enough. Those who advocate regulatory approaches to price and allocation need to understand that there are inherent biases, limitations, and sometimes serious failings in regulatory solutions that arise from the nature of the regulatory process and are inherent in it.

To make the case for government intervention, one should have to demonstrate that the proposed intervention is a good one. One should have to show that the regulatory failure will not be worse than the market failure, since both regulators and markets will depart from the theoretical ideal.

Market failure has been overemphasized. Too many people now believe that markets do not work at all rather than that they work imperfectly, and too many are oblivious to the very disappointing record of government regulation in many areas. So I respond with enthusiasm to Breyer's observation that

> many arguments made in favor of government regulation view regulation, at least in principle, as a perfect solution to a problem of market failure. Indeed, regulation is a "perfect" solution, if one simply states the problem . . . and then views regulators as persons who will order those who pollute too much to stop. "Perfect" regulation would tell firms to arrange price, output processes, and quality so as to cure whatever defect is present in the

275

market. . . . Regulation suffers from typical problems and defects, just as free markets.[2]

A good catalogue of the typical problems and defects of regulation would be a valuable guide to would-be regulators in the field of health services. Roger Noll did a brilliant job of that back in 1974,[3] but unfortunately his paper has not had the circulation and impact it deserved. I wish more people had read Breyer's discussion of the problems of allocation of a scarce resource under a public interest standard before proposing Certificate-of-Need (CON) laws and the National Health Planning and Resources Development Act of 1974. Similarly, the Carter administration might not have proposed the Hospital Cost Containment Act of 1978 if it had read and reflected on Breyer's discussion of price controls based on historical price. While "health care is different," as people specialized in that field like to remind others, it is not so different as to render all other political and economic experience irrelevant. As Breyer puts it, "Persons considering creating or administering systems of regulation must be able to learn from the experience of others in administering a vast variety of other regulatory schemes."[4]

Finally, a survey of the difficulties of regulation reminds us what a marvellous institution the competitive market can be. Charles Schultze noted some of the advantages of the marketplace as a form of social organization in his Godkin Lectures:[5]

> In the first place, relationships in the market are a form of unanimous consent arrangement. . . . [They] minimize the need for coercion as a means of organizing society. A second advantage of the market . . . is that it reduces the need for hard-to-get information. A third advantage . . . [is that] those who may suffer losses are not usually able to stand in the way of change. As a consequence, efficiency-creating changes are not seriously impeded. The final virtue . . . is their potential ability to direct innovation into socially desirable directions.

To these Breyer and I would add that markets allow for continuous individual balancing of costs and benefits by consumers and producers, and markets can adapt quickly, even in anticipation of future changes. Thus, Breyer's study can remind us that, in some cases, a valuable social innovation may be to create a competitive market where one does not exist.

OVERALL REACTIONS: THE NEGATIVE SIDE

On the negative side, Breyer's study reminds me of Isiah Berlin's study of Tolstoy, *The Hedgehog and the Fox*.[6] Berlin took his theme from the Greek poet Archilochus who said, "The fox knows many things, but the hedgehog knows one big thing." Tolstoy wanted to be a hedgehog with his theory of historical inevitability, but he achieved immortality as a fox with his marvelous power of descriptive detail.

It is interesting to trace the evolution of Breyer's thinking through successive drafts. It seems to me that he might have originally intended

to be a hedghog, to make "mismatch" his "one big thing". However, even in his own first summary, he admitted that he is really a fox, for "the value of this paper lies far less in any overarching theory of regulation than in the descriptive details provided in each section." Later, at the end of his first draft, he raised the fox manifesto: ". . . a detailed analysis of the possible advantages *in light of the specific facts related to the relevant industries and* problems must be undertaken before one can reach a firm recommendation [italics added]." Certainly in the refined summary contained in this volume, it is clear that Breyer is proposing an orderly way to examine regulatory alternatives. I think Breyer is a fox, and that that is an honorable and useful breed in the land of regulation.

"Mismatch" suggests "plug in *B* instead of *A* and everything will be okay." Breyer uses the example of rate regulation and rate allocation by the CAB. However, considering his role in CAB deregulation, Breyer does not really offer evidence of "mismatch." The former CAB regulatory style did just what it was supposed to do. It was a cartel run for the airlines by the federal government. To use George Stigler's phrase, the CAB supplied the airline industry's "demand for regulation."[7] It kept the fares above their competitive level, it assured the airlines enough profit and freedom from competitive entry to secure their continued existence, and it supplied members of Congress representing districts with a population inadequate to justify good scheduled airline service with still one more tool by which they could be of assistance to their constituents and thus assure their reelection. In fact, viewed in relation to its real purposes, airline regulation was probably quite a good match.

The problem arose because one consequence of the system was that consumers on many well-travelled routes were forced to pay twice what they would if there were competition. The remedy for that is not some other direct economic control scheme, a "better match." The remedy was abolition of CAB control altogether and the setting of fares and routes in a competitive market, as they first were in California and as is now happening around the country thanks to Breyer's activities.

In a sense, "mismatch" is a truism: If there is an attackable problem, there is a mismatch. If the weapon-problem fit is the best possible— though the results are in some sense poor—then there is no "attackable problem." There is a "problem" if one can hypothesize a better way. The fact that practically everybody dies before age 100 is not a "problem" because nobody had a good idea what to do about it. If someone discovered a fountain of eternal youth at which each drink cost $1 million, then we would have a "problem."

In another sense, the "mismatch" idea is useful. It suggests that one should think through the problem and how things might be made better, examine the experience of various regulatory approaches to see how they have fared in similar circumstances, and pick the best fit. Under other names, that idea has been around for a long time. For example, economists have recommended using taxes to correct for ex-

ternalities for at least 50 years, since the days of Marshall and Pigou.
And 100 years ago the Lord High Executioner in the Mikado was
seeking "to make the punishment fit the crime." So I find no significant
new insight in "mismatch."

Moreover, "mismatch" may inspire an unjustified optimism as to
what can be accomplished with economic regulation. It suggests that
the mere correction of mistakes will solve a lot of problems and make
things better for consumers. I doubt this. I see fewer mistakes and more
underlying reasons than does Breyer. For example, in a memorandum
for then Secretary of HEW Califano on national health insurance,[8] I
observed:

> *Government responds to well-focused producer interests; competitive markets
> respond to broad consumer interests.* People vote their pocketbooks and other
> issues of decisive personal importance. People specialize in production,
> diversify in consumption. To a dairy farmer, a rise in coffee prices is a
> minor irritant, but an increase in milk price supports is a "make or break"
> issue. People are therefore much more likely to pressure their representa-
> tives on their producer interests than on consumer interests, and their
> companies and unions provide a natural organization for doing so. To get
> reelected, members of Congress must respond to well-focused producer
> interests.
>
> In competitive markets, companies get their revenues from satisfied cus-
> tomers who have alternative choices. So in product and pricing decisions,
> business must seek to serve the desires of consumers. Thus, the choice
> between government "command-guided" versus private, competitive,
> market-guided national health insurance is a choice between service
> mainly to providers or to consumers.
>
> Government protection of providers against consumers has been illustrated
> nicely by the typical responses of state legislatures to the so-called "mal-
> practice crisis." That is, they have defined the problem as one of excessive
> judgments and time limits rather than one of excessive incidence of medical
> injury or negligence or inadequate medical quality control. And the reme-
> dies have typically been limits on awards and tighter statutes of lim-
> itations, all to protect providers rather than consumers.

Thus, I find the Breyer paper weak on political insight. Breyer suggests that the reasons for regulation are to correct economic market
failures, and then goes on to see how well it serves these ostensible
purposes. But the reasons for the growth of regulation are far more
complex. For example, George Stigler suggests that there is an economic
demand for regulation: An industry with power to obtain governmental
favors will seek to limit entry by new rivals or by producers of substitute products, and it will seek government help in fixing prices above
competitive levels.[9] Roger Noll offers a "political-economic theory" that
assumes:

> Regulators try to serve some concept of the general public interest, rather
> than act as conduits for the interests of regulated firms. The problem

regulators face is to identify this general public interest in a milieu in which information is uncertain, expensive and biased, and in a society which contains numerous groups whose interests are conflicting rather than harmonious. The political-economic theory focuses on the success indicators available to regulators to assess their own performance. . . . First is the extent to which its decisions are overridden by appeals to the courts. Second is the response of legislators to agency decisions. . . . A third . . . is the performance of the regulated industry. A cataclysmic service failure . . . is likely to be blamed at least in part on the regulators . . . . All three success indicators lead to serious biases in regulatory outcomes. More subtle is the bias inherent in the methods by which agencies collect information for reaching decisions and by which groups dissatisfied with agency decisions appeal to the courts or the legislature for a reversal. . . . All these factors cause regulators to devote most of their attention to the effects of their policies on regulated firms and other well-represented special interest groups.[10]

If Breyer still wants to become a hedgehog, I suggest that he follow the path of other successful social scientists and begin by assuming that there are systematic reasons for things being the way they are and then seek to find them. "Mismatch," i.e., things are what they are because of random mistakes or ignorance, is a fox in hedgehog clothing. A real hedgehog would complete the political-economic circle.

PROCOMPETITIVE REGULATION

Breyer missed a distinction and a policy instrument that I consider important: procompetitive regulation as opposed to direct economic controls. Roger Noll and I developed the idea for the Sun Valley Forum as follows:

A great deal of regulation is inevitable in health care. The debate over regulation is not a matter of all or none. The key issue regarding medical care costs is this. Is the purpose of regulation to stop or reverse the forces determined by the basic financial incentives in the system, or it is to channel those forces into socially desirable forms of competition? Will it attempt to overcome grossly inappropriate financial incentives, or will it merely modify the direction of financial incentives that are already close to being appropriate? Will regulators attempt "to make water run uphill," or merely attempt to channel the stream in its downhill course?

The significance of the distinction is this. The managers of regulated firms will make judgments about the benefits and costs of attempts either to change regulatory rules to their benefit or to evade them. If a regulator attempts to make the regulated behave in a way that is directly opposed to their financial interests, regulated entities will have strong incentives to attempt to bend, fight or evade regulations. This will force regulators to deal with many individual cases and subject them to continuing pressure to grant exceptions to their general policies. If, on the other hand, the regulators attempt merely to modify the behavior of the regulated at the margin in such a way that the financial benefit to the regulated of changing or evading the rules is small, then one can expect fewer, less ferociously battled attempts to change the rules and fewer skillful attempts to evade regulation, for the simple reason that there will be less potential gain if these strategies succeed. In this case, regulators are rarely if ever directly threatening to the financial survival of firms, and can manage these cases by exception.[11]

Antitrust, described by Breyer, is one example. Another is the regulation provided by the Securities and Exchange Commission (SEC)—requirements for audited financial statements, registration statements, publication of material information, limits on insider trading, etc.—all intended to make the securities markets approximate perfect competition and to maintain public confidence in the markets. Another is the requirement in Section 1310 of the Health Maintenance Organization Act of 1973 that most employers must offer their employees membership in one or two health maintenance organizations (HMOs) as part of their health benefits plan.

In September 1977, I recommended to then Secretary Califano establishment of a Consumer Choice Health Plan which includes a procompetitive regulatory framework designed to create competition among health plans that hardly exists today.[12]

It would be useless to argue whether the SEC's program is "procompetitive regulation" or "an alternative to classical economic regulation." Call it what you will. I believe the Breyer paper passed over too lightly a whole range of possible government actions to create or enhance competition, or to design rules for competition in particular industries that will channel their efforts in socially desirable directions.

NATIONALIZATION

I would like to reinforce Breyer's remarks concerning nationalization. The decision to develop the Concorde was exceedingly unwise from an economic point of view. From the onset it was clear that it would never pay back its development and initial production costs if it had to engage in a fair economic competition with contemporary subsonic jets. And it has since become clear that it needs a subsidy to cover operating costs. The plane was developed for reasons of international politics and prestige, a technological spectacular that fit in with General de Gaulle's visions of the leadership role of France. Then, the two national airlines were forced to bail out their governments and spare the political leaders embarrassment by buying and flying some. Thus, nationalization makes an industry into just one more tool that politicians use to get themselves reelected. While private companies have also been known to act on the basis of emotion or prestige, "bottom line responsibility" forces them to be much more dispassionate about promptly burying their mistakes.

I should point out that Breyer probably only included nationalization for the sake of completeness, not because he wanted to engage in a serious discussion of it. Nevertheless in his first draft he wrote "the behavior of governmentally owned airlines, such as British Airways, differs in no significant way from that of private firms such as Pan American or TWA." I found this too uncritical and apparently so did he after the discussion at the conference.

In this country, it is pretty clear that two of the least efficient health care delivery systems are both government-operated: those of the Defense Department and the Veterans Administration.[13] The issue is worth commenting on because there is serious support in this country for government monopoly approaches to national health insurance.

COST-OF-SERVICE RATEMAKING AND NATURAL MONOPOLY

I also do not accept Breyer's preliminary conclusion "that cost-of-service ratemaking is reasonably well suited to the problem of natural monopoly."[14] Where is his evidence?

Here is what Roger Noll found:

> Economists have analyzed demand and cost decisions by regulatory agencies. Except in the case of regulation of natural gas prices at the wellhead, no depressing effect of regulation on prices has been found. For example, retail electric and gas prices do not differ between the group of states that regulates retail power and the group that does not. Airline fares in the intrastate markets in California, where minimum price regulation has not been practiced, are less than half the fares charged in interstate routes of similar length and passenger density that are regulated by the CAB. Pipeline tariffs in regulated interstate markets are not only higher than in the unregulated intrastate markets, but apparently in some cases even somewhat higher than an unconstrained *monopolist* would charge. Either regulation performs no function at all . . . or regulation succeeds, not in lowering prices so that profits will resemble those in competition, but instead in raising costs so that the potential profitability of monopoly pricing is eroded away.[15]

That costs should be raised by cost-of-service ratemaking should not be at all surprising when one considers that it is, as so ably described by Breyer, little else than cost reimbursement in the long run, with its cost-increasing incentives. If our choices are: (1) prices at monopoly levels and profits dissipated in increased costs and (2) prices at monopoly levels, costs minimized, and profits maximized and shared 48 percent/52 percent with the federal government, it would appear to me that the latter alternative is preferable.

CONTROLS ON HEALTH CARE COSTS

The very rapid increase in health care costs in recent years has been straining public finances at every level of government and placing a heavy burden on employers and consumers. While many factors are involved in the cost increases, the main cause is the complex of perverse incentives inherent in the tax-supported system of fee-for-service for doctors, cost reimbursement for hospitals, and third-party intermediaries to protect consumers. Fee-for-service rewards the doctor for providing more and more costly services whether or not more is necessary or beneficial to the patient. Cost reimbursement rewards the hospital with more revenue for generating more costs. Indeed, a hospital administrator who seriously pursued cost cutting, e.g., by instituting tighter controls on surgery and laboratory use and avoiding buying costly diagnostic equipment by referring patients to other hospitals, would be punished by a loss in revenue (Medicare and Medicaid would cut him or her dollar for dollar) and a loss in physician staff and, therefore, patients. Third-party reimbursement leaves the consumer with, at most, a weak financial incentive to question the need for or value of services or to seek out a less costly provider or style of care.

In recent years, the main line of government policy has been to attack the problems created by inappropriate incentives with various forms of regulation, e.g., planning controls on hospital capacity, controls on hospital prices and spending, controls on hospital utilization, and controls on physician fees. The weight of evidence, based on experience in many other industries as well as in health care, supports the view that such regulation is likely to raise costs and retard beneficial innovation.

A great deal of regulation of health services is inevitable. And, as noted *supra*, in some fields, regulation is used to maintain competition, e.g., the SEC. The issue, then, is not regulation in general; it is the specific types of regulation and their likely consequences. The point here is that direct controls on costs, in opposition to the basic financial incentives, are not likely to make things better.

In the long run, price regulation amounts to cost reimbursement and has the same incentives. Regulation tends to protect regulated firms whenever competition or technological change threatens established positions within the industry. The main reason some hospitals favor regulation is that it would function as a cartel to protect them from buyers who want to cut costs. They know that the approved rates will be based on their costs.

Medical care has many characteristics that make it a particularly unsuitable candidate for successful economic regulation. Basic to the problem is the subtle, elusive, and indeed almost indefinable nature of the product. In the health care sector to date, the only economic regulation that has been thoroughly tested is regulation of hospital capacity. And it is clear that CON regulation has not helped control the problem of overbedding. A fixed legislated limit on total capital spending by hospitals might offer a temporary illusion of effectiveness, but it is vulnerable to a number of countermeasures such as "unbundling."

Physician fee controls have been advocated and were tried in the Nixon administration. In judging their likely value as a cost-control device, one should be aware that the "doctor visit" is highly compressible. And the need for doctor visits is impossible to test objectively except in extreme cases.

Overall controls on hospital spending face similar prospects: circumvention, unbundling, exceptions. The Carter administration proposal was quickly emasculated by the wage pass-through, despite the fact that hospital workers now earn more than their counterparts doing similar jobs in other sectors. But even if it were ultimately successful at controlling total hospital spending at the stated growth rate, there would be no force in the system to assure efficiency or equity in the allocation or production of services. At best, we would have frozen the hospital industry in its present wasteful and inequitable pattern. To motivate efficiency and equity, one must address the fundamental financial incentives in the system.

HEALTH CARE AND THE CLASSICAL ARGUMENTS FOR REGULATION

Finally, it is worth noting that the classical arguments for economic regulation for the most part do not apply in health care.

With the exception of small, isolated communities, health care is not a *natural monopoly*. And even in the case of small, isolated communities, there may be "competition for the field" where there cannot be "competition in the field." There are economies of scale in the production of costly specialized services, but generally people can be transported to receive them. There is sufficient demand in California for as many as 30 hospitals producing heart surgery at an efficient volume (500 cases per year).

Some may perceive a need for *windfall profit control* in the case of physician incomes because of limitations in the output of medical schools. As far as I know, the case for control of physician fees for this purpose has not been made and documented. And there is evidence that we are heading toward an oversupply of physicians. Controls on fees are likely to be ineffective in controlling incomes for reasons I explained earlier. Moreover, there are other ways to recapture any excess windfall profit, such as raising tuition to cover the full cost of medical education (accompanied by loans).

Spillovers or externalities are the exception in medical care. Most of the benefits of medical services accrue to the individual patient and his family. The exception is communicable diseases which can be dealt with by various combinations of direct controls (e.g., immunizations required for passports, jobs, school enrollment, etc.) and incentives.

Poor or inadequate information is a serious problem in health care, and the case for regulation to require production of information appears strong. The government could usefully require development and publication of data on qualifications of providers and indicators of quality of care and consumer satisfaction. However, at this point, it appears extremely difficult to develop numerical indicators that are not perverse. For example, use of case-specific fatality rates for heart attacks would penalize providers that take more difficult cases. Frequency of complaints is likely to penalize those who encourage complaints by making it easy to register them and by acting on them positively. So even here it is by no means obvious that a regulatory intervention would make things better.

Finally, the problem of *moral hazard* is not an inescapable and uncorrectable aspect of health care financing in the context of a system of competing private health plans in which providers, as well as consumers, can benefit from economizing choices. While medical insurance must lower the cost of care to the patient below the actual cost at the point of service, the element of provider influence is strong, and an appropriate set of provider incentives can reduce the incentive of physicians to provide care yielding a low marginal value.

NOTES

1. F. Bator, "The Anatomy of Market Failure," *Quarterly Journal of Economics,* (Aug. 1958).

2. Excerpted from *Regulation as an Instrument of Public Administration,* vol. 2, p. 202, the original manuscript of Breyer's forthcoming book as presented to the Harvard Conference (Feb. 27–28, 1978). See Breyer, Chap. 5, "Proposals for Regulatory Reform: An Introduction," *supra* at 202 and n. 1. Also see 92 *Harvard Law Review,* 550. Enthoven's paper, revised 29 April 1979, is based on the book draft presentation at the Conference. It has been updated by the editor to reflect the version in this volume.

3. R. Noll, "The Consequences of Public Utility Regulation of Hospitals," in *Controls on Health Care* (Inst. of Medicine, NAS, 1975).

4. See "Editor's Note," p. 201.

5. C. L. Schultze, *The Public Use of Private Interest* (Brookings Inst., 1977).

6. I. Berlin, *The Hedgehog and The Fox* 1 (Weidenfeld & Nicholson, 1953).

7. G. J. Stigler, "The Theory of Economic Regulation," *The Bell Journal of Economics and Management Science"* (Spring 1971).

8. A. C. Enthoven, *Memorandum for Secretary Califano on National Health Insurance* (Sept. 22, 1977).

9. Stigler, n. 7 *supra.*

10. Noll, n. 3 *supra* at 29–30.

11. A. Enthoven and R. Noll, *Regulatory and Nonregulatory Strategies for Controlling Health Care Costs,* GSB Research Paper, No. 402, (Sept. 1977) (prepared for Sun Valley Forum, Aug. 1977).

12. Enthoven, n. 8 *supra;* see also "Consumer-Choice Health Plan," 298 *New England Journal of Medicine,* 650–658 and 709–720 (Mar. 23 and Mar. 30, 1978, respectively). Also "Consumer-Centered vs Job-Centered Health Insurance," *Harvard Business Review* (Jan.–Feb. 1979).

13. DOD, DHEW, OMB, *Report of the Military Health Care Study* (Dec. 1975); NAS, *Health Care for American Veterans* (May 1977).

14. See Breyer, Chap. 5, "Market Defects" *supra* on page 208.

15. Noll, n. 3 *supra* at 32–33.

REGULATION, HEALTH CARE, AND "MISMATCH"[1]

Lawrence D. Brown, *Governmental Studies Program, The Brookings Institution*

Discussing the application of Stephen Breyer's account of classical regulation to regulatory programs in the health field is difficult, because so little is known about the workings of these latter programs. Until health regulatory programs have been carefully investigated in the field, they cannot usefully be compared with classical counterparts, and sensible policy lessons cannot be drawn. It is important to underscore at the outset the limits of our knowledge about health regulatory programs because the belief has grown up in some quarters that students of public policy command knowledge so vast and insights so deep as to equip them to teach policy makers and administrators when to regulate, when to refrain from regulating, how to regulate when this is the proper course, and how to construct workable policy alternatives when it is not. Indeed this view has taken hold so strongly that some universities now bring practitioners within their walls where they are supposed to learn in courses of greater or lesser length, how and what to do and not to do. In my view this elevated image of the practical wisdom of social scientists and policy analysis is quite mistaken. Academic knowledge and insights about regulation and alternatives to it in the health field at least are in fact rudimentary. As a means of clarifying broad questions and issues, joint scholar-practitioner conferences perform a useful function. However, practitioners who look to scholars for behavioral precepts readily applicable to daily administrative life in the health field delude themselves. Scholars should take pains not to encourage this delusion.

STRUCTURE OF REGULATION

Not least among the many virtues of Breyer's piece is his sensible insistence upon qualifying the noun "regulation" with the adjective

285

"classical." By doing this Breyer shows awareness, often missing in such discussions, that regulation of private firms and public utilities by independent regulatory commissions in Washington is but one mode of regulation among others.

This point is basic, for as much as I admire Breyer's paper—and I know no other treatment of the subject which explains the character of classical regulation so carefully, explores its politics so skillfully, demonstrates its pitfalls and limitations so insightfully, and examines alternatives to it so systematically—I believe that it has very limited application to regulatory programs and problems in the health care field. The classical regulatory agencies, processes, and problems have only a very limited factual and analytical correspondence to contemporary health regulatory efforts.

There is no single regulatory process in the United States; rather, there are several regulatory processes. Classical regulation has dominated the policy literature because: (1) Most of this literature has been written by economists, and (2) economists are fascinated by the market conditions that encourage the resort to classical regulation and by the economic effects that follow from it. In fact, however, *most federal* regulation in the United States does not result when *independent regulatory commissions* hand down rules and specific decisions about the routing, pricing, and other requests of *private firms* and *public utilities*. It results when *line agencies of the federal executive branch* attach regulations as a condition of the receipt of grants-in-aid by *state and local governments*. This latter widespread regulatory process has hardly begun to be studied.[2]

Many health regulatory measures are of this latter type, for example, HEW regulations defining who is eligible for Medicaid benefits and what services Medicaid will cover. In the last few years, however, the federal government for various political reasons that cannot be explored here[3] has played a variation on this theme. It has required, as a condition of receipt of grants, that state and local governments (and in some cases private institutions) establish regulatory processes of their own. By delegating health regulatory tasks, the federal government has deliberately set the process down amidst the distinctive political and administrative environments of the states and their localities. Understanding health care regulation today is an exploration in state and local politics and the politics of federalism.

Health care regulation is not confined to separate delegated health regulatory programs. These delegated programs are the most visible sources of regulatory action in the health care field, however, and the rest of my comments will concentrate upon them. Four programs are of central importance: (1) state rate-setting efforts, which establish prospective charges for hospitals and other institutions; (2) certificate-of-need (CON) processes, which require that hospitals and perhaps other institutions gain approval from state government before significantly expanding their facilities and/or equipment; (3) Professional Standards

Review Organizations (PSROs), which have the power to disallow

certain federal reimbursements for "inappropriate" physician services; and (4) the health systems agencies (HSAs), which construct area-wide plans to be integrated at the state level, and give advice about CON applications and about health-related state and federal grant applications for their jurisdictions.

Two of these programs—PSROs and HSAs—were federal creations. Two—rate-setting and CON—were state innovations now enjoying federal support. Each of the four embodies a distinct structural, political, and administrative approach to regulation. All of them deviate from the independent regulatory commission approach in important ways.

First, rate-setting powers *may* be conferred on a state independent regulatory commission, but in most states they are not. As of December 1975, only four states (Massachusetts, Connecticut, Maryland, and Washington) set rates by independent commission, and only one of them (Massachusetts) provided for full-time commissioners. The rest set hospital rates (if they set them at all) in the departments of health, insurance, social services, or some combination of these, occasionally with the participation of Blue Cross.[4]

A second approach is to vest regulatory powers in some division of a line executive agency of state government. The agency is part of state government, not a commission, much less an independent commission. Most state hospital rate-setting is organized in this way. Similarly, CON offices, usually placed within the state department of public health and usually subject to challenge or reversal by department superiors, the governor, the legislature, the courts, and perhaps some type of public council, partake of this second approach to regulation.

Third, regulation may be entrusted to bodies of professional peers presumed to be uniquely suited to control one another by virtue of special, shared expertise. PSROs, nonprofit associations of local physicians supported by federal funds, come under this heading.

Fourth, regulation may be carried on by local political bodies such as the HSAs. These area-based agencies each include members representing diverse functions (providers, consumers, unions, and so forth) and social groups, and thereby combine a real with functional representation. They reach decisions by supposedly democratic processes and stand subject to the authority of statewide bodies located within but ambiguously related to line agencies of state government.

In short, health care regulatory programs embody four distinct processes conducted at the state and local levels. The four processes—decision making by independent commission, by agency staff, by peer review, and by representative local bodies—represent four distinct normative approaches toward regulation. These are respectively: (1) control by politically insulated "experts," (2) control by politically accountable administrators, (3) control by colleagues, and (4) control by grass-roots citizens. (See Table 6-1.) In view of these differences, it would be extraordinary if any "intrinsic regulatory process" were shared among them, and it is inconceivable that such a process would closely resemble classical regulation at the federal level.

ORIENTATION OF HEALTH CARE REGULATION AND CLASSICAL REGULATION

Many of the characteristics of these health regulatory programs do in fact diverge sharply from classical regulation. In his article "Different Modes of Classical Regulation," for example, Breyer lists four similarities among classical regulatory efforts. These similarities, he argues, explain why it is "possible to group programs of economic regulation into forms which are characterized by certain features and attendant problems. . . ."[5] These areas of similarity are: (1) the bureaucratic character of the regulator, (2) the tendency for new regulatory programs to copy older ones, (3) the applicability of the requirements of administrative law to regulatory decisions, and (4) the adversary relationship between regulator and industry. It may be useful to consider briefly how far these similarities extend to the health regulatory programs.

Bureaucratic character   Rate-setting and CON processes are indeed carried on by an institutional bureaucracy, although in many states this description of a few health department employees is grandiose. On the other hand, the PSROs and HSAs reach decisions by peer interaction and majority rule, respectively. They have their little bureaucracies attached, but all four bodies are institutionalized quite differently from the independent regulatory agencies of which Breyer writes.

For this reason, drawing analogies from the organizational and bureaucratic literature on the federal independent regulatory commissions to health regulatory bodies may be extremely misleading. To understand rate-setting and CON processes, we should look first to studies of public administration at the state level. Unfortunately, very little is known about the behavior of state agencies. For PSROs we might usefully look to the literature on small group theory, on professionals in organizations, and on collegial administration. Better still, we might look to Eliot Freidson's *Doctoring Together*, a splendid study of peer review in a prepaid group practice, which draws careful and balanced implications for PSROs.[6] Lacking good analytical studies of the Comprehensive Health Planning (CHP) agencies, we might seek insight into the HSAs in (for example) the experience of the old farmer committee system or Model Cities or some similar effort to plan by means of local organizations composed of area and interest group spokesmen.[7] None of these orientations owes any important debt to the theory and practice of classical regulation.

Copying old programs   Whereas the classic regulatory programs tend to copy older analogies—"Thus the framers of the Civil Aeronautics Act (1938), precursor of today's Federal Aviation Act, copied the language of the Interstate Commerce Act (1887), which in turn was modeled on the British Railroad Act (1845),"[8]—the health regulatory programs tend to be evolutions—incremental adaptations—or well-established state and

TABLE 6-1   An Overview of Health Care Regulations

Program	Structure	Target	Locus	Powers	Principal
1. Rate setting	Independent commissions State agency	Hospitals (etc.)	State	Set prospective charges	"Expert" decision making
2. CON	State agency	Hospitals (etc.)	State	Control institutional expansion	Decision making by political executives
3. PSROs	Physician review bodies	Physicians	Local	Disallow federal reimbursement	Peer review
4. HSAs	Local representative bodies	"Resources," especially public grants and CON applications	Local	Review, plan, comment, sign off	Grass-roots democracy/interest-group liberalism

local approaches in the health field itself. Rate-setting is an extension of and variation on traditional state insurance regulation. The CON process updates and expands longstanding state accreditation and licensing procedures for hospitals. PSROs extend established hospital utilization and quality review activities. The HSAs increase somewhat the planning and review and comment powers of their predecessors, the Hill-Burton and CHP agencies. Incremental variations on health-related activities well-established in the states themselves may match problem and weapon more effectively than interfunctional, even international analogies.

Applicability of administrative law   Whereas classical decisions "are made subject to the requirements of administrative law, chiefly the Administrative Procedure Act (APA) . . . ,"[9] the health care regulation programs have a more ambiguous legal and administrative status. A judicial and legislative battle is presently underway over whether the PSROs are or not "federal agencies" and what their status implies about the public's right to see their data. The bearing of state administrative procedural law on the HSAs which are partly federal, partly state, and partly local bodies empowered with an ambiguous combination of planning and review and comment "authority," is far from clear. Rate-setting and CON statutes differ greatly from state-to-state, and so, apparently, does the application of administrative law to them. It will probably take years of adjudication and legislative clarification before a body of administrative law emerges to spell out the status and obligations of the health regulatory programs with thoroughness and stability comparable to that found in the relationship between federal regulatory commissions and the federal APA.

Adversary relationship   A final feature of the classical regulatory programs is the "adversary" relationship they establish.[10] If this description means an adversary relationship between industry on the one hand and regulator on the other, it does not apply well to the PSROs and HSAs, a central feature of which is to incorporate industry and regulator in peer or representative bodies. It applies well enough to rate-setting and CON processes, but similarity, important though it is, is hardly enough on which to hang a theory or on which to base many generalizations.

THE RATIONALE FOR HEALTH CARE REGULATION

It may be argued that these distinctions place too much weight upon structure and process and too little upon function. Are the rationales and activities of these regulatory bodies not very similar to those described by Breyer and susceptible to similar pitfalls and problems? Alas, I must repeat that we know very little about what state and local health care regulators do or about how they perceive their tasks. Nonetheless, I suspect that the answer to the first question (similarity of activities and rationales) is "probably not," and to the second (similarity of pitfalls) "quite possibly not."

In the first place, the problems that the health regulatory programs

address and the aims which they set for themselves differ markedly
from those of their classical counterparts. For example, "A traditional, persistent rationale for price and profit regulation," Breyer tells us, "is based on the need to control the exercise of power by a 'natural monopolist.' "[11] This problem is that, "Where economies of scale are so great as to make it inefficient for more than one firm to supply a product, that firm, if not regulated, would increase its profits by restricting output and charging higher than competitive prices if free to do so."[12] The problem, in short, turns on the preconditions of competition.

Despite the predominance of economists in the health policy literature, amazingly little careful empirical attention has been given to what the terms "markets," "competition," "well-functioning market competition," and the like mean or might mean in health care services, and to what their actual or possible meanings mean in turn for public policy. One analyst will invoke the "private" character of the United States health care system, apparently taking it for granted that "nonpublic" and "market-based" are synonymous. A second will compile long lists of the ways in which health care services deviate from the assumptions that support classical market theory and take an agnostic or highly cautious position on policy "solutions." A third analyst, looking at the very same list of deviations, will offer heated assurances that policy makers can only solve their problems by strengthening or introducing competition, market forces, cost-consciousness, and the like. A fourth will declare firmly that markets and market forces do not and cannot work in a field with the peculiar properties of health care, while a fifth bitterly deplores the fact that in the United States health care is treated as a "commodity" to be bought and sold. Clarification of these terms, investigation of how they (thus clarified) apply to the United States health care system, and sober reflection on what these findings might mean for public policy would be highly desirable.

For present purposes it is enough to postulate that the cost and composition of health care services in the United States result from interplay among variables which may be grouped under five general headings: (1) the expectations and demands of *consumers*; (2) the state and diffusion of *technology*; (3) the number, distribution, and professional norms of *physicians*; (4) the number, distribution, and organizational character of *hospitals*; and (5) the behavior of *third-party payers* (including government).[13] The last three variables are the ones of greatest direct interest to regulators.

Insurers, hospitals, and physicians display an odd mix of disparate competitive processes, about which we badly need to know more. In most places, health care insurance is quite a competitive business; the competition occurs between nonprofit Blue Cross and Blue Shield and profit-making "commercial" plans, and it is carried on in the economic medium of premiums, costs, and benefits purchased.

Hospital costs, on the other hand, are usually fueled by competition of a very different type—among predominantly nonprofit institutions which meet their organizational maintenance and enhancement needs by competition not in the currency of price but, instead, of "quality," or at any rate the trappings of quality.

Physicians engage in yet a third type of competitive dynamic, little studied and understood. Although physicians are sometimes said to "monopolize" their services, this usually refers to quite a different problem—the fact that the physician-supplier often determines the consumer's demand—and indeed those who charge "monopoly" often assert in the next breath that medicine in the United States is a "cottage industry."

The three different but interdependent competitive modes create a distinctive economic context for regulation in the health field. Whereas the aim of classical regulation is to keep price near cost as a method of inducing the regulated firm to expand its output, in health care the aim is essentially the reverse: To induce providers to contract (or alter the nature of) output as a means of curbing both price and cost.

One aspect of health care to which the traditional rationale seems to apply is rent control. Breyer says that windfall profits may occur as the result of sudden increases in the price of a commodity without a simultaneous change in cost.[14] Superficially analogous is the increase in physician incomes and hospital revenues that followed the introduction of Medicare or Medicaid or that would probably follow the enactment of national health insurance. Yet whereas the examples Breyer offers— "those who owned large stocks of oil earned huge rents when the Arabs raised the price of new oil; owners of old natural gas earned rents when the costs of finding new natural gas rose; and those who own existing housing earn rents as long as construction costs rise faster than other costs . . ."[15]—follow from restrictions on supply, the "explosions" following new government entitlements follow largely from new demand by disadvantaged groups. And whereas classical windfall profits are "undeserved," meaning that they "do not reflect any particular talent or skill on the part of the producers," higher health care charges are *fees for services* rendered by highly trained professionals whose reasonable and fair rate of reimbursement is precisely what is at issue.

The political context in the health care case thus differs greatly from the classical. Neither taxing away the windfall (one possibility Breyer points out,[16] nor bargaining over fee schedules (the Canadian and European continent approach) are politically acceptable when government leverage is noncomprehensive (confined largely to federal reimbursements for care of the elderly and poor), when the cooperation of the providers of an intimate human service is thought to be essential, and when fear of turning government programs into a system of second-class care is strong. As a result, the least among evils has seemed to be acceptance of "usual and customary" fees, adjusted to be "reasonable," and modified incrementally and quietly over time in administrative regulations accompanying the Medicare and Medicaid programs.

The other traditional rationales are at most minor motives for regulation in the health care field. Some analysts hope that "correcting for inadequate information"[17] on the part of consumers if, for example, doctors were permitted to advertise their fees, would enhance price competition, but few expect such innovations to alter greatly the many forces that subordinate a patient to his or her physician's judgment.

Some argue that we suffer from "excessive competition"[18] among physicians and that the proper antidote is government measures to limit the number of physicians we train. Others argue, however, that the true solution is to increase drastically the number of physicians in the United States in order to make them "really" compete, and thereby drive costs down. That eminent economists may be found on both sides of the question illustrates how little we presently know about competition among physicians.

Rationalization, unequal bargaining power, scarcity, and paternalism[19] have not been major motives for the new health regulatory efforts. "Correcting for spillovers"[20]—meaning reducing the ability of consumer, physician, and hospital to pass along costs to third-party payers—is sometimes adduced as a rationale for regulation, but this is simply an imprecise way of pointing to the one rationale which does play an important role in the health care programs: "Moral hazard."[21] "Escalating medical costs" is the "most obvious current example" of the moral hazard rationale, Breyer observes. Significantly, he cites no other example, current or classical,[22] a fact which may support the argument that the rationales for health care regulation are distinct.

The key and distinctive features of health care regulatory rationales are: (1) that they aim to constrain medical care prices which become "excessive" for reasons that have little to do with classical economics and classical markets; and (2) that they are themselves prohibited from addressing directly the problem of moral hazard, that is, they are not allowed directly to restrict consumers from demanding care without due regard to price. In sum, the regulatory rationale calls for programs to constrain the growth of charges by providers of health care services. This rationale owes little to the classical theories of market breakdown, is more political than economic, and more pragmatic than theoretical. It reflects above all the politician's need to "do something" about a public "crisis."

POLICY WEAPONS

A reader might accept my distinctions between classical regulation and contemporary health care regulation with respect to structure, orientation, and rationale, and yet nonetheless argue that these distinctions simply provide ironic confirmation of Breyer's mismatch hypothesis, that is, that we may well be pursuing policy problems—in this case health policy problems—with inappropriate tools. Differences in structure, orientation, and rationale aside, are the specific policy weapons employed in the two regulatory fields not remarkably similar? Is hospital rate-setting anything other than a subtype of cost-of-service ratemaking and historically based price-setting? What is CON determination but a variant of public interest allocation? And do PSRO and HSA reviews not amount to standard-setting and all that goes with it?

These questions cannot be answered without a detailed comparison of the nature of the "weapons" in the two fields. Such a comparison should examine five variables: (1) the *goal* of regulation, (2) the *object* of regulation, (3) the nature of the regulatory *task*, (4) the nature of the regulatory *organization*, and (5) the distinctive *problems* to which regulation gives rise. Although a thorough discussion cannot be attempted here, the following remarks will suggest that regulatory activities in the two fields are sufficiently different to be in no clear sense analogous.

First, hospital rate-setting deviates in many respects from the cost-of-service ratemaking and historically based price regulation which it seems to resemble. The goal of cost-of-service ratemaking, Breyer writes, "is to replicate those prices that would exist in well-functioning competitive markets."[23] In the hospital sector, a "well-functioning competitive market" is neither a clear nor a useful standard, and the rate-setter's objective therefore differs. In Maryland, for example, the goal is to "certify that total costs are reasonably related to total services offered, that aggregate rates are set in reasonable relationship to aggregate costs, and that rates are set equitably without undue discrimination."[24]

The difference in goals reflects a difference in objects of regulation. Classical federal cost-of-service ratemakers deal mainly with profit-making firms. State health rate-setters deal mainly with nonprofit hospitals. Whether or not precise differences in organizational behavior correspond to the difference between "profits" and "revenues" is unclear, but the two cannot simply be equated. There is a sizable economics and a smaller sociological literature on how hospital structure and behavior differ from those of classical firms and generalizations should take account of these differences.

Not surprisingly, differences in goal and object produce differences in the regulatory task. Breyer's classical cost-of-service ratemaker

> chooses a test year, adds to that year's operating costs, depreciation, and taxes, and adds to that sum a reasonable profit (determined by multiplying a reasonable rate of return times the "rate base," i.e., investment, which is determined by taking historical investment and subtracting prior depreciation), thus giving the firm's "revenue requirement." Prices are then set to yield revenues that equal this revenue requirement.[25]

When the profit variable can be disregarded in computing revenue requirements and prices, the exercise, although not simple, is simpler. For instance, the first two problems Breyer finds in classical ratemaking—"determining the investment upon which the firm is allowed to charge a profit"[26] and "determining the 'just and reasonable' rate of return"[27]—seldom bedevil the hospital rate-setter.

Hospital rate-setting appears to be a much more eclectic and improvisational enterprise than its classical counterpart. Katherine Bauer explains that

There is no established wisdom to guide hospital rate-setting. Most programs are still struggling to develop a satisfactory process, they make changes in their methods almost yearly. . . .

In practice, Bauer notes, the rate setters arrive at the future year's rate by examining the current year's rate in light of special features of the individual hospital's costs, budgets, and volume; comparisons among institutions; the movement of economic indicators; and recommendations of planning agencies, usually in some combination.[28] There is no a priori reason to equate these tasks with those of classical rate-setting. To what extent the agencies do the "same thing" is an open empirical question.

Moreover, the political and organizational character of the regulatory bodies in the two fields differs. As noted earlier, in very few states have rate-setting bodies adapted the independent commission mode of the federal level. In some states, the complex, overlapping responsibilities of state insurance commissioners, state health departments, rate-setting or rate-review commissions, Blue Cross, and others probably politicize rate-setting and facilitate negotiation and bargaining much more than does the traditional federal arrangement.

Finally, the problems to which hospital rate-setting gives rise may well differ too. Of the five classical problems discussed by Breyer, two—those involving profits—are bound to differ. Although it is no doubt difficult to determine "a proper rate structure" for hospitals,[29] it is arguable whether the rates constructed by regulation—which may diminish or remove cross-subsidies among services and departments, for example—are more or less "proper" than those that evolve when the hospital is left alone. Whether the rate-setters have adequately adjusted rates "to reflect likely changes in cost or demand" is likewise an empirical question.[30]

As for efficiency considerations, some impressive statistics can be marshalled in the rate-setters' behalf. A recent review of rate-setting in Maryland, for instance, pointed out that whereas hospital costs rose 15.6 percent in the nation as a whole in 1976, the increase in Maryland was only 11.8 percent. In 1977, the national increase was 14.9 percent but only 9.7 percent in Maryland. The study remarked that the differences "amount to $72 million in savings for Marylanders over two years."[31]

The central question over the longer term, however, concerns the effects of rate-setting on organizational change. Specifically, will the fiscal constraints imposed by rate-setters on hospital managers be translated effectively in turn into managerial pressures-cum-incentives to change physicians' behavior toward inpatient services? The Maryland study is again suggestive:[32]

"It's a doctors' hospital" is the phrase usually used to describe an institution operated on the principle that physicians should be given whatever facilities, equipment, nursing support and ancillary services they want, with no questions asked. Under rate regulation, there are few "doctors' hospitals" left in Maryland . . . [H]ospitals can no longer base their spending decisions primarily on physician requirements. The physician's role, then, is largely one of understanding—a realization that hospitals must now work within a legal and financial framework that they have only a limited ability to change. . . .

But until the sequence of pressures and adjustments is examined microscopically (that is, with interviews and observation, not aggregate data) in a large number of hospitals, the question cannot be answered.

Until careful attention is given to possible differences between classical ratemaking and its health care counterpart with respect to goals, objects, tasks, organization, and problems, it will be impossible to judge whether, for example, the administration's proposed regulatory approach to hospital cost containment will or will not encounter classical pitfalls. On pages 238–240 *supra*, Breyer briefly makes the case for thinking that it would. Unfortunately, he does not discuss how health care might be different, does not draw upon state hospital rate-setting experiences for evidence, does not suggest that these programs might have lessons to offer, and neglects even to mention that these programs exist.

Yet Breyer's own words aptly illustrate the pitfalls of inference. "Firms in a competitive industry, subject to cost-of-service ratemaking," he writes, "will compete by providing excessive service or a higher quality product, giving the consumer more service or quality than he wants, and eventually charging a higher price for doing so."[33] This statement describes quite well the behavior of the non- (price) competitive hospital industry in the *absence* of regulation. The aim of hospital rate-setting is to inhibit the very behavior that, according to Breyer, classical rate-setting tends to produce.

For several reasons, CON regulation cannot readily be equated with public interest allocation, despite the surface similarity that both engage in public licensing of private institutions seeking to provide, expand, or alter a service.

First, in classical public interest allocation, the goal is to compare applicants for a license in order to determine which is "best" able to do a job generally agreed to need doing.[34] In hospital CON processes, the goal is to place a heavy burden of proof on those who allege that the community needs a costly service or facility and that it needs it at a certain institution or location. The objective in the latter case, in short, is first to decide the "what"—or, better, the "whether"—and then decide the "who." The point is to ensure that expectations of expansion and acquisition automatically considered to be institutional prerogatives or rights in the past will be treated now and in the future as problematic.

Second, the CON approach should be examined against the distinctive properties of the regulated object. In a health care system where the services of "doctors' hospitals" are heavily financed by third-party payers, the logic of organizational maintenance and enhancement will lead hospitals to expand facilities and acquire equipment in order to be

first with the best. Thus, whereas debates about whether, for example, airline routes and television broadcasts need be limited for technical reasons and about whether less licensing and more competition will better serve consumers' preferences (as measured in willingness to pay) dominate classical public interest allocations, CON questions turn much less on technical and price-competitive factors than on the combined influence of the organizational character of hospitals and the omnipresence of third-party payment.

Third, the regulatory tasks differ because criteria differ in scope and content. The traditional problem is "too many standards, without clear rules how they apply to individual cases or how they are to be weighed."[35] For example, Breyer lists seven presumably coequal criteria at issue in CAB awards.[36] Analogous criteria come into play in CON processes, but they do so (at least in theory) only after they have been subordinated to one criterion—"the needs of local communities."[37] Moreover, although the CON decision maker may be required to choose among several contending applicants, he or she is often asked to make an "on the merits" judgment of the community's need for expansions proposed by individual applicants. Thus the classical image of a public interest allocator awash in multiple, coequal, ambiguous, and conflicting criteria manipulated and distorted by hordes of clamoring applicants may not accurately capture the regulatory tasks of CON regulators.

Fourth, the two processes are organized differently. Classical regulatory agencies are generally independent commissions. CON agencies (or staffs) are usually parts of the state executive branch, usually the state health department. In public interest allocations, aggrieved interests have recourse mainly to the agencies' own procedures and then to the courts. These appeals take a great deal of time. In CON regulation, disgruntled applicants may try their luck with the agency, the head of the public health department, the governor, the legislature, a public health council (at least in Massachusetts), and the courts. They may also try to bring community, constituent, and media pressures upon any or all of these authorities. They may deploy these political resources before, contemporaneous with, and/or after the decision itself—and they probably will act at all three stages. CON regulation is deeply embedded in the free-wheeling health care politics of the states and localities—and CON regulators know it. For example, Breyer's account of the painstaking steps to change in the CAB[38] contrasts sharply with the CON situation in Massachusetts, where it appears that the process has been drastically transformed overnight simply because a Governor who supported the process was replaced by one who does not.[39]

CONs easily become the occasion, sometimes the stimulus, for bargaining and coalition-building across a wide range of organizations and interests. For example, the proposal of a Dayton, Ohio hospital to expand its beds recently brought on the disapproval of General Motors Corporation (which, a spokesman said, objected to the increased Blue

Cross premiums its Dayton plants would face as a result) and the local health planning agency, which recommended that a CON be denied. When the state health director granted the certificate anyway, Blue Cross of Southwest Ohio terminated its contract with the hospital on the grounds that "The policy of our governing board is not to reimburse hospitals that make capital expenditures contrary to decisions of local health planners." The hospital then appealed the Blue Cross decision to the state insurance director and may turn to the courts.[40]

The community free-for-all surrounding CON decisions may place a check on the major problem in classical public interest allocation: The inevitable, pervasive subjectivism of a process that confers on a few "independent" bureaucrats the task of resolving several unclear, conflicting criteria in favor of one of several conflicting applicants of unclear merit. Or perhaps better put, community health politics produce a different type of subjectivism, one fashioned from the pulling and hauling of affected interests. If one is in search of an antidote to bureaucratic politics as practiced by the classical agencies, the CON approach should not be scorned a priori. If the aim, however, is a decision-making process that reproduces the rigors of the well-functioning competitive market or the rational planner's designs, CON processes obviously fall short.

In sum, classical federal regulatory and state CON processes are differently institutionalized, bureaucratized, and politicized. Interestingly, Breyer seems to come to much the same conclusion. Although he cautions that CON regulators "will be pushed toward public interest allocation,"[41] he then cites a concrete case—CAT scanner policy in Boston[42]—which supports the hypothesis suggested here, that the process is a forum for negotiation and bargaining: "Such negotiation may work to the disadvantage of outsiders, may not be totally [sic] rational, and may reflect political considerations," he warns. "But," he concludes, "the fact that it obtains consensus among those directly affected, that knowledgeable parties make the allocation decision, and that the worst cases of waste are likely to be stopped may make this bargaining solution preferable to any form of classical regulation."[43] That the process lends itself so readily to bargaining solutions may suggest that it is not in fact "any form of classical regulation."

Finally, I shall consider briefly whether the PSROs, which evaluate physician behavior against "profiles" and "norms"—standards, in effect—for the admission of patients to the hospital and their lengths of stay there, and the HSAs, which draw up plans and make recommendations about CON and state and federal grant applications based on these plans, exemplify the standard-setting process described by Breyer.

In essence, classical standard-setting is a process which relies on government regulators imperfectly familiar with the regulated industry to devise standards to govern that industry by means of an adversary process subject to judicial review.[44] In the classical process, the goal is to devise operational, legally defensible standards that address the quality, safety, reliability, or other such properties of some product. The purpose of PSROs is, by contrast, far more limited: To isolate "worst cases"—instances of physician (mis)use of hospital care so blatant as to justify a denial of reimbursement with federal funds. The objective of the HSAs is to draw up plans which do, of course, incorporate standards, but there the similarity ends.

In classical standard-setting, a regulator designs standards and then applies them to an industry usually composed of private firms. In PSROs the object of regulation is physicians, a respected professional group given the luxury of self-regulation precisely in order to avoid the frictions of an adversary process. As for the HSAs, they do not "enforce" their "standards" on an "industry" at all. State and federal officials are expected to take the HSAs' work into account when they make their own decisions, but they need not treat them as authoritative.

The nature of the regulatory tasks differs substantially too. The health standards-setters manage to avoid some of the horrendous complexities that plague classical agencies like the National Highway Traffic Safety Administration (NHTSA).[45] Whereas NHTSA found it very difficult to "prove" associations among product characteristics (such as tire design), environmental variables (such as road conditions), and outcomes (blowouts and other indicators of "safety"), PSROs deal mainly in *procedural* indicators of necessity, appropriateness, and quality, not *outcome* measures. They do this by quantifying prevailing practice patterns for given diseases in given areas and treating them as a "norm." They then permit exceptions when physicians give convincing reasons for large deviation in the course of case-by-case, "on the merits" reactive review by peers. The process is much simpler, much less adversarial, and much less likely to lead to the courts than is NHTSA's approach. For these reasons "the most typical and most serious" of the classical standard-setting problems—that of obtaining accurate and complete information from the industry[46]—takes a nonclassical form in the PSRO case. But the issue is not the (self)-regulator's access to data but rather the public's right to know.

The HSA planners may include in their plans outcome standards—a decrease of a given amount in certain forms of mortality and morbidity in certain areas, for example—but there is no pretense that HSAs or anyone else will *enforce* these standards, that is, impose a definite penalty or go to court if the responsible industry or firm fails to comply with the standard. Most of the HSAs' planning and review activities involve manipulation of reams of statistical data on ratios of *inputs* (physicians, hospitals, and so on) to population units, utilization data, and the like; "enforcement" means patient bargaining and negotiation to win support for the agencies' priorities. The HSAs do not attempt to research and specify elaborate relations among inputs, processes, and outcomes; then formulate operational standards based on these relations; and then enforce and refine them. The regulatory tasks are so different as to be in no useful sense comparable.

PSROs and HSAs are also very different types of institutions from classical standard-setting bodies. Both are local-based, comparatively nonbureaucratic bodies which incorporate regulator and regulated within the organization itself. Indeed the HSAs may be viewed as a type of institutionalized bargaining process in which a perceived imbalance between consumers and providers is offset by the requirement that these and other interests come together to plan around a table at which consumer dominance is, at least in theory, mandated. It would be surprising if organizations based on peer review and interest group bargaining (called "planning") behaved very similarly to classical independent commissions regulating private sector adversaries.

In sum, the health care standard-setters: (1) Set themselves more modest objectives; (2) employ "self-regulation" and bargaining to a large degree; (3) are less preoccupied with precise specifications of relationships among input, processes, and outcomes; and (4) are less bureaucratic and "independent" than their classical counterparts. There are many problems, both in theory and practice with these health care programs,[47] but few, perhaps none, of them could be accurately predicted or usefully discussed on the basis of comparisons with NHTSA or other classical federal standard-setters.

MATCH AND MISMATCH IN HEALTH CARE REGULATION

Some problems of regulation, whether classical or in the health field, are no doubt inherent in the regulatory enterprise itself. Others, however, are intrinsic to assigning values to facts and matching means to ends in complex social systems. Producing useful definitions of "reasonable" hospital charges, "need" for medical facilities, "appropriateness" of physician care, and the like will always be difficult, whether the task is addressed by regulation (classical or other), embodied in legislation, left to market forces, or merely entrusted to "policy analysis" (that is, human reasoning). Fortunately, I may limit myself here to a more modest question, whether health care regulation as now practiced in the United States is more or less likely than alternative policy techniques to achieve desired ends.

As Breyer rightly emphasizes, the choice between regulation and other policy weapons should rest on a careful definition of the problem at hand, just as the decision to "reform" regulation should rest on "a detailed examination of the actual effect of the regulatory program at issue."[48] Policy weapons should be "matched" to the complex characteristics of the problems at which they are aimed. I find this recommendation more correct than useful, for, especially in the health field, it begs the question. The intellectual intricacies involved in discerning a true match—"determine one's objectives, examine the alternative methods of obtaining those objectives, . . . explore in detail all the benefits and harms of and justification for regulation and deregulation, . . . choose the best method"[49]—are basically the same problems that bedevil setting rates, awarding licenses, and establishing product standards in classical regulation. "Matching," it seems to me, is on the same plane of intellectual difficulty as regulating.

The problem is simplified considerably in the health field by the fact that most of the alternative regimes identified by Breyer are obviously unsuited to take on the problems that have fueled the drive toward greater regulation. Specifically, unregulated markets policed by anti-trust,[50] disclosure regulation,[51] bargaining,[52] changes in liability rules,[53] and nationalization[54] are not likely to supplant regulation in the foreseeable future. The list thus dwindles to two alternatives: Taxes and market-based incentives or allocation,[55] which, by virtue of their common focus on consumer cost-consciousness and its effects on providers, are often treated together in the health care field under the heading of "market-based" approaches. And indeed it is often argued that the central policy choice we now face in the health field is that of market approaches "versus" regulation.

Unfortunately, the heuristic maxim that one should seek a "match" between problem and policy offers little useful guidance here. The reason is that we have reached no agreement on exactly what the nature of the cost containment problem is. Of course, coordinating strategies for dealing with this problem with others designed to increase access to care and to improve its quality makes matching enormously more difficult still. Ironically, the most serious conceptual obstacle to perceiving suitable matches in the health care field may be precisely the common view that we must make a "choice between regulatory *versus* market mechanisms."

If we introduce explicitly into consideration the political variables I have been emphasizing throughout these comments, we see that both market and regulatory approaches may be applied in more or less centralized (or decentralized) ways, and the nature of our policy options grow clearer. (See Table 6-2.)

The following argument illustrate how this approach may help the matching process.

First, suppose that our diagnosis of the health care cost problem blames excess hospital beds, overuse of inpatient services, extravagant technological expansion, and the like. This definition of the problem concentrates attention upon patterns of acquisition and use by and within hospitals themselves; it concentrates, in short, upon organizational behavior. If this is the problem we might naturally look to Cell 1—decentralized regulatory strategies—for a solution and this is exactly what policy makers have done. Rate-setting programs to encourage

TABLE 6-2 Policy Strategies and Loci of Application

	Decentralized	Centralized
Regulation	1	2
Market	3	4

institutional thrift, CON procedures to constrain institutional expansion, PSROs to monitor use of inpatient facilities, and HSAs to plan a more defensible areal distribution of resources: all constitute regulatory programs supposed to be close enough to local health care settings—especially hospital settings—to understand their nuances and peculiar needs, but are strong enough to restrain their excesses.

Second, although, as I argued at length above, one should not dismiss this approach out of hand, it is quite possible, perhaps likely, that experience and research will show that local expansionist pressures are simply too powerful for state and local regulators to contain. Perhaps, then, the problem posed by the organizational maintenance and enhancement of hospitals should be viewed in a broader perspective. After all, hospitals in the United States are not only "health care" institutions but also community monuments, chips in local philanthropic and other political games played with great energy and enthusiasm by local notables. Also, it is only natural that regulators who work closely with and sometimes grew up with and live among spokesmen for these health care interests should gain sympathy for their needs and institutional perspectives in the course of interaction. As regulator and "interest" come face-to-face to debate reasonable rates, discuss CON applications, review inpatient use, and assemble an areawide plan, the regulator may acquire an insider's view of the rigors of running a hospital, the merits of new technology, the incredible complexity of professional judgment, and the multiplicity of deeply felt, sincerely held values surrounding health care. For policy purposes, the health care cost problem may be much more than the sum of individual institutional aggrandizements. Our hospital "system"—that is, the way we think about, build, and use hospitals (and other institutions)—may be the problem.

If so, it may seem logical to take many regulatory decisions out of local and perhaps even state political arenas. We might elect to move into Cell 2, centralized regulation, by means of, for example, federally imposed revenue and capital-expenditure "caps" like those proposed by the Carter administration. We might even conceivably choose to make the proper and real division of labor among hospitals a national decision, and distribute and redistribute activities according to a central plan matching function and form to need.[56]

Third, some analysts, however, may argue that hospitals, whether viewed organizationally or systematically, are secondary elements of the cost containment problem. When all the sources of hospital-charge inflation, from wage and salary "catch-up" to excess capacity, have been given their due weight, the "real" problem may turn out to be profligate use by physicians of expensive inpatient care. The average physician, the argument goes, has strong incentives to admit patients to the hospital too often, to keep them there too long, and to run too many tests and procedures on them during their stay. These incentives flow from professional norms, third-party reimbursement rules (which often pay for inpatient but not outpatient procedures), defense against future malpractice claims, the "technological imperative," the convenience of

both doctor and patient, and more.

Canada and many European nations contain more beds-per-10,000 persons than the United States; in these nations admissions tend to be more numerous and hospital stays longer than is customary here.[57] Detailed and widely accepted fee schedules, however, give Canada and much of Europe a measure of control missing in this country. Europe and Canada have adopted universal national health insurance programs and it is apparently accepted that whoever pays the fiddler (government), bargains with providers, unions, sick funds, and others over the tune. In the United States, where government financing of health care extends only to a portion of the population, federal controls on the fees and practices of "private" physicians in the "private" sector would stir great resentment and seem to be another insupportable federal regulatory usurpation. In the United States, at least at present, strong regulatory approaches to physician behavior are unlikely to emerge.

Some therefore have argued that we should address this problem within Cell 3—a decentralized market strategy—designed to change physician incentives. HMOs, local group practice plans operating on prospective budgets with physicians responsible for both inpatient and outpatient care rendered to subscribers enrolled by prepayment, are the major policy effort along these lines.

Although the economic logic of HMOs is undeniably appealing to those whose first concern is cost containment, HMOs cannot be viewed simply as a bundle of economic laws. They are complex organizations which require that an extensive set of contributors—sponsors, subscribers, physicians, and hospitals—be brought together under skillful management and induced to work harmoniously together over time. This organization-building task—attracting the right number of the right contributors at the right time—is extremely difficult and has only been made more complex by the fact that HMO experts and government enthusiasts for HMOs disagree widely and deeply over the design of federally supported HMOs. For these and other reasons, despite almost 10 years of federal efforts to encourage them, HMOs today enroll less than 4 percent of the United States population. As a practical matter, decentralized market strategies are not likely to prove very forceful in the cost containment struggle.

Fourth, apprised of the limitations of Cell 3, we might move to Cell 4 and contemplate centralized market incentives such as changes in federal tax treatment of medical expenses and benefits, and revisions in the deductible and copayment provisions of federally financed programs. But it is unclear whether changes in tax policy would change insurance purchasing practices significantly, and the fact that the federal government, in the absence of national health insurance, enjoys limited political leverage over much of the health insurance system severely limits the efficacy of the latter approach.

Under the present "mixed" system of financing in the United States, the politics and economics of medical benefits steadily weaken price consciousness among consumers. The economic logic of competition among health insurance plans and the political logic of collective bargaining for health care benefits work in the same direction. Both processes succeed by expanding benefits while reducing direct consumer costs. The consequences, of course, are very expensive to society and so, an economist might argue, insurance plans should emerge to compete by combining high deductibles and/or copayments with much reduced premium costs. Such a plan would be a poor bargain, however, as long as consumers can pass along the costs of their medical benefits plans to employers. And as long as employers can pass their costs along to society in higher prices, they lack an incentive to add to their collective bargaining headaches by insisting on higher deductible and/or copayments in the employee health benefit policies which provide most of the nation's protection. The obvious answer is an "optimally" designed national health insurance plan that places firm but not crushing first-dollar responsibilities on the consumer. Even if such a plan could pass Congress, however, to preserve the incentive effect it must prevent consumers from supplementing their expanded public insurance benefits with private first-dollar coverage, which is surely politically infeasible. In short, it is unlikely that any politically acceptable approach to national health insurance will redress the moral hazards of third-party payment sufficiently to contain costs.

Even if tax and market provisions could be made somehow to reduce present rates of inflation, their impact would be largely undone if we also enacted new legislation entitling the population to broader medical care or insurance benefits. The United States achieves a worrisome rate of medical cost inflation with limited public entitlements and correspondingly limited public controls on providers and consumers. Continental Europe achieves a worrisome rate of medical cost inflation with extensive public entitlements and correspondingly stronger measures of public control, especially over provider reimbursement. The only "answer" lies in measures to oblige consumers to bear a larger out-of-pocket share of the costs of benefits held constant, so to speak. This answer is probably poor policy, and unquestionably poor politics. Thus the real question may be, do we prefer to continue along our present all-American road to inflation or do we wish to exchange it for the European approach: broader entitlements, stronger controls, and continuing inflationary worries?

To sum up: The approach outlined here suggests the following hypothetical candidates for problem/policy matches:

Organizational behavior of hospitals	Decentralized regulation (e.g., rate setting, CON, PSROs, HSAs)
The American hospital "system"	Centralized regulation (e.g., revenue and capital caps; central planning)
Physician incentives	Decentralized market strategy (e.g., HMOs)

| Consumer demands | Centralized market strategy (e.g., tax-code changes; changes in cost sharing in publicly financed programs) | |

The approach also suggests three observations on the merits of the candidates. First, it is unlikely that we will solve or even significantly reduce the medical care price problem by any policy weapon or combination of weapons within the bounds of political feasibility. At best we can hope not to lose ground or can hope to lose it less rapidly. Second, despite their theoretical beauty, the major market approaches are as a practical matter not only insufficient by themselves but also comparatively weak weapons in the arsenal. Third, we are likely of necessity to resort to ever-larger measures of regulation for want of cost containment alternatives that are at once theoretically attractive, workable in the real world, and politically feasible.

CONCLUSIONS

All four problems discussed above contribute in some degree to the cost problems that have launched federal regulatory efforts in the health care field. At present we have hardly the foggiest idea of the relative contribution of each to the total problem, and therefore cannot make accurate problem/policy matches. Informed choice must wait upon experience and, one hopes, the sustained field research necessary to make sense of it. In the meantime, practitioners should not seek highly detailed, how-to-do-it advice from scholars; and scholars should resist giving insider views on how to play the game until they have some reasons for confidence that they have found their way to the right ballpark.

The likely future prospect is continued activity in all four cells, with shifts of emphasis among the four with accumulated wisdom and, still more important, shifting political currents. Thus the present frustrating mélange of approaches and its attendant administrative chaos should remain with us for some time to come. Whether this policy approach— good old American "mishmash"—is also a case of mismatch remains to be learned.

While sitting about thinking of the research we would like someone (else) to do, scholars can make a contribution by challenging some currently accepted nostrums and by scrutinizing some language and concepts in heavy use. These comments have suggested four areas of scrutiny. First, we ought to be more self-conscious about what we mean by "regulation." In particular, we should avoid facile analogies between classical regulation and whatever it is we are doing in the health care field. It would be unfortunate too if the present fad to polemicize about the nature and effects of social regulation discourages scholars from examining on their own merits the various and diverse programs often lumped indiscriminately under this heading.

Second, we should devote more sustained attention to what precisely we mean by "market alternatives" to regulation in the health care field. To what extent do "markets," "competition," "well-functioning market competition," and the like exist in the health care system? Where precisely do we see them amidst the interplay of consumers, technology, physicians, hospitals, and third-party payers? What roles might they potentially play in these complex interactions? What can and should public policy do about it? A policy-relevant market alternative must be at once theoretically and normatively attractive, workable in the real world, and politically acceptable. Certainly the complexities briefly noted above in building HMOs and introducing cost consciousness in a largely private, partly public financing system suggest that market alternatives that meet all three criteria will be hard to devise.

Third, we should recognize that the familiar formulation of "regulation versus the market" as alternative, exclusive policy orientations impedes understanding of their deeper interdependence. As Rosemary Stevens has observed, to American eyes the British national health service appears amazingly underregulated whereas the British wonder at the degree of detailed regulation we impose upon health care providers in the United States.[58] It may be that the British, willing to dismantle most of the medical marketplace, can afford to minimize regulation for precisely that reason, whereas an industrial democracy like ours, which insists upon preserving significant market elements in medical care, must for that very reason resort increasingly to regulation in order to redress inequities and retain public confidence. As a political matter, the resort to regulation may vary positively and appropriately with the scope of the medical care market.[59]

Our real choices do not lie *between* the market and regulation; still less do they lie between the market and "classical" regulation. Our major options concern the appropriate degree of centralization and decentralization of both market mechanisms and those distinctive and largely nonclassical regulatory strategies we are employing in the health field. My fourth moral, therefore, is that we ought to begin giving *political* variables the analytical prominence they deserve.

Although economics, history, and law have much to contribute to the understanding of the health care regulatory programs, the first and basic need is to analyze the organizational politics of the regulatory bodies. We should begin with research into intraorganizational processes: How do rate-setting bodies, CON agencies, PSROs, and HSAs interpret statutory goals, recruit leadership, develop a structure and a staff, and translate general goals into operational goals and operational goals into concrete policy strategies and administrative patterns? Next, we should examine patterns of interorganizational bargaining and coalition-formation by which these organizations seek allies and are in turn opposed by other organizational coalitions. To ask these questions is to ask what are the goals and consequences of the current mode of indirect federal regulatory intervention in state and local health care politics? Because the central policy questions turn on age-old debates about the proper distribution of powers among three levels of our political system, we cannot expect to get an accurate fix on the nature of regulation in the health field until we start examining the real world organizational politics concretely in its empirical setting, the politics of American federalism.

NOTES

1. A revised version of comments prepared for the conference of the J. F. Kennedy School of Gov't, Harvard Univ. on *Regulation as an Instrument of Public Administration,* Cambridge, Mass. (Feb. 27–28, 1978). Revisions were prepared with the support of grant No. HS 02932 from the Nat'l Center for Health Serv. Research, OASH.

2. For studies of the regulation process in several federal agencies see 7 *Policy Sciences* (Dec. 1976). A useful study of the Social Security Administration's implementation of Medicare is J. M. Feder, *Medicare: The Politics of Federal Hospital Insurance* (Lexington Books, 1977).

3. I have explored the politics of the formulation of federal health care regulatory programs in an unpublished manuscript, *Health Care Coalitions and Public Policy: An Introduction.*

4. K. G. Bauer, "Hospital Rate-Setting: This Way to Salvation?" 55 *Milbank Memorial Fund Quarterly: Health and Society* 117–158 (Winter 1977), especially p. 126, table 2. Data compiled by the AMA and published in 11 *Review* 12–13 of the Am. Fed'n of Hosps. (Dec. 1978), show that twenty-eight states now have "rate regulation" programs. The list indicates that Colorado, Kansas, and New Jersey have joined the ranks of states regulating rates by commission, although it does not state whether the commissions are "independent" or the commissioners fulltime.

5. This quotation is from S. Breyer, Chap. 5, "Different Modes of Classical Regulation," *supra* on page 216.

6. E. Freidson, *Doctoring Together: A Study of Professional Social Control* (Elsevier, 1975); on PSROs, see pp. 248–249.

7. On the farmer committee system, see M. Grodzins, *The American System: A New View of Government in the United States,* Chap. 14 (Rand McNally, 1966). On Model Cities, see L. D. Brown and B. J. Frieden, "Rulemaking by Improvisation: Guidelines and Goals in the Model Cities Program," 7 *Policy Sciences* 455–488 (Dec. 1976).

8. See n. 5 *supra* at 217.

9. *Ibid.*

10. *Ibid.*

11. *Ibid.,* Breyer, Chap. 5, "Market Defects," *supra* on page 208.

12. *Ibid.*

13. For elaboration, see L. D. Brown, "The Scope and Limits of Equality as a Normative Guide to Federal Health Care Policy," 26 *Public Policy* 503–505 (Fall 1978).

14. See Breyer, n. 11 *supra* at 208.

15. *Ibid.*

16. *Ibid.*, Breyer, Chap. 5, "Alternative Regimes and the Framework Applied," *supra,* on page 235.

17. *Ibid.* See n. 11 *supra* at 209.

18. *Ibid.* at 209–210.

19. *Ibid.* at 211–212.

20. *Ibid.* at 208–209.

21. *Ibid.* at 210.

22. *Ibid.*

23. *Ibid.* See n. 5 *supra* at 217.

24. This is the charge of the Maryland Rate Setting Commission, cited in H. Cohen, "State Rate Regulation," Institute of Medicine, *Controls on Health Care* 124 Inst. of Medicine, Nat'l Academy of Sciences (1975). See also Cohen, Chap. 2 *supra.*

25. See Breyer, n. 5 *supra* at 217.

26. *Ibid.*

27. *Ibid.* at 218.

28. Bauer, "Hospital Rate Setting," p. 136.

29. See Breyer, n. 5 *supra* at 219.

30. *Ibid.* at 218.

31. Md. Hosp. Educ. Inst., "Preface," *A Guide to Rate Review in Maryland Hospitals* (Lutherville, Md., 1978).

32. *Ibid.* at 95.

33. See Breyer, n. 16 *supra* at 240.

34. See n. 5 at 221.

35. *Ibid.* at 222.

36. *Ibid.*

37. *Ibid.*

38. See Breyer, n. 16 *supra* at 243–244. Also see Appendix 5-G: "Regulatory Reform: The CAB Example" *supra* at 268–271.

39. I am grateful to Don Cohodes of Urban Systems Research and Engineering, Inc., Cambridge, Massachusetts, for information on the status of the Massachusetts CON programs since the gubernatorial election of November 1978.

40. My account of the Ohio battle comes from S. B. Enright, "HSAs vs. Doctors: The War Is On," *Medical Economics* 108–109 (Oct. 30, 1978) (quotation at p. 109), and *The Plain Dealer* (Cleveland, Oct. 10, 1978).

41. Breyer, n. 16 *supra* at 239.

42. *Ibid.* at 239, n. 24.

43. *Ibid.* at 239.

44. See Breyer, n. 5 *supra* at 223–227.

45. *Ibid.* Also see Appendix 5-B: "Example of Regulation by Disclosure Standard" at pages 250–251.

46. See Breyer, n. 5 *supra* at 224.

47. On PSROs see Freidson, *Doctoring Together*, especially pp. 248–249, and J. A. Winsten, "The Utah Professional Review Organization as a Prototype for PSRO's," in *Assuring Quality in Medical Care: The State of the Art* 213–239 (R. Greene, Ed., Ballinger, 1976), especially pp. 231–238. On the HSAs, see B. C. Vladeck, "Interest-Group Representation and the HSAs: Health Planning and Political Theory," 67 *American Journal of Public Health* 23–29 (Jan. 1977).

48. Breyer, n. 16 *supra* at 243. See also Appendix 5-F, "Accomplishing Regulatory Reform," 264–267.

49. Breyer, "Proposals for Regulatory Reform: An Introduction," *supra* at page 204.

50. Breyer, n. 16 *supra* at 234–235.

51. *Ibid.*

52. *Ibid.* at 236–237.

53. *Ibid.* at 237.

54. *Ibid.*

55. *Ibid.* at 235–236.

56. For thoughts on what an appropriate distribution of hospital functions would look like in Great Britain, see A. L. Cochrane, *Effectiveness and Efficiency: Random Reflections on Health Services* (Nuffield Provincial Hospitals Trust, 1972).

57. See M. Lalond, *A New Perspective on the Health of Canadians* 27 (Gov'nt of Can., Apr. 1974), and W. A. Glaser, *Health Insurance Bargaining: Foreign Lessons for Americans* (Gardner Press, 1978).

58. R. Stevens, "Government and Medical Care," in *Medical Education and Medical Care: A Scottish-American Symposium* 170–171 (G. McLachlan, Ed., Oxford Univ. Press for the Nuffield Provincial Hospitals Trust, 1977).

59. Experience on the European continent generally falls somewhere between the largely public British system and the largely private system of the United States. Continental systems usually maintain intact the "private" system of fee-for-service physicians, unlike the British, but pay them mostly with public funds, unlike the United States, which lacks national health insurance. What appears to the casual observer to be "governmental regulation" in these systems (fee schedules, for instance) in fact arises from complex bargaining procedures among government, providers, sick funds, and other interests. The procedures are explained and analyzed in Glazer, *Health Insurance Bargaining*, n. 57 *supra*.

REGULATORY CHOICE IN HEALTH[1]

Theodore R. Marmor, *Professor of Political Science,*
Chairman, The Center for Health Studies, Yale University

INTRODUCTION

This paper is an extended comment on Professor Breyer's detailed study of regulation. Certain features of his presentation require preliminary comment if this reaction is to be useful. First, reactors preparing papers received both the draft of a forthcoming book by Breyer and his own summary of that draft. The book manuscript itself raises so many questions, and weaves its various themes together with such skill, that it is difficult to comment on it while doing justice to the subtlety of its analysis and the complexity of its arguments. As he himself warns, the summary is only a substitute for the longer work and for that reason I shall be responding to the fully developed longer effort. In so doing, I shall have to ignore a number of issues for obvious space reasons and shall not try to review one by one the topics Breyer himself summarizes for this book.

Breyer's work is difficult to come to terms with. It is hard to know just what kind of effort it is. It has a central thesis: namely, that certain kinds of traditional direct regulation are ill-suited to certain types of socioeconomic problems and the result is what he terms a regulatory mismatch. In this respect, the work is geared to negative instruction: Look very hard at alleged mismatches before proceeding. And the implication is that the health industry can learn from that exercise as well as any other. The manuscript has a central line of argument as well, one not restricted to identification of leading "mismatches" between problem and regulation. The argument is that every classic regulatory weapon has its own set of implementation problems. To put a regulation into effect means dealing with, implicitly or explicitly, a set of distinctive tasks and issues. Pursuing this line of argument, Breyer brilliantly summarizes the principal justifications for regulatory intervention, identifies three major types, and explicates the operational

310

difficulties of putting each type into practice. In this respect, the work is
a valuable guide to implementation; it foreshadows what problems
health regulators will face if they employ one of the classic tools of rate
setting, allocation, or standard-setting.

The claims of mismatch might be thought of as a special case of the
broader implementation forecasts. That is, for those problems likely to
be intractable for particular regulatory weapons (given an efficiency
objective), the term *mismatch* might be rightly applied. But the effort is
not extended to identifying the implementation problems in detail or to
delineating alternatives to direct regulation. And, quite consciously,
Breyer excludes from his analysis the political environment and personnel that would affect the way in which implementation problems
would be confronted. So, in this sense, the work is truncated. Nevertheless, it is both an illuminating set of warnings about operational problems and a forceful denunciation of using some weapons in some
problem contexts.

All of this is quite abstract so far, and, in that way, consistent with
the abstract level of the central thesis. But the discussion of implementation problems in regulation is vividly concrete and detailed and much
would be lost if that were ignored in pursuit of using the mismatch
thesis alone to illuminate the health industry. Finally, since the volume
and extent of regulation in health—both indirect and direct—has grown
considerably in the past decade, Breyer's work has another benefit for
health industry students and practitioners. His account of the traditional justifications for regulation is as lucid and comprehensive as I
have found and is an ideal source for reviewing the claims made on
behalf of large classes of regulation.

This comment will proceed first to review the implications of Breyer's
classification of typical regulatory problems for health issues. The second section will identify some problems in health regulation for which
Breyer's scheme is only of partial help. The concluding note will try to
appraise the usefulness of the whole exercise Breyer has introduced.

IMPLICATIONS OF REGULATORY
PROBLEMS FOR HEALTH CARE

Cost-of-Service Ratemaking

Breyer spends considerable time explicating the problems public utility
regulators have in implementing cost-of-service ratemaking. Beginning
with the assumption that such regulations are called for by circumstances of natural monopolies, he shows how difficult it is to (1) substitute replacement for historical costs in estimating the base for price
setting, (2) use the test of comparable earnings to assist the process, (3)
allocate joint costs in rate review, and (4) administer different prices for
peak and off-peak use of the service in question.

The first thing that strikes one in the health field is the difference
between patients and users of public utilities. As Seidman has pointed

out, the role of health insurance makes the health market dramatically different from that for telephones.[2] The health market is increasingly one in which patients receive care, another party pays the bill, and a third regulates. In the case of telephones, consumer payment is central, and regulation, as Breyer himself points out, is justified to prevent these consumers from paying the monopoly prices an unregulated telephone company could charge.

It is precisely the conditions of natural monopoly that distinguish the telephone industry from, say, the hospital industry. It is not clear that it is more efficient to have a single hospital in a community than to have competing ones. As a factual matter, there are competing hospitals in most urban areas. It is not that hospitals lack competition that calls regulatory attention to them. Rather, it is that price competition in the wake of extensive hospital insurance is not the way they seek more patients. Whether that price competition could be made dominant—by restricting insurance, by forcing large deductibles on hospital policies, or by encouraging the growth of health maintenance organizations, (HMOs) that use fewer hospital services—is quite another topic. But it is not a topic that arises naturally in connection with discussing the problems of administering cost-of-service ratemaking.

What has in fact arisen in health regulatory debates is whether the institutional facts of insurance and reduced price sensitivity to health expenses are most usefully addressed by creating cost-conscious patients or monopsonistic financiers of health services, a case of countervailing economic power against the health institutions' inclination for most costly production of care.

Is this difference so fundamental that Breyer's whole discussion of ratemaking need not delay those who must set rates (as in state rate commissions) or decide reimbursement levels (as with Medicare, Medicaid, and many other financing programs)? I think not, and for reasons in the Breyer summary: The search for precision, he argues, has not proven sensible in public utility ratemaking. The reasons why are worth pondering before one duplicates in medical care the energetic pursuit of such precision of other fields. Secondly, the problems of administering such ratemaking systems are considerable and the problem to be addressed, he warns, must be very serious to warrant the administrative burdens. While there may be argument from some, the concern about medical care inflation is considerable. It does not look as if this caution from another field would lead health policy analysts to forego serious consideration of regulatory, among other, solutions.

And yet one wonders if that is all to be said just now. Can one take so seriously the other side of Breyer, the wonder about mismatch between problem and solution. The causes of the inflation in health are themselves part of the regulatory dispute. The consensus is that inflation is a worrisome problem, not, as in the case of public utilities, that the cause of the result to be avoided is natural monopoly and hence monopoly pricing. The argument about the causes of health cost inflation is pre-

there is concern about how rate-setting would be enforced—with what degree of industry capture—that leads to further disputes about whether separate rate commissions should be designed, whether consumer cost-sharing is the answer, or whether a British style national fixed budget is called for. Breyer's question—whether the regulatory cure is likely to be better or worse than the disease — is surely the correct evaluative one. But it is questionable whether the answer will be found by investigating the operation of public utility rate-setting and how it deals with the internal implementation problems of administering rates for consumers who pay utility bills monthly.

Public-Interest Allocation

A second type of regulation Breyer discusses is termed *public interest allocation*.[3] His examples are the airline and communication industries; his focus is how the CAB and the FCC allocate the particular licenses in short supply: "government-created licenses to operate television stations or fly airline routes." He goes on to distinguish licensing from allocation by the following example:

> Compare the licensing of doctors, lawyers, or airline pilots with the awarding of television licenses or airline routes. In the former cases, the object of licensing is to prevent unqualified persons from doing business . . . persons meeting the standards can be awarded licenses (and others denied them) regardless of the number of licenses awarded. . . . An award of a license to A is unlikely to require that it be denied to B. In the latter cases, standards are insufficient to determine who will receive the license. Rather, the agency is charged with choosing the best applicant from several. . . . Awarding the license or commodity to A is likely to require that it be denied to B.[4]

From that point, Breyer goes on to discuss the lengthy, adversarial process by which the CAB and the FCC deal with allocation "in the public interest."

At first glance, there seems an obvious analogy to CON regulation in the hospital industry. CON bodies, to be sure, are more restricted in authority than the CAB and FCC; in almost all cases the scope of CON is restricted to evaluating new investments, not renewing the license to use the beds and equipment now in place. But, otherwise, the temptation to make a straightforward analogy is great. But there is reason to believe that CON operates as an example of what Breyer calls licensing rather than allocation. Looking at the instrument will not tell us the answer, whatever it is. If CON bodies review each application serially, if a plausible case of "need" can be met, and if there is no limit on the total beds or investment that can be made in an area, the practical result may be close to licensing decisions. If, as Breyer argues, the standard of the best applicant results in flourishing adversary processes in the case of airline routes and television licenses, one might find both that consequence and further political pressure, in appeals to other bodies, from applicants claiming adequate "qualifications" for their investment aspirations.

Breyer stresses the likelihood of adversarial contests in allocation settings, a lesson that no doubt CON authorities have already learned. Whatever the differences between licensing and allocating, the lesson may be that lawyers' work is increased by either. Breyer goes on to predict another feature of regulatory habit in this area: The appeals to fairness, procedural or historical. He suggests these appeals will not settle the persistent questions of what is to be allocated, who is to get it, and how to find clear standards that will dissuade endless litigation.

There is no substitute for reviewing Breyer's detailed explication of how regulators in classical independent agencies have dealt with these issues and the ways in which administrative law conventions have shaped the behavior of the regulated as well. He uses the FCC example particularly to point out the recurrent difficulties which students of the agency highlight. One is coherence of the standards themselves, the conflicting bases for deciding which applicant is best qualified for a particular television license. One can immediately think of similar problems in certifying hospital expansion where there are many applicants. Making procedures manageable presents serious problems, as CON regulators must face. Inconsistency in the grounds of awards—a third area—define what critics of the FCC emphasize and students of CON will usefully note. Finally, when the stakes are economically large, the potential for corruption is present, an issue which health regulators must deal with as well. In all these areas, Breyer notes questions with which health allocators have to deal and, in that way, offers a forecast of topics requiring familiarity. Whether these will be the central questions for CON allocations is another matter. That is, these problems will face CON regulators, but the central uncertainty facing them may be whether to deal aggressively with allocation at all. And that would depend on political and personnel considerations that Breyer rigorously excludes from his analysis.

There is another point worth noting about allocation and present health concerns. It may be that a large number of allocative health decisions are excluded from the purview of Breyer's work. His subject is reform of specialized regulatory agencies more than reform of government regulations. But a good deal of government health resource allocation arises, so to speak, on the coattails of subsidy programs. Capitation, grants to medical schools, grants for research centers and individual research projects, and Hill-Burton funds in the past—all have had regulations added to them which condition the receipt of scarce resources. It is these regulations that many have in mind as parts of the "explosion" of regulation in health. The application of Breyer's perspective to such regulations is limited by his focus on regulatory agencies.

Standard-Setting

A third class of regulatory tools, the setting of standards for permissible products, services, or procedures is very broad. He identifies several typical problems with standard-setting and suggests they arise naturally out of the process itself. That process is one "which must rely upon government administrators, not perfectly familiar with an industry, to create standards to govern that industry through the use of adversary procedures that comply with legally oriented administrative standards." He lists the five problems that seem typical, all of which seem quite applicable to disputes in the diverse health industry.[5]

This seems an unambiguously fruitful area for health regulators to study. Such health regulating does rely "heavily on existing political debate for determination of the problem and the causal elements" seen as the object of control. There is "heavy reliance upon existing precedent for the creation of initial standards," as anyone familiar with the early history of Medicare's certification of hospitals eligible for reimbursement knows. Negotiation with "interested parties" rather than cost-benefit analyses to formulate standards likewise seems typical for health, whether one thinks of fire safety codes or retroactive Medicare payment denial as the examples. Such rulemaking is, as well, subject to lengthy delay, as those familiar with HMO programs will attest. And, as he says, it appears to produce standards which "prove surprisingly inflexible and difficult to modify after further experience."

What this comment suggests is that such nonhealth analysis is exceedingly valuable in identifying the "costs" of such standard-setting processes. Breyer goes on to argue that one should try to identify mismatches, to select cases where alternatives to direct standard-setting is likely to be more efficient. He is particularly anxious to replace standard-setting with more incentive-based alternatives where possible.

The topic of consumer representation in health planning struck me as one for which these considerations might be exceedingly relevant. At the moment, HEW sets standards of minimum consumer participation in the governing boards of HSAs. The process of certifying HSAs on this count has exhibited all of the features Breyer mentions, from delay to negotiation to reliance on precedent from CHPs and the War on Poverty experience. What Breyer does not take up is whether experience with consumer participation in other regulated industries offers useful guidance for health planning. The question arises about the applicability of recent Federal Trade Commission legislation where funds are provided for consumers to have legal experts in the rulemaking process. Does that suggest that consumers on HSA boards be given funds to seek expert advice in bargaining with providers on HSA boards? Can standards be devised so that representation of consumer interests (and accountability) is induced rather than extended litigation about statistical representation of demographic groups?

The last example is but one of many where questions of regulation in health are at some distance from the reach of Breyer's analysis. Partly, that results, as I have suggested, from the work's focus on regulatory agencies, not regulations, but much of what one worries about in health regulation are the rules themselves. Let me cite two striking illustrations of this point.

One is the fact that health regulation disputes centrally raise the question of who should do the regulating and, if public, at what level of public authority. Those are subjects which are contested throughout the health industry, but Breyer's theoretical stance excludes the question. What follows, it is often asked, from joining facility and rate regulation to budgetary responsibility for health expenditures? Related to that are problems that arise not so much from a regulatory tool as the combination of regulations, coming from different governmental bodies, that bear upon the same health actor. Hospitals do not face a regulatory agency; they face many, and deal with regulations tied to all sorts of subsidy and reimbursement programs on which they depend. The reform of this regulatory problem in health could not proceed by identification of mismatches between tool and problem. It will have to proceed by taking into account the net of regulations that affect the industry. Saying that Breyer does not illuminate that problem means only that he has not begun with the problems of the health industry. The worth of his effort is not measured solely by the important subjects outside his scope.

There is another issue beyond the multiple sources of regulations in the health industry. I have alluded to this in passing, but here want to make the point explicitly. The fact that Breyer did not have the health industry in mind when writing importantly affects the character of what one can learn from him for health regulatory reform. First, it means that much of what concerns the health industry is excluded or tangentially related. In rate-setting, there is the obvious connection between hospital rate commissions and Breyer's discussion of public utility setting of rates. But the regulations that accompany the major government health finance programs—Medicare and Medicaid—arise from a process for which the rate commissions are not close analogues. The subsidy programs and their accompanying regulations importantly affect the health industry, but are difficult to interpret on the model of FCC or CAB procedures. Finally, the health industry is preoccupied with meeting government standards and the economic costs of compliance raise issues for which some of Breyer's discussion is relevant. But a substantial portion of those standards arise from paternalistic concerns, a category which Breyer develops, but not with its enormous salience to the health industry in mind. It is particularly in this area that the multiple impact of regulatory interventions by different authorities become crucial for health. But Breyer's focus on the fit between a regulatory agency's tool and the problem it addresses leads away from the problem of multiple, overlapping regulatory burdens.

For those health regulatory efforts that resemble the examples of the
classic regulatory agencies, Breyer's work will be extremely useful. For a review of the justification of government regulatory intervention, Breyer's summary will be illuminating. But for a large proportion of the regulatory issues in health—including the questions of what organizational form and site should prevail—the Breyer work will be tangential. For those topics, however, the conference can usefully turn to the Feldman/Roberts paper in Chapter Two *supra*, which emphasizes precisely the question of how health regulators might do better, not when they should be out of the business altogether.

The question is what can one learn for health regulation from experience in other industry regulation. Breyer's essay is of use, but it cannot be a substitute for a wider look at both the health industry's current concerns and the lessons from government regulatory efforts outside the classic agency model.

NOTES

1. Marmor's reaction paper is based on the manuscript draft of Breyer's forthcoming book as presented to conference participants for review and discussion. Breyer's more recent work, such as "Analyzing Regulatory Failure: Mismatches, Less Restrictive Alternatives, and Reform," 92 *Harvard Law Review* 549–609 (Jan. 1979) and Chapter 5 *supra* of this volume essentially summarize the main points of the proposed book. In general Breyer's book will reflect certain input of the conference discussion and analysis.

2. I. S. Seidman, *Health Sector vs. Public Utility Regulation: A Comparison,* manuscript (Oct., 1977).

3. See section on Allocation Under a Public Interest Standard in Chapter 5, "Different Modes of Classical Regulation," *supra* at pp. 221–223. Also see generally Marmor, D. A. Wittman and T. C. Heagy, "The Politics of Medical Inflation," *Journal of Health Politics, Policy and Law;* and Marmor, Wittman and Heagy, "Politics, Public Policy, and Medical Inflation," *Health: A Victim or Cause of Inflation,* (M. Zubkoff, Ed., Milbank, 1975).

4. Excerpted from original manuscript of forthcoming book. See Breyer, n. 3 *supra.*

5. *Ibid.* at 223–227.

GOVERNMENT'S ROLE IN HEALTH CARE REGULATION

Howard Berman, *Vice President, American Hospital Association*

Lawrence Brown makes the following observation toward the end of his paper with more wisdom than "tongue in cheek:"

> At present we . . . cannot make accurate problem/policy matches. [That] informed choice must wait upon experience and, one hopes, the sustained field research necessary to make sense of it. In the meantime, practitioners should not seek highly detailed, how-to-do-it advice from scholars; and scholars should resist giving insider views on how to play the game [at least] until they have some reasons for confidence that they have found their way to the right ballpark.[1]

I will come back to the portion of the comment dealing with research, but first let me attempt to do two things. I will try to add a piece to the puzzle before us all which may well serve to increase understanding of at least a portion of health regulation. Second, let me try to narrow the focus of debate and problem solving to the realism of the current major regulatory initiative which is facing the country—namely the administration's "Cap" proposal—which is a cost-of-service ratemaking, or probably more accurately, a historical price-setting proposal.

Like Enthoven, I find Breyer's approach basically sensible and useful—particularly if we accept it for what it is and not try to stretch it beyond its designed bounds. Obviously, health is different—it is not so different, however, as to render all other political, economic, and therefore regulatory experiences irrelevant.

In the context of government regulation, the other commentors have described many of the operational as well as socioeconomic and political distinctions between health and other regulated industries. A fundamental distinction, however, deserves further emphasis. In the case of health, the regulator or potential regulator—government—is obviously neither a marginal economic force nor a disinterested party.

We are all familiar with the government health spending data. The

history of more than a decade can be summarized in a realization that
about one-half (54.9 percent) of hospital revenues are paid by government, that about 40 percent of total health costs are paid by government, and that the health component of the federal budget has been
growing at double-digit rates. Importantly, the budgetary increases have
not all been for more staff or new programs. Rather, they have been
driven by nondiscretionary program expenditure requirements which
are beyond the administrative control of governmental managers. Only
about 15 percent of federal health expenditures are within the Secretary
of HEW's control. Put that 15 percent in the context of the HEW budget,
which will be about one-third of the total federal budget, and that will
require about 50 percent of the total to be spent on health.

The bottom line of all this has two entries. First, government is
clearly a major party, force, payor, contributor—or call it what you
will—to meeting the country's health care bill. Secondly, and the point
is just as clear though perhaps less discussed, the government's social
welfare budget and program plans are increasingly being held hostage
to its compulsory health expenditures. The fact that government, therefore, wants to control its health benefit costs is understandable. The
question which we are really confronted with then, can be simply
stated. How does or should government move to control its health
expenditures?

The answer gets shaded by the proposition that we do not want to
provide impetus for a two-class health system—a point which I think
we all appreciate—and that if government were to act using just a
portion of the hospital payment system as the lever, that the result
would be a two-class system. This latter point, I would argue, is not as
clear as the first and demands some careful scrutinizing before it is
accepted.

The current distillant of all this is a legislative proposal for hospital
price controls implemented through a revenue cap mechanism. An
approach which, while perhaps not providing a precisely tailored fit,
falls in the arena of cost-of-service ratemaking and historical price-
setting.

Given both the proposal and the nature of the goal to be achieved,
the question that we have to answer is which approach is the most
productive way to proceed in attempting to control, or if you prefer
contain either hospital costs or government's hospital expenditures?

Obviously, in attempting to answer this question, we have to recognize the limits of our knowledge. Even so, we are neither totally ignorant nor inexperienced. Thus, I think we can proceed to formulate some
answers. Breyer takes us a step forward in this direction. Marmor and
Enthoven move us ahead by several more steps. Without fully rehears-
ing the material which has already been presented, let me go quickly
through several key points.

With respect to historically based price regulation, Breyer suggests that it is only practical when price controls are imposed throughout the entire economy. Clearly, in the case of the present proposal, we are not contemplating general price controls.

Breyer further suggests that historically based price regulation tends to evolve toward a system of cost-of-service ratemaking. In this regard he notes that cost-of-service ratemaking seems reasonably well-suited to the problems of natural monopoly. I should point out that Enthoven does not agree with even this degree of usefulness. Even so, the hospital industry with its 5,800 or so firms, multiple staff privileges, transfer agreements, alternative physician choices, and so forth does not fit the classical definition of a natural monopoly. Thus, what we may have is the potential for a mismatch.

The point is well made by Marmor when he notes that it is not that hospitals lack competition that calls regulatory attention to them, but rather that price competition in the wake of extensive hospital insurance is not the way hospitals compete.

The import of this observation is that not only does it bring into focus one of the ways in which health differs from the telephone, electric power, and other industries, but also it leads the way to recognizing that a solution to the cost containment issue involves more than just supply side controls. The "demand side" of the equation is fundamental to the solution.

Enthoven builds on this with his notion of procompetitive changes. He in effect moves us from symptoms to causes by focusing us on the forces determined by the basic financial incentives in the system. Enthoven's point is largely aimed at health payment plans. The same arguments are applicable, however, on both the supply and demand side of the issue.

Obviously, more than just classical procompetitive changes are needed. For example, increasing supply (such as the stock of physicians) is likely to drive total expenditures up. Similarly, such procompetitive forces as antitrust laws may have to take on new interpretations in the health arena. That is, these laws should not be allowed to prevent horizontal, cooperative activity among providers—*if* that activity takes place in the context of the proper incentives and *if*, as Breyer notes, "the agreements . . . achieve legitimate economic objectives."[2]

The next step is to move from these sets of touchstones to deduce some not only potentially productive but also practicable solutions to the issue.

In closing, let me go back to an earlier point. Brown highlights the challenge most sharply when he talks about the limits of current research knowledge and the future research which is necessary. Bearing in mind Breyer's comments about industry's role in providing information, I still would like to offer an invitation.

If nothing else, we can at least all agree that there is much that we do not know. In response to our mutual needs to know more, we are prepared to make our data and staff available to join with you and others in joint ventures which begin to find more answers. The invitation is open.

NOTES

1. See L. Brown, "Regulation, Health Care, and Mismatch," this chap. *supra* on page 305.
2. Excerpted from *Regulation as an Instrument of Public Administration*, vol. 2, the original Breyer manuscript presentation to the Harvard Conference (Feb. 27–28 1978). Also see Breyer, Chap. 5, "Proposals for Regulatory Reform: An Introduction," *supra* n. 1 at 204 and "Market Defects" *supra* at 206–212.

THE "SELF-PROPELLED BED" SYNDROME

Caspar W. Weinberger, *Vice President and General Counsel, Bechtel Corporation*

Any discussion of the regulatory process and health care must inevitably come to the question of the high (and going higher) costs of hospitalization, and any scheme or regulation must be tested by asking if it can do anything to reduce that cost.

If the regulatory process could do anything about that central problem of health care, even dedicated opponents of government regulation might be willing to think about what kind of regulation might accomplish a reduction in the cost of going to a hospital.

Everyone knows the dimensions of the problem: From 1950 to 1976 while the consumer price index as a whole was going up 125 percent, and while medical care costs as a whole rose 240 percent during the same period, hospital costs increased by a bit over 1000 percent during these years. The average cost per patient day in 1950 was $16. In 1976 it was about $175,[2] and I suspect it is perilously close to, if not over, $200 a day now. If it is not, it will be shortly.

Clearly, if more government regulation would improve those dismal statistics, we should try it. But a large part of the problem is too much government intervention now.[3] The basic design of Medicare and, to some extent, Medicaid, and the way those programs have been administered are principal causes of this ruinously high inflation.

Of course there are many other areas of health care that are regulated, including health planning, trained manpower supply, quality control, and many others. Also there have been numerous efforts to try to correct some of the worst features of Medicare in the interest of reducing the amount the government has to spend for health care costs of all kinds. For example, we have seen since 1973 utilization review committees, PSROs, maximum allowable credit for drugs, attempts to curtail unnecessary building, and many other efforts to cut costs.

Breyer's imaginative and creative paper provides a most appropriate backdrop against which to consider whether at least this one major problem in health care—the costs of hospitalization—is caused by a mismatch of regulatory weapons, and thus whether a change of regulatory weapons would help contain these soaring costs, or whether something quite different than a more choice of regulatory weapons is required.

Breyer begins, commendably, by indicating that regulation is really only appropriate when there has been some failure of the market mechanism. The Council on Wage and Price Stability reached the conclusion that there is "an unacknowledged potential of the private sector to exert influence and control in the area of health care cost inflation."[4] But at the moment, and for at least the last twelve–to–fifteen years, there have been and are such government restraints on what is left of the market mechanism in this area that it can properly be said the market mechanism is not working now.

Health care does not fit precisely into any of Breyer's categories or examples. Thus, it is not really the classical "monopoly power" that is causing high hospital costs or failure of the market mechanism. Indeed with some 75,000 surplus hospital beds, we are missing one of the most obvious and essential factors of monopoly power.

Nor does hospital care lend itself to a "rent control" analysis. It is not a "windfall profit" that a few are experiencing. The great bulk of hospital room charges are about the same within a given community; and usually up to 40 percent of the beds are empty at any given time.

Nor is the broad set of problems which Breyer sums up under the term "spillovers" really applicable to hospitals or their costs. Thus, the justification of regulation to correct pollution is said to be the fear that automobiles, etc. will be sold without antismog controls, and so the marketplace must be corrected by insisting that only cars with smog-control devices can be sold, even though it adds a cost the public might not have to pay if the fully free market mechanism were operating. In the case of hospitals, the government or private insurers pay most of whatever is billed.

Nor does regulation to provide adequate information to consumers seem helpful: With all the extra hospitals and beds available, additional government information is not really going to lower the daily room charge because, as we know, you as an individual are in no position to choose your hospital anyway.

And if a lack of competition is not the problem, it certainly cannot be said that excessive competition provides the rationale for regulation.

But clearly something in the market is wrong if the price of one of the services rises 1000 percent during a period when other items are going up a mere 125 percent. Without spending too much time now on causes because it is more important to look at the choice of regulatory weapons or other cures, it seems enough to say that at least the design of Medicare with the enormous increase in demand which it injected into the system—a demand for which providers were guaranteed payment by the government in virtually any amount for which claim was made—had a lot to do with it. Also this helped to produce an unrestrained (because there were no incentives for restraint) demand in the hospitals for more and more new technologies which more and more government-sponsored research was helping to develop. Finally, as will be mentioned in a moment, the government's tax policies cannot be overlooked when we hunt for villains.

One of the other major causes is the vast and vastly expensive new machinery, equipment, and new technologies of all kinds that all hospitals feel compelled to acquire. I used to call this new technology explosion the "self-propelled bed syndrome." It is not hard to imagine a new hospital bed with a small motor on each of the four legs enabling the patient to move his own bed anywhere he wishes. It is not strictly necessary, but it is new and expensive, and since the government will pay for most of it, soon each hospital will decide they need it. Then another charge, payable by the government will be added to the cost of care per day.

The government as well as other insurers must also bear a major part of the responsibility for the heavy overusage of hospitals—("it's all covered by insurance, so while I'm not sure you really need to go to the hospital, we'll put you in for a few days and see how it comes out"). Since the first few days of hospitalization involve the most costs, that too has not only injected more demand for the most expensive form of care, but also guaranteed payment for it.

Whether any of this has significantly improved the nation's health can, I think, be debated, but that is another subject. These are a few things which have so significantly distorted the market that something else must be used to try to lower health care costs.

The point to consider now is *first*, whether the government regulation and intervention we have now constitutes a mismatch of regulatory weapon for the problem which could be cured under Breyer's thesis, by a change of regulation weapons; and *second*, what else can we do?

DOES THE MISMATCH THEORY WORK?

Starting with Breyer's first regulatory weapon, it seems clear that cost-of-service regulation will not accomplish any reduction of hospital charges. There is no real contention that hospital profits are too high. Most are nonprofit institutions, and most could probably prove that the services they are providing actually do cost perilously close to $175 a day.

One of the basic questions is what level of service should be provided? As Professor Martin Feldstein has pointed out, the direct regulation of hospital costs differs fundamentally from public utility regulation because hospital costs reflect not some monopolistic, predatory pricing practice, but simply a dramatic increase in services and equipment, some of which may not be necessary.[5] But if the government is going to regulate the costs of hospital care, it really means it is going to regulate the quality and level of service. And while we certainly may be able to agree that the self-propelled bed is not a necessary level of service, there are others that are more difficult to decide. For example,

CAT scanners are both a status, prestige item and a most useful, albeit expensive, diagnostic tool. Who should have them and how many should there be in one community? I do not believe government regulators can or should determine the proper standard of care in each case.

Feldstein also anticipates and properly refutes the notion that you can solve the problem, as the administration is now trying to do, simply by limiting hospital operating revenues to a 9 percent increase per year [currently, hospital costs are increasing about 15 percent per year].[6]

That is a simple and tempting approach, but it requires that in each case or uniformly (which is as bad or worse) the government determines what is the proper (hence allowable) cost or service for all hospitals to use.

This problem also makes it quite impractical to think of or use standard-setting, the next regulatory weapon. The difficulty, of course, is that our government programs and most available private insurance give first-dollar, or near it, coverage for hospitalization in such a way that restraints and incentives to reserve hospital care for the last resort are nonexistent.

Thus all the pressures to add new services and equipment are unrestrained. Any government standard-setting would have to be designed to decide that some hospitals could be better or better equipped than others, and it would be an exceedingly foolhardy regulator to embark on such a course.

Breyer's allocation-type regulation might be of some help in determining whether CONS should be issued for new hospitals or added wings or even possibly new machinery, but the main trouble is there is no real scarcity or inherently limited supply, as there is with television channels.

It is also difficult to see how present antitrust laws could be used to lower hospital costs. Within their unique and limited systems hospitals do compete with each other and their prices are a function of their costs. The real culprit is the government payment and tax policy and insurance programs which pay more than 88 percent of all hospital bills. Thus far, no one has successfully sued the government for antitrust violations. And it would be hard to convict an insurance company because it offered to pay too much of each hospital bill.

The reason pure competition does not exist is found in the unique nature of the system. Neither you nor I can read the advertisement or talk to fellow sufferers or inspect all hospitals and decide which one we want to use. That is why ideas such as giving the consumer more information are quite unrealistic.

We can only be admitted to hospitals (even in dire emergencies) if we use a doctor who has previously been admitted, in the sense of being allowed to send patients to that hospital. It is, of course, possible for doctors to practice in several hospitals, and some do, but usually each physician (and almost always each surgeon) prefers one hospital because he knows its staff, nurses, equipment, etc. and because he has persuaded the hospital management to admit him to practice there.

Carrying it one step farther, we cannot all use any doctor we wish. Our choice is limited by whether he has any time left for us, or whether he considers our case one he wants to treat, etc.

Some would say that if we just nationalized all health care all these problems would disappear, but even in nationalized health countries, you do not shop for your doctor (unless it is to find one willing to take you whether you want him or not) or your hospital.

HOW TO RESTRAIN HEALTH CARE COSTS

We could indeed make some significant regulatory changes by means of tax changes (another of Breyer's alternate weapons), but whether these would reduce prices in hospitals is by no means assured. Taxes are skewed in favor of more hospitalization because the cost of premiums for private insurance are favorably treated for both individuals and business by our tax system, and we have seen how much overemphasis on hospital care there is in most insurance. And what the government does not encourage by taxation, it pays for directly through Medicare and Medicaid.

So, we could help discourage some of this artificially induced stimulus for more usage and hence higher costs by revisions in the tax system. But I believe it would take far more than this to restrain the ever-increasing cost of hospital care.

That is why I favored the national health insurance plan developed under and submitted to the Ford administration. Under that plan each employer would have to furnish a broad policy of privately procured health insurance to each employee who wished it. The government's role would be limited to prescribing the coverages required in the insurance policy to quality. Each policy would have to offer comprehensive care, including home health care and treatment for alcoholism, drug abuse, mental illness, and ailments not usually covered. The government also would help pay the premiums for the unemployed or those with low incomes.

The result would be only a small increase in current federal government costs initially, and (using 1974 figures) a saving of over $1 billion a year for state and local governments, which would be relieved of much of their direct health care costs.

The most important aspect of this return to reliance on the market in place of the regulatory mismatch we now have, would be that insurance companies could compete with each other by lowering the cost of their policies. And to do that successfully, they would have to scrutinize each payment they made to medical providers. Quite soon unnecessary services and unneeded hospitalization would be substantially reduced because no longer would the government pay for everything whether the patient needed it or not. And by thus reducing the artificial stimulus now inserted into health care costs by the government's present programs, the market mechanism could have at best some chance to operate and to produce lower costs.

I end simply with the basic feeling that Breyer's imaginative and creative analysis of regulation mismatch will be most helpful if it leads us to the conclusion that there is no regulatory tool that can reach the causes of health care inflation. Rather, I think it will take root and branch change by reviving the private sector through use of the insurance plan mentioned above, or through some combination of other plans that make use of the private sector and attempts to revive market mechanisms, now so sadly neglected and indeed blocked. As Professor Havighurst put it, "the report that the market (for health care) cannot be restored to health is greatly exaggerated."[6]

Breyer's framework for analysis will have performed a most valuable service if it leads others to realize that the best regulation for health care cost inflation may well be the limited return to the free market principle exemplified by numerous insurance companies engaged in vigorous competition with each other to offer the lowest cost health policy meeting the government's standards for comprehensiveness.

NOTES

1. Reactor paper presented at the J. F. Kennedy School of Gov't conference on *Regulation as an Instrument of Public Administration* (Feb. 27–28, 1978).

2. M. Feldstein, "The High Costs of Hospitals," *The Public Interest* 40 (Summer 1977).

3. R. Kessel, "Ethical and Economic Aspects of Government Intervention in the Medical Care Market," in *Market and Morals* (Wash., 1977).

4. Council on Wage and Price Stability, "The Problem of Rising Health Care Costs" (Wash., Apr. 1976). Quoted in Havighurst, "Controlling Health Care Costs," in 1 *Journal of Health Politics, Policy and Law* 74 (1977).

5. M. Feldstein, "The Medical Economy," *Scientific American* 151ff (Sept. 1973).

6. Feldstein, n. 2 *supra* at 47.

7. Havighurst, n. 4 *supra* at 488.

MATCH AND MISMATCH—RATE SETTING AND NURSING HOMES

Harold Cohen, *Executive Director,*
Health Services Cost Review Commission, Maryland

Breyer in Chapter 5 *supra* argues that cost-of-service ratemaking seems reasonably well-suited to the problem of natural monopoly. Maryland's nursing home industry is pressing for such rate setting by the Commission. Since the Health Services Cost Review Commission (HSCRC) is an independent agency and subject to judicial review, the nursing home industry expects to get more money through it than by having Medicaid rates set by the state's budgeting process. The suggestion is that Medicaid list the services it is willing to buy and the Commission cost them out. The Commission would prefer not to set nursing home rates but let Medicaid and the homes bargain collectively while the marketplace determines the rate for self-paying patients. Given the near absence of insurance and many providers, there is no evidence of "a serious market failure."

Consumer groups such as the Legal Aid Society want the Commission to set nursing home rates so as to improve quality of care. They would have us set rates even though those rates would not be binding upon Medicaid. The Commission deliberately chose not to exercise its power to set nursing home rates because it agrees with Breyer (see pages 238–239 *supra*) that rate review is not the appropriate tool for solving problems of quality. The Legal Aid Society, in the name of two clients, filed suit.[1] The Commission supported legislation to delay its power to set nursing home rates until the state government asks and the federal government grants a waiver such that Commission-set nursing home rates are binding upon Medicaid without jeopardizing federal matching funds. The case was dismissed after the bill became law. Similarly, the commission has introduced and secured passage of legislation eliminating its jurisdiction over many miscellaneous "related institutions" and has successfully fought hospital and planning efforts to give us authority over HMOs. True to the regulatory image, however, we have attempted to expand our jurisdiction to certain hospital-based physicians on the grounds of their monopoly power. The courts may give us that power (Holy Cross Hospital):[2] The legislature will not clarify our law so as to give clearly (or take away) that authority.

RATE SETTING OR TAXATION—THE QUESTION OF CROSS-SUBSIDIZATION

As mentioned above, the Commission is to assure the public that "rates" are set equitably among all purchasers or classes of purchasers without undue discrimination or reference. (Section 568V(a)).[3] The Commission has basically adopted the position that it will not approve cross-subsidization unless it appears likely that not to do so will severely curtail access or will raise the costs of the health care delivery system. We have argued that a redefinition of medical indigency under the Medicaid law, coupled with higher Medicaid payments to primary care physicians (all tax matters) and full-cost pricing of clinic visits, is preferable to subsidized clinics. (This could be in addition to a minimum deductible for Medicaid and a prudent buyer contract for clinics.) I am convinced that the long-run marginal costs of clinics are only slightly lower than fully allocated costs as developed by our system.

We have had several requests, mostly by obstetricians and hospitals (mostly upon the urging of obstetricians), to subsidize obstetrical and related services. Their arguments concern the absence of insurance and the poor economic circumstances of the typical person involved. We argue that if the legislature wants to subsidize obstetrical services, a tax and subsidy is clearly the appropriate tool. The Commission's staff, in developing its case, routinely has the Commission take Official Notice of Posner's *Taxation by Regulation*.[4]

The Commission's staff is informally reviewing a request for a subsidy of the emergency-room rate at a small hospital on Maryland's eastern shore. The hospital has suffered a significant drop in emergency-room patients who are going to another hospital. This is causing a shift in inpatients which is putting pressure on the other hospital's facility. We have advised the first hospital to request a letter from their local HSA indicating both that their emergency room is needed despite its small volume and that shifting patients back from the second hospital will lead to more efficient use of current capacity and delay or eliminate the need to expand the second hospital.

NOTES

1. Mary Louise Root et al. vs. Health Serv. Cost Review Comm'n, in the Superior Court for Baltimore City, Docket 1975, Folio 895, File No. 5781.

2. Holy Cross Hosp. of Silver Springs, Inc. vs. Health Serv. Cost Review Comm'n, in the Circuit Court for Montgomery County, Md., Law No. 46598.

3. Art. 43, Ann. Code of Md.

4. R. Posner, "Taxation by Regulation," *The Bell Journal of Economics and Management Science* (Spring, 1971).

CHAPTER SEVEN
Issues in Health Care Regulation

Richard S. Gordon, *Kennedy School of Government*

INTRODUCTION

This book began with a quick look at very recent events in North Dakota. There voters, by referendum, directed state authorities to assume responsibility for setting all future health care prices, including physician fees, hospital charges, drug costs, etc.

The question was then raised, if cost control is such a national priority, why was the 1978 Cost Containment bill proposed by the administration ultimately defeated in Congress? Obviously many factors conspired toward this result. Chapter One *supra* discussed just one: The 1978 bill proposed relying on existing Certificate-of-Need (CON) procedures to allocate the amount of capital being spent for health care facilities within a state. If the Massachusetts experience as outlined in Chapter One is at all typical, when stringent cost control is seen as a goal of the CON process one can expect a sizable cross-section of influential voters to doubt the effectiveness of the proposed measure.

What have we learned in the preceding chapters concerning the possibility of success of a referendum such as that passed in North Dakota? Can CON programs be used to reduce capital expenditures? Federal economic regulation has generally been used to control segments of the private business sector. Even in cases where government rules require that citizens, institutions, and/or agencies come together only to establish priorities, what can be expected from such government intervention in the health care sector?

The search for a forum where such questions could be discussed led to the organization of the conference, *Regulation as an Instrument of Public Administration*. To recap, the broad purpose of the conference was to develop approaches which would lead to the overall improvement of

331

health care regulation. In order to stimulate the thinking of the participants (a cross section of the leadership of the health care sector), three
major papers (by Breyer, Feldman and Roberts, and Weinstein and
Sherman) as well as two case studies ("Certificate-of-Need in Massachusetts" and "The HMO Case: The Reimbursement of Chronic Alcoholism") were prepared through a somewhat unusual interactive process: Participants were asked during the period it took to plan and
organize the conference to suggest improvements in proposals for and
drafts of the papers and case studies. Several persons were directly
commissioned to prepare written commentary on the papers for the
conference. Much of this material was substantially reordered, rewritten, and reedited for this volume.

One important feature of the conference is not directly reflected in
the preceding chapters—the always lively and sometimes heated discussions that took place. This chapter summarizes the gist of these
discussions, considering, in particular, the following question posed by
the HEW sponsors of the project: What can health care regulators learn
from the experience of regulators of other sectors of society? Because the
conference took place at the same time as the congressional debate over
the 1978 Cost Containment bill, the discussions began by considering
the then current justification for increased regulation of health care—
cost control.

MARKET INCENTIVES AND COST CONTROL[1]

The main problem in the health sector for which regulation continues to
be proposed is the need for control of health service costs. There is also
the correlative problem of preventing these high costs from creating a
health care system in which only the rich or fully insured can afford a
complete medical care program. Costs of health services are escalating
quickly. From 1950 to 1976 the cost of living rose 125 percent, but
medical costs rose 230 percent and hospitalization costs, 1000 percent. It
is often suggested that inefficient provision of services is causing enormous amounts of waste. However, not all cost increases stem from
inefficiency. There is also a large increase in total demand for health
care services—a demand which, through third-party reimbursement
mechanisms, allows prices to rise and the level of inputs (e.g., technology, surgical interventions) to increase, with no ensuing cutback in the
amount of medical care.

The cost control problem is complex in the health sector because most
costs are not paid for by the consumer but rather by insurance or
government agencies. The federal government thus compounds its
problems as regulator by also being the major purchaser of health care.

Therefore it can be argued that market failure correction involves
more than just regulating prices; it must also be directed at limiting the
demand which allows prices to rise. As L. S. Seidman points out in a
recent article, "Any market will fail if a 'third party' pays 100 percent of

the bill for most consumers. . . . Today nearly 95 percent of the national
hospital bill is paid by insurers."[2]

Lack of consumer information and third-party payment prevent consumers from questioning the value of expensive technology. Thus, Weinberger's "self-propelled bed" syndrome—the phenomenon of innovation for its own sake—so far appears always to increase cost-of-service. Meanwhile, medical insurance encourages the most expensive care (hospital care in lieu of outpatient care), because until very recently only hospitalization costs were typically covered by insurance.

Therefore, even if health maintenance organizations (HMOs) are a long-term answer to cost control, continuing cost escalation and other problems will generate pressures for government action and intervention now. It is in considering the government's regulatory alternatives that Breyer's analytical framework most usefully illumines problems and consequences associated with particular courses of action which future health care regulators may select.

AN ANALYSIS OF HEALTH CARE PROBLEMS
BASED ON BREYER'S APPROACH[3]

In his summary of problems associated with economic regulation, Breyer furnishes numerous examples of particular regulatory approaches that are not suitable for a given class of problems. He formulates generalizations concerning the strengths and weaknesses of the regulatory tools used in areas as unrelated as airline regulation, natural gas pricing, and environmental protection. His aim is to categorize the likely consequences of pursuing one mode of regulation versus another. Breyer suggests how a policy problem can best be "matched" with an appropriate intervention tool. In order to do this, he outlines the justifications for government intervention in private markets, e.g., natural monopoly, windfall profits, etc. Breyer then explores the range of traditional regulatory responses to these situations, including cost-of-service ratemaking, public interest allocation, standard-setting, and antitrust among others. Breyer's analysis generates some vital questions when applied to health care regulation which need to be confronted by regulators. Does the increased pressure to limit revenue and capital expenditures mean that health care resource allocation is headed in the same direction as allocation of radio and television licenses by the FCC? What alternative approaches are worthy of consideration that would accomplish the same ends as the administration's cost containment proposals? Is the only choice the "piggy backing" on the CON process?

Health Care Applications

The purpose of Breyer's work is not to suggest minor changes in regulatory programs but to identify regulatory "basket cases." In so doing, he wishes to stimulate thinking about the purposes and processes of regulation. Utilizing his framework requires ordering one's thinking so as to ask these three questions:

1. What is the problem that requires government intervention?

2. What are the alternatives?

3. Which (regulatory) weapon or alternative approach best fits the problem?

First, the objective to be accomplished by regulation should be examined skeptically. Breyer would ask: Why do we want to regulate health care? If the general response is to control costs, then Breyer would stress the importance of looking deeper. Cost control without judgment of quality or determination of quantity may not be the objective. There is no assurance that the quality and quantity of care received today are not worth the current inflated costs of providing them. If, in fact, Congress, the administration, and state and local agencies are unwilling to lessen the quality and quantity of services provided, and if the current levels of access and quality of service bear a direct relation to cost, Breyer would argue that the overall purpose in much of present and proposed health care regulation must be called into question.

In light of the fact that no national health policy exists, it becomes difficult to resolve questions such as whether the purpose of regulation is to reverse the financial incentives inherent in the present health care system or to channel health delivery resources into more socially desirable forms of competition. The state of health care may be such that we are willing to spend still more to provide needy people with the quality and quantity of services available to those with high incomes or with comprehensive coverage provided by a large employer.

Another problem in regulating health care is that it is difficult to define the desired output of a physician, a hospital, or a clinic. Distributional questions concerning *who* should provide *what* and *to whom* are all variable within a health system and are obviously affected by health care regulation. However, since economic regulation usually influences outputs and because there is no agreement about what the desired outputs of the health care system should be, health care seems to be a poor candidate for direct economic regulation. Yet many signs point to the increasing use by all government levels of regulatory tools drawn directly from the economic regulation of other sectors. If this trend continues, then Breyer's analysis of probable consequences of and desirable alternatives to economic regulation might be more specifically applied, as the following two examples indicate.

COST-OF-SERVICE RATEMAKING[4]

Cost-of-Service ratemaking would involve the government in the setting of rates for medical services. In the past, government-determined rates have been based on the calculated cost of provision or, more usually, on past (historical) rates. As Breyer points out,[5] this was true

because of the administrative impossibility of measuring replacement costs of assets in the rate base. Furthermore, in any determination of the cost of health services, levels of quality and quantity must also be ascertained. Yet because "quality" and "quantity" of health care elude definition, it is not at all clear how the government can be involved in setting standards—let alone cost standards for hospital quality—or in regulating the quantities of services to be offered. Generally, rate-setting revenue limitation leads to examination of individual items, a cumbersome product at best. Choices have to be made. Some hospitals have only X services; others have Y services. On the other hand, it can be argued that if quantity and quality levels are set independently, the government's supply projections used in cost-setting procedures may not meet the demand. Since demand all too often depends on decisions of individual physicians, the government would have to regulate further in order to:

1. Assure that consumers had the necessary market information.

2. Achieve predictable choices and estimates of demand.

3. Adjust return or replacement of capital levels and resource allocation to methods used by health care providers.

In short, cost-of-service ratemaking seems to lead to more government intervention than is desirable.

In any case, although the reasons to use cost-of-service ratemaking in health care might be different from the reason Breyer advances to regulate utilities (to control monopoly power), problems attendant on calculating the cost base for utilities (i.e., difficulty in calculating replacement costs and in allocating share of capital and overhead to each service rendered) appear likely to occur in establishing the cost base for a health care facility or service.

Notwithstanding the defeat of various federal cost containment proposals in 1978 and 1979, the North Dakota referendum to regulate all health charges has become law. Persons interested in health care regulation should follow its success and problems. This is a specific case with which to test Breyer's analysis. If he is right, cost-of-service ratemaking for the diversity of health care enterprises in North Dakota should devolve into the perverse situation Breyer describes in Chapter Five:[6] In the long run, cost-of-service ratemaking amounts to cost reimbursement and provides incentive for continuing cost increases.

PUBLIC INTEREST ALLOCATION AND CERTIFICATE-OF-NEED (CON)[7]

In the past, public interest allocation was not completely applicable to health care because there was no inherently limited resource in the provision of medical services analogous, for example, to the allocation of radio frequencies by the FCC. If capital or total revenues become limiting, as was proposed in the 1978 Cost Containment bill, and choices have to be made between competing institutions, then Breyer's description of allocation difficulties would have application. Breyer points out that the main problem that arises in the allocation of a scarce resource under a public interest standard is that it is impossible to separate *what* is being allocated from *who* is going to do it. It is like the bureaucratic art of writing job descriptions. One can decide the *what* in such a way that the *who* is decided also. It has proven difficult to develop clear standards, especially with respect to the process of trading off one attribute versus another. This, in turn, has made it difficult to devise simple, efficient allocation procedures. The results have frequently been open to charges of randomness, inconsistency, and corruption. The renewal process clearly favors incumbents (as in the case of radio and TV licenses). It is not clear whether this is good or bad. Breyer points out that "it reflects a more deep-seated tendency apparent throughout the law to protect the identifiable investment or identifiable persons who act in reliance upon the continuance of the existing administration or legal regime."[8]

Unfortunately the 1978 legislation (for example, see S. 1371) did not outline a simple or efficient allocation procedure. Rather it relied on enforcing the capital expenditure ceiling through use of the CON process as it now operates in the several states. In Chapter One it was estimated that this bill would reduce annual capital expenditures in Massachusetts by some 40 percent based on a proposed national allocation system related to population. In short, controversy arising from denial of CONs for hospital facility expansion (as summarized for Massachusetts in Chapter One) could only be expected to increase if the Congress should pass a bill similar to the 1978 Act.

The inflation-fighting mood of recent years will obviously carry forward into the next decade. The next ten years should witness continuing attempts to restrain rising costs in the health care sector. At this writing, a ceiling on capital expenditures by health care institutions has not yet been considered by the Ninety-Sixth Congress although proposals for such limits are to be found in various committee drafts. In order to examine what might happen when and if such legislative proposals become law, it is useful to recall what the CON process tries to do.

When is CON really allocation of a scarce resource under a public interest standard? To date, CON review has been conducted on a case-by-case basis, focusing on evaluating the "necessity" of specific capital projects proposed by individual institutions. CON agencies have not been constrained in the total number or dollar value of projects they can approve, and only in selected instances (such as the review of applications for installation of CAT scanners summarized in Chapter One *supra*) has the approval of a proposal from one institution at one time required the denial of similar proposals submitted by other institutions. Hence, up to the present time, the CON program has served

only a limited allocative function.

Nonetheless CON programs have been created to help "rationalize" the health care delivery system by avoiding duplication and assuring that only "necessary" projects are undertaken. Persons involved in the process have therefore had to confront such issues as the definition of "necessary" for various categories of health care facilities, equipment, and services, and the development of criteria for the selection of "qualified" institutions to offer such services. Use of CON regulation thus seems to bear many of the characteristics of "allocation under a public interest standard" categorized by Breyer and exemplified by the function of agencies such as the FCC. The expenditure ceiling will further cast CON regulation into this mold, for it will force CON applications during any given year into competition with each other (at least as long as the total exceeds the state's ceiling).

The CON process Without a limit or capital lid on expenditures, CON is a process which pits an applicant against a standard. There are several problems which exist under a CON process without a capital lid:

1. CON enforcement and effectiveness varies within and among the states.

2. Need is hard to measure, and this is not a standard for a project's eligibility.

3. Quality of health care is hard to measure, and the effect of an individual project on the health of a region is unclear.

4. Health systems agencies (HSAs) are planning bodies organized to make priority decisions among projects rather than to be able to set the size of a regional expenditure pot.

5. The CON process stretches over a great deal of time, creating a sense of uncertainty and unpredictability for health administrators and planners over which project will be approved.

6. There is an increasing tendency to use the CON process as a vehicle to "piggy back" other legislative or regulatory agendas.

In general, one is inclined to agree with a statement Breyer made concerning the current CON process: Judging qualification of "need" against a standard can be expected to weed out only the bizarre and/or the obviously unqualified.[9]

The CON process with a capital lid: pitting applicant against applicant Once a lid is placed on expenditures, Breyer's public interest allocation model predicts other problems will result. First, not only must health care providers demonstrate that their proposals are worthwhile, but they must also make a case for the fact that their specific plan or proposal is the best one available. It follows that increasing amounts of money will probably be spent in competitive case building, involving lobbying and public relations. Second, any capital expenditure ceiling would be set at a level less than the present level of demand. As a result, entry by new institutions would be discouraged. Third, HSAs and providers would, as in other fields, probably unite with state governments to push for higher expenditure ceilings and thus presumably thwart cost-control efforts. Besides predicting the foregoing from Breyer's analysis, one might also predict a certain number of positive results from placing an expenditure lid on capital projects:

1. Program growth rates could be forecast with greater ease.

2. Applicants' perceptions of fund limitations might cause them to file only what they believed to be the most important proposals.

3. HSAs and the states would have to cooperate in enforcing CON decisions.

4. Priorities would become more uniform among the states.

5. The CON process would include more social factors in decisions.

6. Administrative or programmatic decisions would be more likely to be upheld by the courts.

Unexpected or untoward consequences of using CON for capital funds allocation Several possible side effects of placing an expenditure lid on the CON process must be considered. First, buildings and equipment will probably be used longer before replacement (and there can be no assurance that this will improve or decrease cost-effectiveness). Second, CON begins with the premise that technology is the cause of increased costs of medical care; this may not be the case. The effect of a CON capital ceiling may be to shift money into the labor sector—a shift which may result in higher total health expenditures.

Finally, it is hard to visualize a regulatory process without some exemption-granting procedure. Yet, the granting of exemptions to the CON regulatory process would create another predictable but separate set of problems. Providers of health service would surely attempt to channel their applications into exempted categories, and this could prove to be a discouragement to the provision of other, more-needed but nonexempt facilities. It is also predictable that those institutions which acquired CON exempt status would fight regulatory challenges affecting their exempt status.

The Fielding plan Jonathan Fielding, as commissioner of the Massachusetts Department of Public Health, presented a plan that a typical Public Health Council might follow if it were informed that a capital lid was going to be set. His nine-step plan suggests:

1. Determine exactly what the legislation will mean—what will be included, and any standards or criteria for selection of projects.

2. Finish already existing expenditure plans up to a given date.

3. Build on existing planning regulations and group planning agreements; require all applications to come in at once so that all applications are ranked together.

4. Set up a task force for setting priority criteria; include doctors, administrators, interest groups, and HSAs in the task force.

5. Speed promulgation of standards for all types of applications.

6. Estimate how much money is needed for maintenance of the quality of the health care system at its present level.

7. Coordinate priority projects among HSAs.

8. Plan with other agencies—HSAs, rate-setting agencies, insurance agencies—to be sure of congruence of plans.

9. Get more participants involved in health planning to be sure that resources are allocated in the public interest.

Despite careful planning, however, allocation problems cannot be avoided. For example, Fielding said that he could not see any good way to make exemptions; very quickly projects get channeled into "exempt" areas and one loses the ability to change whatever exists. Furthermore, granting exemptions usually undermines enforceability of standards and erodes public support.

Policy issues In short, two public policy decisions are made when dealing with a lid on capital expenditures: (1) How much money should be spent in each planning region; and (2) what services are desired in each region? Given the expenditure lid and list of services desired, providers, consumers, and local officials will have to work together to meet whatever the legislative requirements are for limits both on hospital capital expenditures and on total year-to-year hospital revenue increases (also proposed by the Congress in various bills under scrutiny in 1978–1980). Yet the most troublesome and key issue undergirding all the rest is rarely discussed in detail: Just exactly how does one decide *how* and *by whom* final decisions concerning the allocation of local health care resources should be made? Working together and then going through the state system to the commissioner and the courts has not proved completely satisfactory in Massachusetts. In fact, the situation is already plagued by the problems that Breyer describes.

As Blendon points out in his introduction to Chapter Two, until very recently the cry in health care was to increase access to reduce scarcity or shortage of service, not to deal with "surplus" or overlap. Consequently, procedures such as bidding for "market rights" (services to be offered) have not been used to resolve competing claims between health care institutions. There are other options to command-and-control regulation which emerge from a careful analysis of different modes of government intervention in health care.

An alternative approach to health care regulation adopted by Weinstein and Sherman is based upon a typology these authors developed to describe the different ways government can intervene in health care. It does not lead to conclusions that differ dramatically from Breyer's. Weinstein/Sherman are concerned with identifying alternative modes of public intervention in the health sector. Their premise is that many of those who debate and design programs are unaware of or give insufficient consideration to the rich array of policy alternatives available. Weinstein/Sherman have, therefore, constructed a detailed framework exploring the important dimensions of choice in health care regulatory design: the specification of regulatee and regulator; the particular point in health care delivery at which regulation is applied; the various alternatives for enforcement and monitoring systems; and the choice among measures of performance. These choices are subdivided in detail to generate a comprehensive, organized set of optional policy objectives.

Assuming that a capital expenditure lid for health care is still favored, the Weinstein/Sherman approach could be used to test alternatives in the detailed design of a CON program to foresee and alleviate the allocation problems predicted by Breyer. Finally, the framework could be used to ask whether the basic CON approach was or continues to be the ideal practical means of pursuing the program's several objectives (see Figure 7-1).

The Weinstein/Sherman Framework as Applied to CON

People react variously to the Weinstein/Sherman framework shown in Figure 7-1. This framework should be seen as a useful tool in disciplining one's thoughts and in thinking through what the various combinations of regulatory alternatives might accomplish in furthering programmatic ends. In many cases, the performance of a regulatory agency depends on how administrators work their way through the maze of

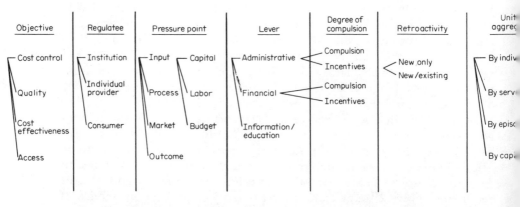

FIGURE 7-1   Regulatory Options (Levers) Available for Use in the CON Process.

options such as those shown in the framework. This, in turn, depends on how precise they are in defining their objectives.

Underlying the discussion of CON is the current federal assumption that control of capital expenditures could become an important means of cost containment. At the very least, Figure 7-1 suggests that, disconnected from total cost, capital limitation is unlikely to *control*, let alone *reduce* total expense. The question is, can the categories in Figure 7-1 be used to outline alternatives to applying CON to capital allocation?

The Weinstein/Sherman analysis illustrates how complicated and ill-defined the issues are with regard to CON with a capital lid. Assuming that the objective of health care regulation is cost control, an argument can be made that CON regulation will only minimally reduce cost of service by limiting capital investment.

This conclusion does not differ that much from Breyer's conclusion that "capital expenses" and "need" are often terms which are hard to define in practice. However, unlike a capital intensive utility, CON with a capital expenditure limit may encourage substitution of unregulated capital and labor for regulated capital. Obviously this seriously sidetracks efforts to reallocate capital that might be inefficiently deployed. It almost certainly would not result in cost savings or improved cost-effectiveness.

The diagramming of the CON/cost containment choices, using a typology such as that developed by Weinstein/Sherman, reveals another major weakness in the CON-process/capital-lid proposal: The CON process can only be applied to proposed expenditures; ineffective distribution of existing facilities and expenditures is not considered. Any gains obtained by limiting new equipment may be lost through failure to address already existing economic excesses (something regulatory commissions should—and do—inquire into all the time). For example, closing excess beds is difficult to achieve if an expenditure cap is imminent, but such a bed reduction could save more money in the long run than that saved by preventing an institution from purchasing some new type of equipment which has proven to be diagnostically useful but whose cost effectiveness is uncertain.

A particular problem is that when objectives are unclear, standards can conflict with whatever objective is introduced into the determination of need. For example, while increased or full utilization of capacity may be an important factor in cost control, utilization depends on demand for treatment of medical problems that can only be handled inside a hospital. Since CON penalizes institutions with low occupancy, higher utilization can be stimulated only if doctors create demand by increasing the number of admittees (which means including those patients who would benefit medically if treated as outpatients), thereby increasing total costs in the short run (although perhaps reducing cost per patient). It becomes apparent that regulatory alternatives to achieve the goal of cost control would have to involve extensive and drastic changes in incentives that would have unpredictable consequences in the health care system.

The use of the Weinstein/Sherman framework makes it easy to see the solution to the problem of substituting unregulated capital and labor for new capital that would have to be approved via the CON process. An expenditure lid on the total budget could prevent the predictable distortions that are sure to occur. It also suggests ways one could address the other problem of more efficient deployment of existing facilities. When focusing on cost control, alternative approaches to be considered could include: (1) franchising hospitals on the basis of cost-effectiveness; and (2) billing patients for what a service *really* costs. There are many "combinations" that one group or another might find appealing (i.e., paying physicians on the basis of years of useful patient life gained from their services), but although many combinations of variables might even be feasible from an operational or professional point of view, it is probable that some workable options would not survive the political process.

What are some of the options which are difficult politically? The Weinstein/Sherman categorization suggests that it might be useful to redefine institutional purpose or even change institutional character i.e., from acute to chronic care. Another alternative suggested by the more general Weinstein/Sherman approach is to redefine the regional area ("market" in economic terms) served in order to achieve a better allocation of capital. Probably the most politically difficult question is how to allocate capital that recognizes differences in mission.

Breyer reminds us that politically acceptable alternatives to centralized regulation (or "top-down" administrative rulemaking) are beginning to be employed in some sectors. These include such legislative incentives as taxes, fines, and subsidies. However, the important question that Weinstein/Sherman raise is why are less radical, quite modest in fact, alternatives not more widely employed? Here are two alternatives that flow from their analysis which are generally widely discussed:

1. Incentives associated with reimbursement should be changed so that outpatient care is favored over (the more expensive) hospitalization. Reimbursement for outpatient care, as compared with only inpatient care, will lessen the expenses associated with short hospital stays.

2. The formation of private health plans must be greatly accelerated. Such plans should compete with one another in price and scope of services offered (most proposed could exist under some form of national health insurance). For each plan, the employer would have to furnish a policy providing broad coverage of privately procured health insurance to each employee who wished it.[11] Government's role would be limited to prescribing the scope of minimum coverage required. Each policy would have to offer comprehensive care including, for example, home health care; treatment for alcoholism, drug abuse, and mental illness; and dental care, some of which currently are not usually covered. The government would also subsidize the payment of premiums for the poor and unemployed.

After viewing all the options for intervention, the regulator must
remember that doing nothing is also an option which should be considered. In short, some of these alternative approaches to hospital cost control certainly appear to be as desirable as placing a lid on capital expenditures or mandating arbitrary limits on year-to-year increases in revenue.

What inferences can be drawn from the Weinstein/Sherman framework? While the approximately 4,000 possible alternatives available by concatenating each level or option of the framework decision tree might seem an unprofitable exercise (many combinations could never be tested and analyzed rigorously), there are simplifications and political limitations which prune the tree to a more manageable set of alternatives. In any case, people tend to be unclear about what they mean by (or want in) regulation. This lack of clarity leads to disagreements about both means and ends, with resultant miscommunication and counterproductive rulemaking. The framework could untangle such arguments by uncovering the specific differences in fact or opinion which lead to disagreements. The Weinstein/Sherman framework reminds us that every time a regulation is proposed, the goals should be clear and measurable. It also suggests that if one regulatory approach fails in its application to reach that goal, one should not conclude that a different approach to the same regulatory application would also fail. If one is clear about exactly *whom* or *what* one wants to regulate, and if one carefully considers *what degree* of compulsion and *at what point* regulation should occur, then the resultant regulatory process should be improved.

Nevertheless, at this writing, the argument in the Congress for the use of CON for cost containment seems to ignore the substantive difficulties discussed here. As a consequence, one would predict failure or only limited success for such a federal approach using a cost containment standard. Furthermore, so much of the regulation of health care is of recent origin that little is really known concerning the effectiveness, appropriateness, and match or mismatch of problem and regulatory approach (weapon) chosen to solve any particular problem.

APPLICABILITY OF EXPERIENCE FROM THE NONHEALTH SECTOR

Many (particularly those in the health professions) doubt that growing government intervention will improve the practice of medicine. Surprisingly, however, even advocates of greater government control are sympathetic to the difficulties that administrators of health care institutions face in dealing with the numerous regulatory bodies with conflicting or competing mandates. This situation is unique to health care (although some would argue that overlap in other fields between federal and state agencies, or the Justice Department and the Federal Trade Commission, is not all that dissimilar).

The intentional regulation of health care delivery (as opposed, say, to physician licensure) is a new phenomenon. Much original health care regulation emerged, as Marmor suggests, on the coattails of subsidy programs. As a result, it is argued (see Chapter Six *supra*) that many of these older health care regulatory programs have problems different from those Breyer discusses, because they have only a tangential relationship to classical economic regulation. On the other hand, an increasing number of *recent* health care regulatory proposals bear a striking relationship to "classic" regulatory approaches. Thus, as discussed above and illustrated in Chapter One (see "The CAT Scanner Controversy"), the newer proposals should encounter problems and lead to "unintended" consequences similar to those suggested by Breyer's analysis of regulatory failure. Consequently, a major premise of this book seems strengthened: Experience from other regulatory areas can be used by health regulators to predict and hopefully to avoid specific pitfalls and perverse outcomes. Consider some examples from this volume:

1. The problems faced in distributing television station licenses (the rights to build or acquire) among competing claimants certainly represents a close analogy to the CON process.

2. Students of antitrust have noted both the positive and negative effects of government-sanctioned barriers to entry on regulated industries, a problem briefly noted in Chapter One *supra* in the capsule summary of the discussion between HEW and FTC lawyers concerning physician licensure.

3. Even a cursory examination of the proceedings of any utility rate setting commission will convince one of their similarity to the problems summarized in the brief problem statement (Chapter One *supra*) or in Harold Cohen's detailed description of the Maryland Health Services Cost Review Commission's work: All rate setters wrestle with the need to determine how much revenue a regulated organization may receive for a broad array of services, the individual costs of which are problematic. (See Chapter Two *supra*, Appendix 2-C, "Methodology of Computing Prospective Rate Adjustments Under the Guaranteed Inpatient Revenue Program.")

4. The problem most regulatory bodies have in converting "simple" legislative language into a practicable set of rules which would establish regulatory format across the nation is illustrated by the difficulty in drafting regulations for reimbursement for treatment of (chronic) alcoholism (see Chapter One *supra*).

As Dunlop notes in Chapter Four *supra*, it has been useful in some sectors of society to distinguish among the various kinds and purposes of regulation, most notably between *economic* regulation of rates, prices, and fees and *social* regulation affecting conditions of work such as discrimination, health, and safety. (In addition the government invariably develops a regulatory format when it provides funds for a purpose such as welfare, food stamps, research grants, medical schools, and unemployment insurance.) Given the complexity of the health care

field, there is much to suggest that such distinctions may not be very useful. The defining characteristics among options for governmental involvement and/or intervention must be established by using more complex criteria, i.e., the recent pressures for cost containment and the regulation of fees and prices in hospitals bear all the earmarks of an economic regulatory approach to an area of social concern.

Where Is Health Care Different?

Accordingly, while there are obvious analogies between many of the problems addressed (and created) by government intervention in health care on the one hand and intervention, participation, or involvement in other sectors on the other, it is useful to consider some of the unique characteristics of the health care field which could vitiate programs, policies, tactics, and tools that have been successfully applied in other fields.

Among the most important of these characteristics are the following:

1. Rate and fee regulation depends partly on assessment of quantity, quality, and variety of services provided. Yet, there is little consensus concerning acceptable measures or levels of quality or concerning the variety of medical practices required.

2. There are no well-defined, long-existing structures (equivalent to the land-grant colleges or experiment stations) which (a) provide a body of locally based "neutral" parties to interact with providers, consumers, and regulatory and legislative interests, capable of assessing the "results" of various programs; and (b) over a period of time build up a system for priority identification and consensus building.

3. The dynamic state of medical science and technology makes it difficult to write regulations which anticipate technological options not even perceived or contemplated in the legislative or administrative record.[12]

4. The inapplicability of market models, problems of imperfect information, and lack of price competition have combined with third-party payment systems and myriad forms of government interventions to make the health sector quite different from an ideal competitive market. Furthermore, consumer behavior with respect to health decisions is *sui generis* in that balancing financial burden with medical benefit is difficult; consumers avoid making decisions for themselves, relying instead on health professionals. Many argue that we seem to overconsume high-priced medical services (tests, hospital stays) and underconsume regular exercise and healthful diets.

5. The third-sector character of the health system, and the combination of not-for-profit and the past period of relying largely on community support probably produce those features of health care which might cause classical regulation to work poorly or to produce unexpected outcomes.

These five points, taken together, suggest that to regulate by "symptom"—some prominent feature such as capital expense—can have a result no better than palliation and is likely, as in clinical medicine, to permit the underlying pathology and dysfunction to progress.

AFFECTING REGULATORY BEHAVIOR

The result of the recent shift from promotion to containment and cost control of health care has radically changed the behavior of all affected parties. Based on their research into the implementation of recent health care regulation, Feldman and Roberts describe the sociopolitical realities which govern the drafting and implementation of regulation. In a free society, the regulatory process depends on individual behavior and on the interaction among individuals, both as independent professionals and as administrators of governmental or private sector organizations. Feldman/Roberts offer the following interrelated hypotheses which are important to most regulatory activity and which seem particularly important to health care.

Hypotheses Affecting Regulatory Behavior

1. To the extent that publicly available scientific evidence links regulatory requirements to possible ends of regulatory activity, regulation is much more likely to be implemented successfully.

2. The ability of an agency to achieve a change in behavior in a regulated sector depends in part on the costs it incurs in reliably monitoring the behavior in question.

3. The political process will enhance regulatory implementation as a function of a number of factors, including broad public consensus regarding the importance of program objectives, the presence of organized interest groups that support regulatory activity, and key elected officials or political parties to whom program success is important.

Yet, Feldman/Roberts also hypothesize that the organizational context within which a regulatory body operates will inhibit regulatory effectiveness where a number of factors are present, e.g., when regulatory control is fragmented among many agencies, when mechanisms for coordinating agency activity are weak, and when incentives available for altering behavior are limited. Unfortunately, such inhibitory factors tend to be endemic in health care agencies.

Feldman and Roberts examine a number of regulatory outcomes to test their hypotheses:

1. Studies of *entry and capital investment controls* suggest that CON programs have been relatively effective in reducing growth in the number of hospital beds in some states but have had varying impacts on nonbed investments and on hospital costs.

2. Studies of *direct cost and price controls* indicate that such, too, have had mixed results. There is evidence that programs which set *reimbursement rates* through hospital-by-hospital *budget review* are relatively ineffective in controlling hospital costs, while programs making use of *formulas* have had somewhat greater impact on the growth of hospital prices, costs, and inputs.

3. Studies of *utilization* or *"product characteristic" controls* indicate that, in some circumstances, hospital admission rates and lengths of stay have been constrained, but evidently not in all.

Feldman/Roberts conclude that it is difficult to "prove" their hypotheses based on such a wide range of results. They do see their hypotheses as illuminating a number of key factors which influence regulatory outcomes.

In particular, Feldman/Roberts' understanding of the bargaining relationship inherent in health area regulatory implementation suggests that the preponderance of on-site review activities and the general disinclination of review agencies to make use of reimbursement sanctions have weakened rather than strengthened agency resources and agency effectiveness in constraining costs. These observations reflect a more fundamental set of constraints on implementing "product characteristic" controls for the purpose of controlling health care costs. That is, insofar as decisions about "appropriate" or "necessary" utilization entail judgments about the quality and efficacy of medical care itself rather than about how much the public wants to pay for it, such will inevitably depend on medical expertise and medical judgment. Regulators, then, will either have to employ doctors as consultants or be doctors themselves. Doctors who are employed as consultants, however, and who derive their principal livelihood as well as their professional norms from outside the government, wil not have very strong incentives to impose rigorous constraints on the practice of medicine. This is especially the case when there is a dearth of data which might link specified standards of practice to desired medical outcomes. Even if regulators were doctors who derived their principal livelihood from government, their capacity to change the practice of medicine would depend at the most basic level on their ability to formulate reasonable and valid substantive standards for medical care. The difficulty a senior health regulator would have in maintaining a model medical practice is obvious.

Yet it is precisely this ability to maintain medical leadership which is lacking in any part of the health care regulatory system—and without which utilization and quality controls are ineffective. While it is true that the bases for determining need in CON programs and for establishing rates in rate-setting programs are still at an early stage of development, at least there are two areas of growing expert and political consensus concerning priorities and long-term regional needs. In the "product characteristic" area of health regulation this is not apparently the case. The centrality to the medical profession of decisions about quality and its reluctance to subject those decisions to government-sponsored scrutiny (as evidenced, for example, in American Medical Association opposition to government involvement in health technology evaluation) suggest that even incipient consensus is still far off. Short of nationalization of the entire United States health system, then, it is hard to see how regulation which proposes "uniform" utilization or quality standards will be effective throughout the balance of the century.

Consequences of the Feldman/Roberts Hypotheses

Feldman and Roberts reach the following conclusions:

1. Justifiable clear standards derived from well-established methodologies will generally facilitate the enforcement process.

2. Agencies need to encourage more reliable and less expensive monitoring technology. This appears the most practicable means of lowering the cost of detecting violations and of enforcement.

3. Within the broad confines of any program, having enough people with enough expertise may be critical. Better management does make a difference.

4. Developing appropriate political support for a program may be critical to long-term effectiveness.

5. There must be provision for regulators to improve implementation of their programs by developing a more secure scientific basis for their efforts. In particular, problem solving, program-oriented research should become a significant priority to the agencies concerned with the regulation of health care.

6. There needs to be a much greater effort made by both executive and legislative branches concerning program design. In particular, trying to reduce vertical fragmentation, and hence limit the number of indirect and imperfectly manipulable linkages that an agency must utilize, is likely to have a positive influence on program impact.

7. A very helpful way to characterize the relationship between regulator and regulatee is as a complex bargaining process. Much more work, particularly in health care regulation, needs to be conducted to elucidate the usefulness of this concept.

Reaction to the Feldman/Roberts Ideas[13]

According to *Cohen*,[14] a major health policy question raised by the Feldman/Roberts paper is whether prospective hospital rate setting is a necessary or sufficient condition for securing an effective and efficient hospital delivery system. Cohen feels if there were high coinsurance and great HMO penetration, such rate setting would not be necessary. However, under present circumstances, the system is clearly not sufficient; therefore, discussions of prospective reimbursement require

challenging the fee-for-service system. Obviously such challenges **349**
can only be dealt with productively by employing the negotiating *Issues in Health*
approach envisaged by Feldman and Roberts. *Care Regulation*

Noll[15] feels that two observations by Feldman/Roberts are consistent
with all scholarly research on regulation in the past two decades: (1)
Regulation systematically tends to redound to the benefit of groups that
are well-represented in the regulatory process; and (2) regulators generally have too few resources to find good solutions to technically difficult
public policy problems and then to force compliance with the solution.
Noll also feels that in order to provide greater detail in policy conclusions, more concreteness must be added at certain points in the development of Feldman/Roberts' argument. Three additional points might
also be made.[16]

1. In many ways regulators represent a fourth part of government. They act
   almost independently of statute; they seem to have authority to operate
   case by case as they see fit, and it is difficult and costly for an individual
   institution to challenge their actions.

2. Industry is having an increasing problem in seeing the difference between guidelines and standards, let alone acting upon them. Yet industry needs some kind of clear antitrust exemption in order to come
   together to work out its common regulatory problems.

3. It might be fine theoretically to talk about negotiation or bargaining, but
   the health sector does not seem committed to such a process. Furthermore, major reform has to occur within government at all levels, particularly when it comes to making key officials accountable for what is
   proposed and implemented.

Overview of Issues Raised by the Feldman/Roberts Paper[17]

There was agreement among those who reviewed and discussed the
Feldman and Roberts paper that the dramatic growth in health care
costs has spurred the evolution of health care from a system emphasizing access and quality to a mature system equally (and/or contradicto-
rily) concerned with process and cost containment (see Cohen, Chapter
Two *supra*). Furthermore, the regulatory agencies' lack of a substantial
body of objective data concerning the efficacy of most clinical practices
requires reliance on self-regulation with its own attendant problems.
Additionally, regulatory responsibilities are given to so many public
and quasipublic organizations at the federal, state, and local levels, that
the resultant inconsistent requirements and confusion are not unexpected.

Another issue addressed by Feldman/Roberts is the inability of regulation writers or policy makers to decide whether a regulation has any
benefit and to change direction if not. It seems that there is great
difficulty in judging regulatory programs as quickly as Congress would
like. Further, legislators underestimate the decades that are required to
effect change and to measure the results thereof.

One particular question that might confront a regulation writer or policy maker is: Would it be better to have prospective reimbursement rather than historical-based reimbursement of hospital costs? Because much of the current debate in health regulation is aimed at defining the nature of "correct" incentives, finding a mechanism to change incentives which now work against cost containment (and/or greater access to care) seems of high priority.

But, there are some useful general principles that relate choices of regulatory strategy to the resulting implementation difficulties. The question is whether it is the choice of the strategy or its method of operation that matters in successful regulation of health care. It is possible that regulations can be implemented well or poorly. Roberts,[18] in particular, felt that the evidence suggests that the choice of regulatory strategy in health care is not as critical in affecting an outcome as is how well regulations are implemented.

For example, the insurance industry has recently run a series of advertisements praising the work of the Maryland Health Services Cost Review Commission among others in containing hospital costs.[19] It is evident from considering the Commission's approach[20] that despite the difficulties inherent in rate setting, the sophisticated analysis of the cost and rate structure by a dedicated body of public servants can pay off. (Incidentally, note that the use of formulae by the Maryland Commission sustains Feldman/Roberts' second hypothesis on page 347 *supra*).

IMPLEMENTING CONGRESSIONAL LEGISLATION: THE HMO EXAMPLE[21]

If implementation is as important as Feldman and Roberts found, then why does regulatory implementation falter so often? Roberts' answer was that Feldman and he discovered during their study of bureaucratic rulemaking that administrators preferred to argue about data rather than values or purpose. Discussing "data" avoids direct personal or policy confrontation and appears more easily justified—the idea or proposal at issue is a result of an "expert investigation." Consider the difficulties, therefore, that administrators face implementing congressional legislation. The legislative process must, of necessity, require considerable tradeoffs to secure enactment. It must be very difficult to build all relevant political considerations into programmatic activity. Sooner or later an administrator will have to take a stand on legislative language based on his or her views or values as much as on whatever data are on hand.

Yet, this is easier said than done, as the difficulty in drafting regulations for HMO reimbursement in Chapter One illustrates. The multiple problems with which the HMO/HEW task force had to cope were used as a basis to test Feldman/Roberts' ideas. Table 1-2 in Chapter One *supra* shows that the HEW task force was considerably behind schedule in its drafting of a number of regulations, including those which govern reimbursements for the treatment of chronic alcoholism. Over three years of intra-agency and interagency work is summarized here, which took place directly under the congressional gun so to speak, as the original legislation had directed that regulations be issued in a much shorter time period. Why did it take so long? Roberts felt that guidelines failed to issue for a number of reasons.

First of all, even at the federal level there is an almost endless list of key players, including the President, the senators and representatives on the key committees, the Secretary of HEW, and key staffers to all the preceding as well as those in the Office of Management and Budget (OMB) and the National Institute for Alcohol Abuse and Addiction (NIAAA). These key players often interact more on the basis of personality and their overall position in the government hierarchy than on the substance of the matter. Feldman/Roberts predict the resulting fragmentation and conflicting points of view observed.

In addition, there are all the persons, institutions, and organizations with vested interests. Further, Feldman/Roberts (as well as Breyer) report that there is often, as in the HMO case, a lack of expertise; outside experts or consultants have to be relied on. Even when there is expertise, executive branch turnover is such that periodically a totally new approach might be superimposed on some ongoing program or agency, meaning that all levels of staff often have to start all over again. Yet the senior appointees, such as the Secretary of HEW, seem so swamped by other matters that they must rely on subordinates to expose the relevant issues. Even where there have been no longstanding differences of opinion within HEW, it is still difficult to achieve consensus concerning a broad new program from the career personnel in the different agencies and even from the bureaus within one agency. Of course, as Feldman/Roberts indicate, authority over all aspects of guideline drafting is diffuse. Therefore, when the enabling legislation is ambiguous, one has to find a determined and knowledgeable Secretary or very senior administrator who will impose one direction on all the disparate elements through some firm negotiating process, with those overruled waiting their turn to plead their case to a new Secretary or to the next administration. The ambiguity of language (part of the genius in legislative drafting that ensures passage of a complex measure), however, may also reflect another crucial point: That society as a whole is not yet ready to face the issue involved, a barrier no amount of internal or external bargaining can overcome.

In short, as Feldman/Roberts suggest, there are problems with objectives. Most obviously, Congress would like to maintain control over its legislation; it apparently does so by diffusing the power which it delegates and by writing policy guidelines which may be strict or flexible depending on the goal Congress would like the agency to reach. It is thus difficult to imbue the regulatory writing process with a commitment to the legislation or to clear and successful rules. "Copying the legislation" may be the only choice the regulators have. As seen in the HMO example, guidelines and regulations often have to be written so as not to have to confront issues which the Congress had previously refused to act or decide upon.

In sum, factors which influence legislative/regulatory outcomes are the lack of congressional consensus, the personalities of those who interact, institutional limitations, and the lack of experience or expertise of those involved. Given this melange, it is no wonder that Feldman/ Roberts conclude that good administrators do make a difference. Given the complexity of health care, the quality of implementation of a rule can often make a greater difference than the considerations by which the rule or regulation was drafted in the first place.

These findings are not all that new, of course, as the following excerpt from a paper by Drew Altman and Harvey Sapolsky illustrates:

> Some guarded generalizations about the structural context for the development of regulations in health are possible. It is a context that is time-consuming and timetable-sensitive. Pressures to expedite the production of particular regulations often place a considerable burden on operations at lower levels. It is a process that is somewhat detailed, formal, and routinized although, of course, controversial situations or personal interest may increase the impact of informal channels and key officials in particular instances. . . . especially controversial instances high officials may impact the process considerably through direct action, indirect pressures, or prolonged inaction.

> Because the process is so complex, however, and because existing agencies have established roles and functions, excessive reliance on informal channels or intervention from higher levels may disrupt orderly processing of regulations while creating internal conflict. The process involves officials and individuals with different backgrounds and perspectives, including career officials, political appointees, fiscal managers, lawyers, professional specialists, and outside consultants. It formally involves outsiders only at specified stages. Finally, it is a process that, except in special circumstances, limits upper level functions largely to those of review, providing considerable insulation for policy formulation and decision at early stages and at lower levels.[22]

IS CHANGE POSSIBLE?

At the conference where the subject matter of this book was reviewed at length,[23] the question of changing physician behavior patterns was discussed. Without the cost/bonus incentive system that could be built into an HMO, many agreed (with the director of a very large city hospital) that the cost of medical care is unlikely to change as long as doctors are trained only within hospitals.[24] Training in community settings not only helps doctors see real opportunities and problems but might also allow them to put academic medicine into perspective. Certainly they would come to understand the high cost of increasing access only through the big general hospitals.

In a similar vein, one wonders if people will stay so caught up in the daily agendas of their agency or institution as to make disciplinary or professional change difficult. What kind of external pressure or environmental modification would stimulate new administrative, disciplinary, or professional approaches?

Some answer this question by proposing the use of a tax-credit system[25] so that patients will bear part of the cost of their own health care (proportionate to their income). The question then becomes, if households ultimately bear a fraction of the cost of their own hospital care, will regulator, physician, patient, and hospital work together to provide a specified level of care at a minimum cost? Based on what is presented here, it is hard to see such changes actually taking place or even regulations being written and implemented to prevent coinsurance from covering the balance of the cost incurred by the patient.

While we will return to the tax credit proposal *infra*, there is another approach to change based on the presumption that the fee-for-service system, given a "chance," would respond to cost-competitive forces. The point many government officials make in rebuttal is that cost effectiveness of "market" competition has yet to be demonstrated in health care. Save for the development of HMOs, it is not clear what would be required in order to select examples of marketplace implementation as guidelines for the further development of alternatives to classical economic regulation of health care. The Feldman/Roberts' paper and the discussion of the HMO example suggest that the confounding of rational economic, medical, or managerial approaches by political consideration needs greater unraveling and understanding.

It is all too easy to say that more persons, institutions, and agencies would probably be helped in developing and implementing regulations if there were better understanding of the day-to-day workings of the American political system. Even the idea of a bargaining model as a useful way of regarding the health care regulatory process has its problems. John Dunlop, in his discussion in Chapter Two *supra*, reiterates the great advantage a bargaining format possesses in bringing interested parties together to work out what will affect them. Yet, as Judge Wright points out in Chapter Two, this bargaining process has to take place in some open and fair way so that all parties are heard and their interests most equitably represented. A moment's reflection brings to mind myriad difficulties in actually achieving such a combination of bargaining with due process in which, within our political system, all (meaning the general public) can play a part. Clearly new ground will have to be broken to achieve such an outcome.

WHERE DOES ONE GO FROM HERE?

The conference this volume reflects posed the problem of finding a road-map to lead one through the largely uncharted morass of health care regulation. The sudden shift in the health care environment from prostimulation to cost mindfulness has come to a society not generally prepared to regard individual health as a "business." Further, as Breyer demonstrates, classical regulation of business creates its own series of

problems with which our society is currently wrestling. Yet Feldman/
Roberts highlight the point that regulation without regulator and regulatee sharing the same goal is regulation which is largely unenforce-
able.

Weinstein/Sherman develop a typology based on actual and
hypothetical possibilities for government intervention in health care.
Breyer's framework is largely built on the experience of regulatory
agencies in classical economic regulation. Yet the fact that both approaches lead toward convincing parallels regarding health care regulation should not be surprising: Both approaches require careful analysis
of each regulatory situation. It may be frustrating to discover that there
is no simple list of do's and don'ts that will guarantee improved health
care regulation in the future. What Breyer, Feldman/Roberts, and
Weinstein/Sherman all require is that regulators be clear in the questions they ask when considering proposals for government intervention. Specificity and clarity will improve the regulatory process rather
than will platitudinous exhortations to consider choices or examine
parallel experience. In a way, the following list of questions regulators
should ask seems obvious, but as Breyer and Feldman/Roberts suggest,
the record indicates that most regulatory problems arise from regulation
writers or implementors ignoring all but two or three of these fundamental questions.

1. What *exactly* is to be regulated?

2. How will success be measured?

3. What is required to bring all parties involved to a consensus concerning:

    a. The need for regulation?

    b. The regulatory mode or approach most appropriate to secure the ends
    desired?

4. How will activities be monitored to ensure that regulatory ends are
    achieved?

    a. Are budgetary provisions adequate to do the job?

    b. Even with an adequate budget, are there trained persons available to
    execute monitoring programs?

5. What system will be instituted for testing and evaluating alternative
    intervention schemes?

6. What approach will be used to identify and correct problems that
    emerge once the regulatory program takes effect?

7. Can all those involved or with a stake in the regulatory proposal be
    identified? Can their objectives and concerns also be identified?

    a. Regulatory entities?

    b. Executive and legislative branch political overseers?

    c. Executives and administrators with related responsibilities in public or private agencies?

    d. Regulated organizations and associations?

    e. Community and public interest groups including:
      (1) Those with trustee or fiduciary oversight?

      (2) Consumers including their own health resource providers— (employers, insurance companies, etc.)?

Who Is Going to Bell the Cat?

The regulation of health care institutions will probably be a continuing focus of government over the next decade or two. Yet it appears that an increasing percentage of persons involved in regulation and administration of health care does not know enough medicine. Conversely, the medical profession does not know enough economics and management, to quote one of the few young men trained in both medicine and health policy matters.[26] In particular, in the latter case, there is very little evidence that doctors and other health personnel tend to think of themselves as other than autonomous health professionals; they certainly do not think of themselves as members of an industrial or business sector. The questions listed above are designed to help all persons approach health care regulation in a manner appropriate to the problem at hand.

We have presumed throughout this book that the lack of knowledge necessary for successful health care regulation by the above groups of professionals, forced into interacting without understanding each other's fields of interest and concerns, is the reason why senior HEW officials sponsored the conference that led to this volume. This absence of understanding may also explain why so many regulatory approaches applied to health care institutions seem to lack careful analysis, particularly when the value of these same approaches is being questioned in other sectors of society.

As mentioned at the outset, this book has not been concerned with the regulation of individual health professionals, their licensing, their relationship with individual patients, etc. Nevertheless, given the present structure of most of the health care system in the United States, regulation of health care institutions inevitably circumscribes the freedom of the health professionals employed by or associated with any institution. Certainly organized elements of the medical profession have noted that cost containment and allocative schemes will materially interfere with United States physicians' historic prerogative to employ any procedure or acquire any equipment they feel is appropriate to treatment of the problems of any specific patient. Cost, the allocation of scarce resources, etc., have not been central parts of physicians' general training, let alone specialty qualifications. In the absence of credible standards of quality and quantity of services, no "objective" regulatory approach can be expected to emerge. Accordingly, it is not surprising to find many physicians and health professionals joining with those from other sectors in the deregulation countermovement.

Regulation of Health?

In the summary of his work prepared for the Health Resources Administration, Breyer suggests that generally the most serious economic harm that regulation can work on the business sector is to inhibit the attainment of the "advantages of a competitive and unregulated marketplace, particularly those of economic efficiency, production efficiency, and innovation."[27] Even given the differences in the health care sector (i.e., the difficulty in defining "product"), it is still believable that increasing regulation will impair the efficiency and innovative approach with which health services are provided. For example, Seidman,[28] arguing for a consumer cost-sharing alternative to the several proposals for national health insurance, outlines the untoward consequences of the regulatory environment which he feels inevitably will develop if consumer cost-sharing alternatives for health care are not pursued. His concern is that under several proposals for national health insurance, "physicians and patients would have no incentive to restrain demand for hospital services." Accordingly,

> Strict limits would have to be placed on the supply of hospital facilities and technologies to contain cost. Unrestrained demand . . . then would confront limited supply and the result would be shortages with waiting lists established for both hospital admissions and the use of particular technologies, as has long occurred in Britain. Regulators, rather than each physician and patient, would decide what service was urgent, whether a particular use of technology was necessary and whether the length of a particular hospital stay had become excessive.

Yet, as Marmor comments:[29]

> Reliance on cost sharing in national health insurance makes sense only if (1) it can be effectively administered and (2) people do not buy private, supplementary insurance to pay for whatever services national health insurance does not cover. Administratively, cost sharing appears feasible but difficult and increasingly expensive when tied to the income of insurance beneficiaries. The likelihood of extensive supplementation appears high because of a number of factors, but particularly because of strong pressures in collective bargaining to maintain the size of health and welfare fringe benefits. If policy makers fail to take the likelihood of private supplementation into account before adopting a national health insurance plan, their expectations for cost sharing as a cost containment device will probably not be realized.

This book is written at a time when there is no consensus in the United States on how to integrate various and conflicting concerns and priorities into one national health insurance plan. There is not even agreement on how to reduce the previous decade's explosive increase in

health care costs. This situation leads to a very difficult social quandary
which Rabkin and Bloom summarize as follows:

> How to reach the disadvantaged without exercising complete control over
> the distribution and financing of health care, is a dilemma that neither the
> government nor the health care professions are close to solving.[30]

As our society moves inexorably towards greater institutionalization,
the increasing availability of various prepaid health plans offers a
broader array of options than has been available in the past. The lessons
suggested by the work in this volume indicate that competition based
on service and cost can emerge from bargaining among third-party
payors, health care organizations, employers, and labor or consumers,
provided that government does not insist on predetermining the individual outcome of each negotiation. Government may wish to require
some ground rules on which to build these bargaining relationships,
but we have seen that trying to impose one uniform condition, approach, or outcome tends to be inherently unworkable. From a federal
point of view, it may not be neat and tidy to let competition at the local
level be modulated by local organizations, agencies, or licensing
bodies. On the other hand, consider how much regulatory effort can be
tied up by the 5 to 10 percent of regulatees who fall outside the range of
some national norm. Such considerations are gaining increasing acceptance.

The End: Closing the Circle

To end where we began: We are all aware that in recent years local,
state, and federal governments have undertaken sustained efforts to
regulate health care—to control costs, while at the same time attempting
to upgrade the quality of as well as to increase access to medical care. All
recognize the troubles such conflicting objectives can generate. The
challenge is to reduce dollar expenditures per patient so as to be able to
provide better care, in the aggregate, to a greater number of persons.
The germs of possible ways to achieve such a reduction of expenditures
per patient by decreasing demand or by other approaches are probably
already extant in our society (e.g., greater emphasis on fitness and
preventive methods, increased use of paraprofessionals, and greater
understanding by the general population of what it can do to treat
submajor and self-limiting illness itself).

There are signs that the health status of the United States population,
after a decade or more of sustained spending, cost escalation, and the
like, is improving.[31] It may also take one or two generations to accom-
modate within our political system the "right" to health care independent of the means to pay for it. Yet it will be a particularly difficult task
to find some fair and cost-effective way to apply to all the continuing
rapid advances in knowledge of prevention, diagnosis, and treatment
of disease and debilitation. One is often struck by the thought that our

society is officially "against" death and will spend limitless sums to ward off the inevitable . Politically, we have not found a way to deal with lifespan limitations in setting health priorities. The likelihood of doubling lifespan by the next century, for example, is not a goal that seems realistic, and spending increased sums will not alter this. In particular, we have yet to confront the biological and social limitations of our present policy of death postponement as opposed to life enhancement. A shift from one to the other would have profound effects on our allocation of resources.

In any case, the general population must see the outcome of health regulation at present as a bewildering proliferation of acronyms: PSRO, HMO, CON, etc.—all indicative of increased government intervention. The population will not oppose rules which make sure that only treatment of proven benefit is applied to everybody; yet every physician knows that each family will demand, in times of crisis, anything that might conceivably help the loved one in need.[32] At present there seems to be no visible counterforce that will diminish this pressure.

It would be hoped that in the future, persons or agencies proposing major health care regulatory programs will submit them to a forum similar to the one organized at the Kennedy School to review the material in this volume. Preenactment review by such a diverse cross-section might avert many of the difficulties now being experienced in the field. Certainly, there need to be more projects conducted jointly by the public and private sectors to develop data and to develop greater understanding of alternatives to intervention as ways of achieving health care goals.[33]

Finally, during the time between the end of the conference and the final submission of this manuscript to the publisher, it appears that many of the problems and difficulties categorized in this volume are becoming more generally recognized. In particular, as the Ninety-Sixth Congress struggled with various proposals for cost containment and resource allocation, it also passed amendments to the Health Planning Act exempting HMOs from the CON process and introducing competition as a new criterion in order to encourage local initiative and sustain important local differences. In general Havighurst[34] believes that there is much to suggest that Congress is reconsidering its approach to health care, moving away from heavy-handed "command-and-control" regulation. Given the cross-section of the leadership of the American health care community that participated in the work that led to this volume, it is not unreasonable to believe that what is contained herein may have had a positive influence on these developments. As the ideas and arguments presented here are further disseminated, a wider understanding will be achieved of what needs to be considered in both fostering and regulating health care delivery systems.

NOTES

1. Based on conference discussion of Stephen Breyer's preliminary draft for a forthcoming book presented in manuscript form and summary to partici-

pants for review and analysis. Chapter Five of this volume summarizes the **359**
main points of Breyer's book. Don Price, Dean Emeritus of the Kennedy *Issues in Health*
School of Government, chaired the discussion which included panelists *Care Regulation*
Howard Berman, Vice President, American Hospital Association; Alain
Enthoven, Stanford University; Theodore Marmor, then of the University of
Chicago, now Chairman, The Center for Health Studies, Yale University;
and Caspar Weinberger, former Secretary of HEW, now Vice President,
Bechtel Corporation.

2. L. S. Seidman, "Hospital Inflation: A Diagnosis and Prescription," *Challenge,* July–Aug. 1979, pp. 12–23.

3. *Conference Proceedings,* submitted to the Health Resources Administration as Final Report on Contract HRA 230-77-0037.

4. Based on conference discussion I of the CON case, "Certificate-of-Need in Massachusetts," chaired by Harvey Fineberg, Assistant Professor, Harvard School of Public Health. Panelists included Stephen Breyer, Professor, Harvard Law School; Jonathan Fielding, former Commissioner of Health, Commonwealth of Massachusetts; and John Hill, Chairman of the Board, Hospital Corporation of America.

5. See Breyer, Chap. 5, "Different Modes of Classical Regulation," *supra* on page 219.

6. *Ibid.* on pages 217–221.

7. This is extracted from Alain Enthoven's concise summary of Breyer's work as presented in the *Conference Proceedings.* See n. 3 *supra.*

8. See Breyer, Chap. 5, "Different Modes of Classical Regulation," *supra* on pages 222–223.

9. See n. 3 *supra.*

10. This section is based on discussion II of the CON Case chaired by Graham Allison, Dean, Kennedy School of Government. Panelists included James Kimmey, Director, Midwest Center for Health Planning, Inc.; Roger Noll, Professor, Department of Economics, California Institute of Technology; Herbert Sherman, Associate Director for Technology, Center for the Analysis of Health Practices, Harvard School of Public Health; and Milton Weinstein, Associate Professor, Kennedy School of Government.

11. Are private plans going to be permitted as a viable option? Or is their fate to be that of the several "voucher" proposals for educational reform?

12. The dynamic state of medical science also raises one of the original "Hoover Commission" issues: Can a regulatory agency also be a promulgator of policy? How does one instruct the regulatory agency to construe future possibilities in a positive way rather than to view new developments only as having the potential of creating undue risk or cost?

13. This section is based on a discussion chaired by Robert Blendon, Vice President, Robert Wood Johnson Foundation. Panelists included Harold Cohen, Executive Director, Health Services Cost Review Commission, Maryland; Jacob Getson, Assistant Commissioner of Health, Commonwealth of Massachusetts; Lawrence Huston, Assistant Vice President, Group Division, Aetna Life and Casualty; Roger Noll, Professor, Department of Economics, California Institute of Technology; and Mitchell Rabkin, General Director, Beth Israel Hospital.

14. See Chap. 2 *supra*.

15. *Ibid.*

16. See n. 3 *supra*.

17. See n. 9 *supra*.

18. See n. 3 *supra*.

19. Advertisements citing the cost control efforts of the Maryland Health Services Cost Review Commission among others appeared in national magazines in recent months. See *Money Magazine,* Nov. 1979, pp. 32–33.

20. See Cohen, Chap. 2, "Response to 'Magic Bullets or Seven-Card Stud," Appendices, *supra* at pp. 121–130.

21. This section is based on a conference discussion chaired by Marc Roberts, Professor, Harvard School of Public Health, Panelists included Scott Fleming, Senior Vice President, Kaiser Foundation Hospital Plans, Inc.; and Lee Cummings, Alcohol, Drug Abuse and Mental Health Administration; see also Chap. 1 *supra*.

22. D. Altman and H. M. Sapolsky, *Policy Sciences* 7 (1976).

23. *Regulation as an Instrument of Public Administration,* Harvard University, February 27–28, 1978.

24. See n. 3 *supra*.

25. See n. 2 *supra* at 22.

26. *Time,* Aug. 6, 1979, p. 36.

27. See Breyer, n. 3 *supra* at 240.

28. See n. 2 *supra*.

29. Extracted from a draft by T. Marmor and D. Conrad, "Patient Cost-Sharing," Chap. 8, in *National Health Insurance: Policy Issues for the 1980s,"* to be published by the Urban Institute, Washington, D.C.

30. M. T. Rabkin, and T. F. Bloom, *Radcliffe Quarterly* 15 (June 1979).

31. For example, see D. E. Rogers and R. J. Blendon, *JAMA* 237:1710-1714, 1977.

32. Frazier, in n. 3 *supra*.

33. At the time this program was started at Harvard University, it was hoped that one could find a way to establish a permanent, nongovernmental group that would be concerned with maintaining an overview of national health care regulation. This remains a hope, but it is hard to see how to accomplish this practicably other than through the gadfly approach.

34. C. C. Havighurst, *Prospects for Competition Under Health Planning-Cum-Regulation,* Discussion Paper, circulated to the National Health Council on Health Planning and Dev. (Nov. 7, 1979).

Index

Index

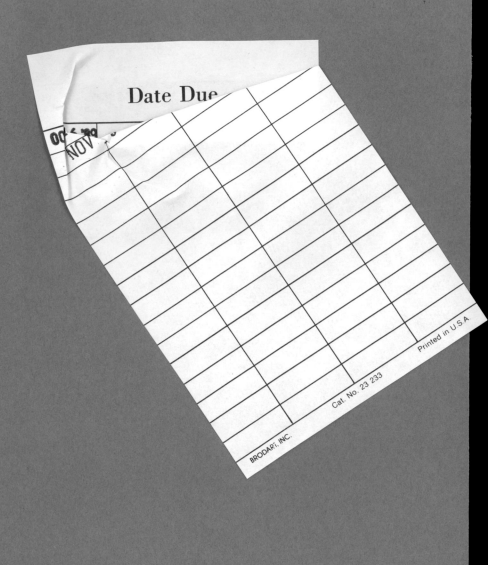

Date Due

NOV

BRODART, INC.   Cat. No. 23 233

Printed in U.S.A.